Panagiota Kotsila

Socio-political and Cultural Determinants of Diarrheal Disease in the Mekong Delta

ZEF Development Studies

edited by

Solvay Gerke and Hans-Dieter Evers

Volume 28

Center for Development Research (ZEF)
University of Bonn
www.zef.de

LIT

Panagiota Kotsila

Socio-political and Cultural Determinants of Diarrheal Disease in the Mekong Delta

From Discourse to Incidence

LIT

Cover image: Panagiota Kotsila

The print is paid by the BMBF and the WISDOM project

This dissertation has been accepted by the Faculty of Philosophy
of the University of Bonn

Bibliographic information published by the Deutsche Nationalbibliothek
The Deutsche Nationalbibliothek lists this publication in the Deutsche Nationalbibliografie; detailed bibliographic data are available in the Internet at http://dnb.d-nb.de.

ISBN 978-3-643-90562 8
Zugl.: Bonn, Univ., Diss., 2014

A catalogue record for this book is available from the British Library

Klosbachstr. 107
CH-8032 Zürich
Tel. +41 (0) 44-251 75 05
Fax +41 (0) 44-251 75 06
E-Mail: zuerich@lit-verlag.ch
http://www.lit-verlag.ch

LIT VERLAG Dr. W. Hopf
Berlin 2014
Fresnostr. 2
D-48159 Münster
Tel. +49 (0) 2 51-62 03 20
Fax +49 (0) 2 51-23 19 72
E-Mail: lit@lit-verlag.de
http://www.lit-verlag.de

Distribution:

In the UK: Global Book Marketing, e-mail: mo@centralbooks.com
In North America: International Specialized Book Services, e-mail: orders@isbs.com
In Germany: LIT Verlag Fresnostr. 2, D-48159 Münster
Tel. +49 (0) 2 51-620 32 22, Fax +49 (0) 2 51-922 60 99, E-mail: vertrieb@lit-verlag.de

In Austria: Medienlogistik Pichler-ÖBZ, e-mail: mlo@medien-logistik.at
e-books are available at www.litwebshop.de

Acknowledgments

This book owes to the support, the guidance and the resources I received from many people and institutions. I would like to express my gratitude to them for enabling this research project and for helping me to successfully complete it. My sincere thanks go firstly to the German Federal Ministry of Education and Research (BMBF), for funding this study under the wider scope of the WISDOM[1] project. I would like to thank my supervisor, Prof. Dr. Solvay Gerke and my tutor Dr. Subramanian Saravanan, for their invaluable academic guidance and support. My appreciation goes also to all the lecturers, researchers and staff in the Center of Development Research (ZEF) of the University of Bonn, for accommodating my research and for opening up my academic horizons. Especially I want to thank Dr. Gabi Waibel and my colleagues Siwei, Linh, Sven, Sarah, Judith, Nadine, Simon and Carmen for the inspiration they generously offered to me through their work and their personalities. This research would also not have been possible without the facilitation offered by the Can Tho University in Vietnam and particularly without the help and advice of Dr. Bui Thi Nga. I want to also send my gratitude to Nhan, for being a tireless research assistant and a positive spirit throughout my fieldwork. Moreover, my thanks go to all the Vietnamese people who shared their time and their experiences, selflessly offering me their hospitality and kindness. Finally, I want to thank my family and friends, for being my mental refuge and a never-ending source of love. Most of all, I thank you Alan, for this work would have never been started or completed without you by my side.

[1] Water-Related Information System for the Sustainable Development of the Mekong Delta, Vietnam (www.wisdom.eoc.dlr.de).

TABLE OF CONTENTS

LIST OF FIGURES

LIST OF TABLES

LIST OF PICTURES

ABBREVIATIONS

ADB	Asian Development Bank
AIDS	Acquired immune Deficiency Syndrome
ASA	American Sociological Association
CARE	Cooperative for Assistance and Relief Everywhere
CDD	Control of Diarrheal Disease
CERWASS	Centre for Rural Water Supply and Sanitation
CHEC	Centre for Health Education and Communication
CHECC	Can Tho Health Education and Communication Centre
CIDS	Can Tho City Institute for Socio-Economic Development
CPV	Communist Party of Vietnam
CTWSC	Can Tho City Water Supply Company
DANIDA	Danish International Development Agency
DARD	Department of Agriculture and Rural Development
DOH	Department of Health
DOLISA	Department of Labour, Invalids and Social Affairs
DONRE	Department of Natural Resources and the Environment
DoPM	Department of Preventive Medicine
DoPI	Department of Planning and Investment
DoPM	Department of Preventive Medicine (of the MoH)
dPHC	district-level Preventive Health Centre
DSO	District Statistics Office
FU	Farmers Union
GDP	Gross Domestic Product
GoV	Government of Vietnam
GPS	Global Positioning System
GSO	General Statistics Office
HELVETAS	Swiss Association for International Cooperation
HEMA	Health Environment Management Agency
HH	Household
HIV	Human Immunodeficiency Virus
HSPI	Health Strategy and Policy Institute
IEC	Information Education and Communication
IHPH	Institute of Hygiene and Public Health

JMP	Joint Monitoring Program (WHO and UNICEF)
MARD	Ministry of Agriculture and Rural Development
MDG	Millennium Development Goal
MoC	Ministry of Construction
MoH	Ministry of Health
MoNRE	Ministry of Natural Resources and the Environment
NCERWASS	National Centre for Rural Water Supply and Sanitation
NTP	National Target Programme
OARD	Office of Agriculture and Rural Development
OLISA	Office of Labour, War Invalids and Social Affairs
OoH	Office of Health
ORS	Oral Rehydration Solution
PATH	Program for Appropriate Technology in Health
PC	People's Committee
PCFP	Provincial Child Friendly Programme
PHC	Preventive Health Centre
RWSS	Rural Water Supply and Sanitation strategy
SEA	South East Asia
SNV	Netherlands Development Organization
SODIS	Solar Water Disinfection
TM	Traditional Medicine
UN	United Nations
UNDP	United Nations Development Programme
UNICEF	United Nations Children's Fund
USD	United States Dollar (currency)
VBSP	Vietnam Bank for Social Policies
VCP	Vietnamese Communist Party
VND	Vietnamese Dong (currency)
WASH	Water Sanitation and Hygiene
WB	World Bank
WHO	World Health Organization
WISDOM	Water-related Information System for the Sustainable Development of the Mekong Delta
WU	Women's Union
YU	Youth's Union

FRAMING THE PROBLEM OF DIARRHEAL DISEASE IN VIETNAM: AN INTRODUCTION

CHAPTER 1

The annual diarrhoea deaths of children under 5 years old in the world are at the striking level of 1 - 3 million (Santosham et al., 2010). Together with pneumonia, diarrhoea is one of the primary killers of children and especially the poor, with countries in Africa and South East Asia (SEA) bearing most of its global burden (UNICEF, 2012b). The SEA region has been generally acknowledged as a "hotspot for risk, with new, emergent, and resurgent infectious diseases exploiting ecological niches that result in large part from man's influence on his environment" (Coker et al., 2011). Vietnam is a country which, despite its official exit from poverty during the 1990s, has been facing an average of over 1.5 million annual documented cases of diarrhoea for the period between 2005 to 2011 (MoH, 2012b). This persistently high incidence[2] of the disease persists despite the existence of known preventions, and thus remains an ongoing development concern. By examining the case of diarrheal disease in the region of the Vietnam's Mekong Delta, the study strives to understand the factors that govern this essentially preventable health risk.

1.1 Holistic views on a globally persistent disease

Diarrheal diseases are some of the oldest and most persistent health impediments in the history of human civilisation (Lim and Wallace, 2004, Hénock Blaise and Dovie, 2007). After centuries of experience, the epidemiological and biomedical knowledge on diarrhoea has grown remarkably, providing us with what has proven to be effective measures for its prevention and control. Nevertheless, diarrhoea is still a widespread disease, in particular affecting those living in environmental conditions that are favourable to its spread, namely: those in poverty and those who, for a multitude of reasons, are not being reached by public health supporting programs. Despite a few remaining questions about what governs the spread of diarrheal diseases, the global health community already possesses enough medical, epidemiological and microbiological information to effectively guide prevention. Seeing how these measures have been successfully used for the control of diarrhoea in the western world, it becomes clear that the real problem is not the existence of pathogens that cause diarrhoea, but the lack of knowledge on how to use the available knowledge and

[2] Incidence (of disease) = the number of new cases within a period of time (Joralemon, 2010).

information for its effective management and control. This chapter discusses the core elements that surround this problem while also introducing the study region in Vietnam's Mekong Delta.

1.1.1 Discourse and context: Why diarrheal disease is not only a medical problem

When one considers a visit Vietnam, much of the information available on web pages and printed travel guides underline the risk of what is termed "travellers' diarrhoea". The extent to which diarrhoea is a problem only for travellers as opposed to people living in endemic regions is not widely documented in literature, being only indicated in a few studies (Grimwood and Lambert, 2009, Levine et al., 1981, Black et al., 1981). Because the types of microorganisms able to cause diarrheal disease are numerous and ever-mutating, the suggestion that local people have developed immunity to some of the pathogens is doubtful. In a general sense, the high numbers of diarrhoea morbidity and mortality[3], especially from the regions of the world considered as hot-spots for "travellers' diarrhoea", point to the fact that diarrheal disease does indeed not only affect travellers; in fact, given their continued exposure, it primarily impacts locals. However, when I narrated my own personal experience with the disease to a local cadre that I interviewed, he was eager to convince me that I, as a foreigner, am different than local people, who "have high resistance to diarrhoea, they are used to the water they drink" (local cadre, rural district, Mekong Delta Vietnam). The opinion of a local farmer from the same rural commune revealed a somewhat different reality:

> "No one can avoid diarrhoea; we can get it from anything. You leave the food unprotected and a fly goes on it, or you touch something around and bacteria get in your system." (Farmer, rural district, Mekong Delta, Vietnam)

Diseases such as diarrhoea are often discussed as owing simply to the lack of modern water infrastructure and are often primarily associated with poor people in underdeveloped countries. While this might be a partial explanation, the reality is unsurprisingly more complex. Vietnam has not only officially escaped poverty but has been experiencing a remarkable economic performance over the last few decades. Modernisation and progress is a vision that the Vietnamese government has embraced and is following through eagerly (Ehlert, 2011: 2ff). The WHO has documented that in Vietnam diarrhoea is responsible for 10% of the deaths in children under 5 years old (WHO, 2012a), suggesting the

[3] Morbidity (rate) = the rate of a disease's occurrence in a certain population (prevalence/pop). Mortality (rate) = the rate of deaths caused by a disease in a certain population (deaths /pop).

continued presence of the disease in the country. The words of the local farmer above, among others, corroborate this. Considering diarrhoea's popular association with poverty and also considering Vietnam's efforts to dust off the stigma of poverty through modernisation and to cultivate a new development image, the statement of the local cadre above can be perhaps be interpreted as part of the effort to protect the image of a state which is successfully acting on behalf of people's health, making sure that "backward" diseases such as diarrhoea do not affect the population.

How do popular views on "traveller's diarrhoea" reflect how the West sees a disease that kills millions of children? Is the local cadre right when he presents diarrhoea as a problem only for those not used to it? Is the usual 3-day diarrheal episode not a global concern when it is silently suffered by those who, in the words of the farmer above, simply cannot avoid it? Does it only turn into a serious health problem when it interrupts our travels or only when it is turned into mortality statistics for the poor? Good health has been declared as a human right (United Nations, 2007) but how can one define it? As this work will demonstrate, despite the tangible reality of disease, it remains an issue highly subjective to people's feelings and personal judgments, as well as a platform for debate and negotiation. Health has often been operationalised through fractional analysis of physiological bodily functions but, according to an Indian proverb, someone's health is also proportionate to "how happy he or she is". The continuum from healthy to ill is being contested and redefined daily and differently in medical circles, private discussions and public platforms. Claims about human health naturally mean a lot for those with the responsibility to implement health-related policy and those in a position to safeguard it, both at the local and global scale. More importantly, claims about health affect those whose health is at stake. Metaphorically speaking, as nothing in this world is naturally sterile, problems of disease are also "infected" by the world's social, institutional and political complexity.

Health is often viewed as paralleled to well-being, which in turn has been –at least in principle- the central purpose of worldwide development. Following Peet and Hartwick (1999), development can be seen as a "belief" and a "project" guided by western thought and the neoliberal paradigms of industrialisation, economic growth and modernity. This type of vision of development has often meant imposing the views and practices of the west on the rest of the world and has thus narrowly and intrusively defined the desired paths of progress *for* people (as supposed to *by* them), yet all the while still acting in the name of *their* well-being. Many critiques of such approaches have argued for a step away from rational knowledge claims (postmodernism), away from looking for structures that govern society and all human existence (poststructuralism) and away from single-sided visions of one, finite development (post-developmentalism), which tend "to subordinate, contain and assimilate the Third World as *other*" (Slatter 1993 cited in Peet and Hartwick, 1999, my emphasis). Instead of seeking to replicate and force western, scientific and discursive "mastery" onto societies which are seen as problematic, one of the core poststructuralist thinkers, Michel Foucault, begged for respect of diversity and to allow "people the freedom to define and solve their own problems" (Best & Kellner 1991 and Peet 1998 cited in Peet and Hartwick, 1999: 132). Similar to the encompassing term of development, well-being can be debated as something that societies should be defining from within rather than being subjected to interventions from outside.

Definitions of health are sensitive to cultural and social context and, in this sense, the concepts of *external* and *internal* can be understood in relation not only to countries and national boarders or institutions, but also to personal bodily boundaries. The work of Mary Douglas is illustrative of how the human body is reflected in and at the same time reflects society. People deal differently and give different meanings to bodily categorisations, paying particular attention to the inner and outer boundaries of the body but they always do so with regard to their cultural and social context (Douglas, 2002: 115ff). This is visible in the execution of cultural rituals as they "enact the form of social relations and in giving these relations visible expression they enable people to know their own society. The rituals work upon the body politic through the symbolic medium of the physical body" (Ibid., 2002: 129). This is also visible in how different cultures use distinct categories to provoke disgust or fear in the face of natural excretions that the body produces, in order to maintain some kind of order in their societies, even though ultimately "pollution rules do not correspond closely to moral rules" (Ibid., 2002: 130). What Douglas tells us is that physical and social processes are materialised and experienced in parallel. In this light, it becomes important to examine disease within personal, social and political spheres, paying attention to the meanings that social and cultural actors give to disease and, in turn, how the definitions given to disease reflect social structures and morals.

Considering what has been described above, taking either the view of healthiness as a fixed and determined bodily state or as a set of logical activities towards the prevention of illness in which individuals or societies engage, would blind observers to the reality that disease and health are also culturally and socially constructed. Of course it can be claimed that certain physical states and bodily reactions cannot be denied and are tangibly causing discomfort, pain, or malfunction, and can prove harmful for the body to the extent of death. Diarrheal disease undoubtedly has these characteristics. Nevertheless, the example of how different the views about a problem of disease such as diarrhoea can be, depending on the originators of that discourse (popular western media, a state representative or a local farmer), already suggests that interpretations of the same phenomenon can vary to a large extent. So on the one hand, if health is thought of in purely biophysical terms, it risks being stripped of social and cultural content. On the other hand, seeing health or disease solely as discursive products would ignore their biological nature and physical consequences. Given this duality, the fact that western medical science has so far dominated over definitions and explanations about bodily functions and experiences, calls for the enrichment of human health studies with accounts from the humanities.

1.1.2 Global efforts and omissions: why re-prioritising diarrhoea needs local relevance

During the UN Summit in 2010, some of the world's leaders together with international representatives of civil society and research, committed to maintain and fortify their efforts in achieving the eight Millennium Development Goals (United Nations, 2010). These goals include bringing down the rate of child mortality (MDG 4) and decreasing the share of people without sustainable access to safe drinking water and sanitation (Target 10). Due to the focus on children and on water facilities, diarrhoea has often been brought to the centre of global health discourse. Targeted efforts for its worldwide control had been climaxing in the 1980s (WHO, 1987) and indeed bearing fruit judging by the decrease in the number of children dying from diarrhoea (Chiabi et al., 2010). However, despite all the experience and knowledge of its prevention that has accumulated over the years, the fight against the disease's incidence has yet to be won. The prevalence of well-publicized and heavily supported measures that see neither committed local implementation nor a positive impact on health has continued to be a challenge for public health policy.

At this point it needs to be acknowledged that the mere description and evaluation of the problem is usually confined to indicators that show how many annual deaths are attributed to the disease (mortality rates). However low the mortality rates might be, however, diarrhoea continues to impact millions of people, constituting a serious impediment to the well-being of children and adults and undermining their quality of life, even when the disease is often self-limiting and non-fatal. Furthermore, the frequent experience of diarrheal infections carries serious health risks in the long-run (Stephenson et al., 2000,

Thapar and Sanderson, 2004)[4] which in the absence of high mortality rates, also tend to be ignored. Guerrant et al. (2002) show that compared to previous decades, morbidity levels of diarrhoea have seen a worldwide increase between the years 1992 and 2005, particularly among the world's poor. It therefore seems that the problem of diarrheal disease is easily mal-assessed to begin with. This may be one cause of its deprioritisation by both national governments and global health initiatives.

Considering that efforts to control diarrhoea have not produced the expected results, one needs to further ask why this has happened. Even though most cases of diarrhoea can be prevented or effectively treated at home, evidence attests to the difficulties adopting proposed curative and preventive measures. The use of oral rehydration solutions (ORS) for example, remains surprisingly low, even though it is the globally most advocated and effective way to treat symptoms of diarrhoea (UNICEF and WHO, 2009, Santosham et al., 2010, Chiabi et al., 2010). The expansion of improved water supply and sanitation facilities has also not been achieved to a satisfactory level, even though it has been heavily pushed by global organisations and local governments as the ultimate preventive medicine (Saravanan and Gondhalekar, 2013). The overall access to both water supply and sanitation (WSS) facilities and anti-diarrhoea medication remains highly problematic, especially for those who are mostly vulnerable to disease in both urban and rural areas of the world (Graham and Selendy, 2011b, Graham and Selendy, 2011a, Bartlett, 2003, UNICEF, 2012b: 33). One of the enigmas in health prevention that development agencies and various research projects have tried to solve is why people do not follow the expert advice that is provided to them, especially when they find themselves to be particularly vulnerable to disease.

Partly answering the above question, one of the things that we do know about diarrhoea is that it maintains a highly stratified nature, with the world's poorer children being the most exposed and most vulnerable to it (UNICEF, 2012b). Poverty leads more easily to disease and disease hampers people's ability to exit poverty (Harriss and Salway, 2009, Bloom and Canning, 2003). Such "vicious circles" persist widely in the context of developing nations and thus disease

---

[4] Thapar and Sanderson (2004) discuss the example of the recurring diarrhoea, which often goes untreated and can permanently upset the nutrient absorption functions of the digestive path, especially in children. Stephenson et al. (2000) refer to the long-lasting diarrhoea which is caused by protozoa for which improper medication is often prescribed in addition to insufficient food intake by the patients. As a result, the disease can lead to malnutrition and inhibit children's growth, or even cause an abrupt life-threatening relapse (Ibid., 2000).

cannot be seen separately from the socio-economic realities that people experience. The role of state mechanisms in fostering equitable and effective public health measures cannot be overemphasized. As seen in the example of the water sector, questioning institutions and governance has revealed that comprehensive access to safe water is often hampered by the lack of political will and by poor transparency when formulating and implementing policy (Bakker et al., 2008, WHO, 2012b: 10). The WHO points to the role and responsibility of particular health institutions in preventing diseases like diarrhoea "through evidence-based advocacy, health promotion and education to improve hygiene practices, and the promotion of affordable interim measures at the household and community level" (WHO, 2001a:2). The reasons behind public "non-compliance" to recommended measures appear connected to the involvement of institutions in facilitating the equitable access to the resources that can foster the adoption of preventative measures and behaviours.

Moreover, although the problem of disease expresses itself at the individual level, it is defined by more than what the individual alone can control, such as household-level infrastructure, medicine provision or the access to healthcare services. Looking particularly at the water and health nexus, where diarrheal disease predominantly exists, Saravanan et al. (2011) underline that "water and health are closely interlinked and complex. In this complexity, one-direction interventions based on the 'cause-effect-remedy' paradigms such as providing drinking water, using toilets and washing hands becomes irrelevant to address diarrhoea when people continuously bath, inhale, work and live in and around polluted water". In other words, in the case of a problem that comes as a result of socio-environmental interaction, the analysis would have to look not only at the equitability of policy implementation, but also at the level of integration of various sectors that need to be involved.

It still holds true, however, that individual behaviours shape the health outcomes that preventive measures are expected to deliver. Everyday hygiene and water practices, for example, are crucial in determining the risk of diarrheal disease prevention, even when an improved water source is available (Curtis et al., 2000, Heller et al., 2003, Jensen et al., 2002, Mintz et al., 2001, Herbst et al., 2009, Curtis and Cairncross, 2003). How far should one go with water treatment or how often should people wash their hands? What is the best way to keep food safe and which defecation habits are jeopardizing public health? Whereas there might exist guidelines that are adopted and provide answers to such questions, their implementation remains, at least to some extent, in the hands of individuals. This is why part of the success or the failure of preventive measures cannot be explained simply by looking at what is advocated in formal policy or how well institutions perform; this success or failure needs to be contrasted with factors that are rooted in local culture and society (Nichter and Nichter, 1996b, Aunger et al., 2010, Joshi et al., 2011, Curtis et al., 2009).

In light of this debate, some socio-cultural aspects have been acknowledged as important and have entered global assessments of sectors such as water supply and sanitation (JMP, 2012b, The World Bank (WB) and International Development Association (IDA), 2006). Nevertheless, these acknowledgments have not yet translated into concrete targets in the general sector of public health. Organisations like the WHO, have been promoting health policy that is socially embedded and acknowledge that addressing the needs of the most vulnerable and enhancing participatory health education is a strong measure against diarrhoea (UNICEF and WHO, 2009: 3). However, such aspects are routinely ignored when reporting on the success of health policies. The typical indicators are blind to social inequalities, assume the same health needs and capacities for each context and, most importantly, largely restrict the concept of health to the absence of death or hospitalisation, monopolising attention with mortality rates and incidence recorded within hospital units (WHO, 2005, WHO, 2012e). For diseases such as diarrhoea, which are controlled by action in multiple sectors, and which present social and cultural particularities (usually institutionally fragmented and socially superficial approaches) fail to capture the reality of the problem and thereby often fail to address it.

This study takes Vietnam as a case in point, bringing together information from social, institutional, cultural and political spheres in order to discover the reasons behind the conundrum of stubborn incidence of diarrhoea and possible solutions. The following sections will describe aspects that characterize diarrheal disease in more detail, provide some necessary background information for the study region and finally pin down this study's research question and objectives.

1.2 Troubling diarrhoea: aetiologies and prevention

Diarrhoea is a waterborne disease. The spread of the disease is thus closely connected to the quality of water that people use, consume and live close to, and as such diarrheal disease is intimately connected to questions of water quality, water habits and water environments. When waters are polluted, mismanaged or appropriated in ways that negatively affect some people's clean water availability, it impacts their everyday lives and their health. As this section will explain however, while the potential of clean water in minimising the risk of disease is promising, and particularly emphasized in the context of the Mekong Delta (Köster, 2008, Soussan et al., 2005), the spread of diarrhoea is governed by a nexus of factors that are not confined to the quality of water resources and, for this reason, deserves a more detailed explanation.

1.2.1 Infection pathways: a web of human and nature interactions

Diarrhoea can be the one of many, or the main, symptom in a number of pathogenic infections. The WHO defines diarrhoea as "the passage of three or more loose or liquid stools per day (or more frequent passage than is normal for the individual)". In this work, by "diarrhoea" or "diarrheal disease" I am referring to the ill status of individuals who have this as the main and most severe symptom. Some common types of diarrheal diseases include cholera, typhoid fever and dysentery. Diarrhoea generally follows a faecal-oral transmission route in which water acts as a medium for the pathogen's survival and multiplication. The disease however can also be transmitted through contaminated food, flies, or dirty hands. Infectious diarrhoea can be caused by bacteria, viruses, protozoa or helminths. Their numerous types and mutations each differ in their epidemiology, resistance and geographical distribution (Dawson, 2005, Karanis, 2006, Nguyen et al., 2007), causing distinct types of diarrhoea that differ in their symptoms, duration and severity.

Diarrhoea can occur as a secondary symptom of other diseases, such as measles or hepatitis. It can furthermore be the cause and the consequence of malnutrition, a very common condition for children growing up in poverty (Fitzwater et al., 2011). It is thus particularly hard to distinguish whether diarrhoea is an indicator of other latent health issues or whether it is a purely gastrointestinal pathogenic attack. Moreover, the life cycles and the transmission routes of many known and emerging diarrheal microbes remain widely unclear (Karanis, 2006). Due to this heterogeneity that characterizes the disease, it is often hard to identify the exact cause of an episode, especially when attempted in conditions of restricted medical capacity and limited laboratory infrastructure. Unfortunately, this lack of capacities is usually encountered in places that are also hotspots for diarrheal disease, hampering its accurate diagnosis and documentation. In many cases, practitioners will follow a clinical syndromic diagnosis as a guide to decide on its medical treatment (Table 1.1). Syndromic diagnoses widely categorize the disease along the following guidelines: acute watery diarrhoea, persistent diarrhoea or bloody diarrhoea (Thapar and Sanderson, 2004, Farthing, 2000, Fitzwater et al., 2011).

Table 1.1: Categorisation of common diarrheal diseases by aetiology, transmission and diagnostic characteristics

Aetiology	Characteristics of transmission	Diagnostic characteristics
Shigella	Person to person, inanimate objects, water, food	One type of dysentery (bacillary): watery diarrhoea maybe bloody, including abdominal cramps, vomiting, fever
Vibrio cholerae	Through food or water	Acute watery diarrhoea
Salmonella group	Water, food, and animal-human transmission	Gastroenteritis or food poisoning: nausea, vomiting, and diarrhoea which may be bloody
Salmonella typhi (severe form)		Typhoid fever (diarrhoea as one of the symptoms): green stools, characteristic smell
Escherichia coli group	Water, uncooked food, cross-contamination	Can vary from watery, neonatal to bloody diarrhoea, including with fever. Might evolve into persistent diarrhoea
Protozoa or Helminths[5]	Contaminated food & water	Watery and maybe bloody diarrhoea, dysentery, persistent diarrhoea, nausea, anorexia and many other variations
Rotavirus	Faecal-oral, dirty hands and objects, food and water	Acute watery diarrhoea, fever and vomiting

[5] Some diarrhoea-causing protozoa include the species *Entamoeba histolytica, Cryptosporidium spp., Giardia intestinalis, Balantidium coli.* Some diarrhoea-causing helminths are the species *Trichinella spiralis,Trichuris trichiura, Stvongyloides stercoralis,* and *Capillaria philippinensis.*

Based on Grimwood and Lambert (2009), Karanis (2006), Keusch et al. (2006) and WHO (2009, 2011). The words in bold indicate the common names (other than "diarrhoea") used for the different diagnoses.

Apart from the generally understood causality between the ingestion of pathogens and the expression of diarrheal disease, it is not easy to pinpoint the path ways that pathogens use in order to infect individuals in each specific context. This uncertainty increases in places with dense population and an abundance of hydro-social interaction, such as the Mekong Delta (Soussan et al., 2005, Herbst et al., 2009), making the control of diarrheal disease particularly challenging. As a result, it is also difficult to conclude whether changes in human behaviour, health policy or environmental sanitation have actually produced changes in the disease's incidence (Blum and Feachem, 1983). Nevertheless, research has provided some useful insights, which suggest positive potential in prevention measures.

1.2.2 Challenges in the prevention of diarrhoea: the factor of human behaviour

Establishing systems that deliver water of good quality and provide for the safer disposal of sewage has undoubtedly helped considerably in the control of disease (Cairncross et al., 2010b, Thompson et al., 2003, Young and Briscoe, 1988) and are, in any case, considered "essential for human life, dignity and human development" (WHO, 2012b). The results have been very encouraging when the health impacts from both water and sanitation improvements were studied together (Fewtrell et al., 2005, WHO, 2012d) as well as when sanitation was studied in isolation (Daniels et al., 1990, Cairncross et al., 2010a). However, evaluating the implementation of projects during the years from 1997 – 2007, the World Bank admits that, overall, "evidence of improved water quality is rare, as are indications of the improved health of project beneficiaries" (World Bank (WB), 2010: xiii). It is thus worth looking at when and how such improvements can really be a powerful preventive measure against disease.

Poor environmental sanitation has long been identified as a risk factor for human health (Manderson, 1987: 261) and thus there is no doubt that improving the sanitary conditions of people's living environment can surely deter the transmission of disease. However, it is important to stress that the success of protecting human health through environmental sanitation, is not adequately represented only by the presence of improved toilet constructions at the household level (Saravanan et al., 2011). Disease-exacerbating factors that are related to environmental sanitation also include aspects such as the "presence of wastewater in the street; refuse storage, collection and disposal; domestic water reservoir conditions; feces disposal from swaddles; presence of vectors in the house and flooding in the lot" (Heller et al., 2003). These aspects of *community* or *public* sanitation, in particular, were found to contribute to the spread of diarrhoea (Ibid. 2003).

With regard to clean water, Clasen and Cairncross (2004) emphasize that positive health impacts of improved water quality remain ambiguous when looking simply at the water source, drawing attention to the fact that pathogens can reappear by the time water is actually being used or consumed (Ibid. 2004). This is corroborated by Sobsey (2002) and Wright (2004), who demonstrate that intra-household behaviour often determines the quality of consumed water, for better or worse. The review study of Fewtrel et al. (2005) also supports the contention that the proper treatment and storage of water in the households can significantly contribute to the prevention of disease. As the diagram of Wagner and Lanoix from 1985 depicts (Fig. 1.1), most of the pathogens causing diarrhoea are waterborne, but not all cases are due to dirty water consumption (Jensen et al., 2004) and, in fact, apart from fluids, the main transmission routes of diarrhoea involve faeces, fields, flies, fingers and foods. Cairncross (2003) also finds that a large portion of endemic diarrhoea is actually transmitted from person to person, through dirty hands or feet and through practices of non-hygienic behaviour.

Curtis et al. (2000) underline the need for better community hygiene, which apart from the construction of toilets, also stresses the importance of extending or maintaining the practices of hand-washing with soap after defecation or after handling infants' stools. The assumption that the key ingredient in the fight against disease is merely the construction of WSS facilities ignores aspects of maintenance and sustainable use, which depend both on people's perceptions of safety and hygiene, as well as on the institutional support that they receive to maintain and use such facilities (Cairncross, 2003, Carter et al., 1999). Recently updated data from the WHO (2012d) show that even if improvements in water supply and sanitation might reduce the levels of diarrhoea morbidity up to 30%, it is the combination of those improvements with hygiene education that can lead to a worldwide reduction of diarrhoea cases up to 45% (WHO, 2012d). What literature tells us, in a nutshell, is that water and sanitation need to be looked at both in the community and in the household level, both in institutional and in behavioural terms, and most importantly need to be looked at in relation to each other, via integrated systems of delivery and treatment.

Figure 1.1: The F-diagram, depicting the main transmission routes of diarrheal diseases

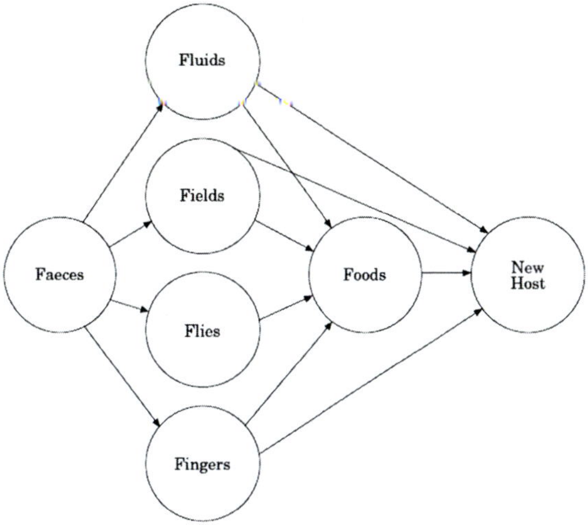

Wagner and Lanoix (1959) adopted from Curtis et al. (2000)

A central message that has emerged after years of dealing with and studying diarrheal diseases is that tackling the problem necessitates action on many fronts and not just with respect to improved water supply and sanitation. Practices of good nutrition and preventive Rotavirus vaccination can both help in building resistance and immunity in the population. Better hygienic practices and the correct use of oral re-hydration treatments can assist in recovery and in the avoidance of the disease's spread. As Feachem et al. (1983) have rightly pointed already in the 1980s, it is necessary to have a "multifaceted approach in which oral rehydration is one of several anti-diarrhoea measures that are implemented simultaneously with mutually reinforcing and complementary impacts". UNICEF and the WHO (2009) conclude that the concurrent adoption of the following six measures, can not only reduce the number of diarrheal deaths but also significantly control the disease's incidence in the medium to long term:

- Vaccinations against Rotavirus and measles
- Promotion of early and exclusive breastfeeding and vitamin A supplementation
- Promotion of hand-washing with soap

- Improved water supply quantity and quality, including the treatment and safe storage of water used in the household
- Community-wide sanitation promotion
- Fluid replacement therapy (Oral Re-hydration Therapy, ORT)

The use of ORT has been strongly advocated by the WHO since the 1980s as it reduces the loss of liquids and prevents the disease's severe stages, which can effectively saving children's lives. Chiabi et al. (2010) review the latest improvements of oral rehydration solutions and conclude that using "reduced osmolarity ORS and zinc supplementation have proven to be the cornerstone for the management of diarrhoea in children", bringing down the levels of diarrhoea mortality and morbidity. Together with Rotavirus vaccination (one of diarrhoea's main causes), ORT is one of the strongest biomedical tools to treat the disease and prevent its spread. Despite its huge potential, however, its use has not been as widespread and consistent as hoped for (Chiabi et al., 2010). Apart from not being promoted enough, its use has also been hampered by public uncertainty and confusion regarding its distinct and unique effect when compared to other type of home-prepared fluids. Moreover, people have been often resistant to adopt advice concerning the continued breastfeeding or solid food intake of patients during a diarrheal episode, both of which practices are known to reinforce the positive effects of ORT (Santosham et al., 2010, Thapar and Sanderson, 2004).

It is clear how many of the key preventive measures depend on behaviour and choices at the household level. Practicing hand-washing with soap, breastfeeding children, seeking timely medical advice, using ORS correctly, treating water carefully, keeping sanitation facilities hygienic and so on, all depend on individual judgments and choices. However, access to vaccines and medication, or to information about their availability and use, is not easily attained and can become particularly hard for people living in poverty. The same types of constraints might prevent people from improving their WSS situation, with direct consequences for their health. It therefore becomes clear that people's behaviour is not independent from the social and political spheres within which it takes place. The Mekong Delta presents a dynamic constellation of social and environmental characteristics which makes interaction between such spheres particularly interesting to study.

1.3 The Mekong Delta: diarrheal risks in an environment of intense hydro-social interaction and change

The process of transforming Vietnam from a planned to a market economy began in the 1980s and led to what today could be described as a system of socialist capitalism. The legal policy reforms that were initiated in 1986 marked the official beginning of the "□ ổi mới" reformation era. Since then, the country's markets have become open to private activity, foreign investment and external capital. One consequence of this shift appears to be the increase in the national GDP levels, as well as the improved picture of the country when observing indicators of well-being, such as the Human Development Index (Trading Economics, 2012, Nguyen Thang et al., 2006). Nevertheless, economic growth and a free market have not come without consequences. A closer look at the wealth distribution in the country shows that poverty elimination is still far from being achieved (Varis, 2008, World Bank (WB), 2013). Moreover, the increased agricultural and industrial production in Vietnam has come at the cost of severe environmental degradation. Human-induced pollution is currently endangering the sustainability of the country's rich water resources (Molle and Hoanh, 2008, Nguyen Thi Phuong Loan, 2010b) and has become particularly evident in the Mekong Delta (O'Rourke, 2004). The Delta is a hub of agro-activity and a region where industrial growth has also been strongly promoted. At the same time, water pollution control and wastewater treatment are two deficient and controversial sectors, in which inaction poses serious health risks to the local population. One of these is diarrhoea (Herbst et al., 2009, Reis and Mollinga, 2012).

1.3.1 Economic growth, polluted water environments and growing health disparities

A first glance at Vietnam's economic growth during the last 20 years shows a continuous rise of the country's GDP since the □ ổi mới era (from 6.3 to 103 billion USD), accompanied by a fluctuating but consistently positive annual economic growth (Trading Economics, 2012, IMF 2010 cited in Priwitzer, 2012: 78). Poverty levels have improved in the country, with the percentage of poor people dropping from 37.4% in 1998 (GSO, 2012a) to 11.1% in 2012 (GSO, 2013). The poverty indicators used in Vietnam however, are as low as 400,000 VND[6] monthly for the upper threshold to be considered impover-

[6] This amount is equivalent to about 20 USD and was reported by local cadres of district offices in Can Tho City. Informants distinguished a threshold of 400,000 VND for rural areas and 500,000 VND for urban areas (see also Box 4.2 in chapter 4.2.2). In the

ished, a sum that can barely cover the basic needs of food and clothes (MARD, 2010). In a recent report, the World Bank indicates that the use of newly-calculated and more appropriate poverty indicators would lead to a 27% poverty rate, more than doubling the officially-reported values (World Bank (WB), 2013). In comparing the rise in GDP and the performance in reducing poverty, there appears to be growing disparity. Leaving aside the argument of how much (extreme) poverty has been avoided due to economic growth, the question that is perhaps more worthwhile to examine is for whom this growth has been beneficial and who has been left behind.

Indeed, modern Vietnam is characterized by large disparities and an unequal distribution wealth. The average monthly income per capita for the richest household quintile in 2008 was 8.9 times higher than that in the poorest (GSO, 2008). The national Gini coefficient has risen to 0.43 during that same year (Ibid. 2008). Persisting inequalities in poverty and deprivation are mostly felt in the country's rural parts and particularly in areas where ethnic minorities are concentrated (Taylor, 2004, UNDP, 2011: 47). This stratification of access to wealth is bound to reflect on people's general well-being and health. It is indicative, for example, that the highest under-five mortality rates and the lowest high-school education levels are being noticed in regions that contain high ethnic diversity, such as the Northern midlands/mountainous areas and the central Highlands (GSO, 2011b: 90, GSO, 2010b: 78). Minh Nguyen Thang and Popkin (2003) observe the changes that took place after the renovation period (1993 – 1998) and underline how aspects of health appear to be closely linked with poverty:

> "The health status of the Vietnamese people has improved substantially in recent years but not for the poor (citing Pham et al. 2000) [...] The poor suffer a greater disease burden, have greater health needs, are less likely to seek health care services, and are less able to afford user fees." (Minh Nguyen Thang and Popkin, 2003)

The authors find links between poverty and health indicators that are closely related to diarrhoea, like infant mortality and children's malnutrition. Moreover, they point to the problem of people's access to healthcare that remains unaddressed in the country (Ibid. 2003). Fritzen (2007) describes how even after positive improvements in the health sector's organisational status, healthcare continues to be experienced differently by the poor, who mostly utilise low quality local health services. Despite significant improvements in legislation and

---

databases produced by the GSO of Vietnam, it is stated that, for the year 2011, the limits were adjusted by inflation and moved to 480,000 VND for rural areas and 600,000 VND for urban areas (GSO, 2012a).

efforts to increase the rate of health insurance among the population, the Vietnamese government has, according to Fforde (2013: 103), "failed to deal with major political questions [...] such as reforms to public health".

The rural areas and the poor are facing growing disparities regarding their access to resources and health, and at the same time are disproportionately experiencing the effects of water pollution, as rivers and canals nearby near to their work and life contain increasing levels of agrochemicals, pesticides, residual waste and faecal material. The Mekong Delta is a region where the local culture is closely connected to the waterscape and the services that water offers to people. Wet-rice cultivation, annual cycles of flooding, and river-based transportation and trade are almost synonymous with the Delta. Surface water from the rivers and canals has been traditionally used for daily activities like bathing, washing vegetables and drinking, but such habits are gradually being abandoned due to fears of water pollution and water-transmitted disease. Frequent flooding is known to contribute to the spread of waterborne disease, especially in a context of rapid urbanisation and water pollution, such as in the Delta (Saravanan et al., 2011, WHO, 2012d, Confalonieri et al., 2007: 400). The Hau River, which crosses the central Delta and flows through Can Tho City, "is heavily polluted by organic, chemical and microbiological substances, despite its high ability to self-clean (citing Nuber et al. 2008), and the related drainage canals suffer from untreated wastewater discharges" (Waibel et al., 2012: 181). People try to understand the risks and adapt to the changes that take place in their hydro-environments, but the consequences of those changes are complex and hard to cope with, especially for those with limited options at hand.

The problem of water pollution is not confined to the Delta; untreated wastewater is being discharged to the network of streams and canals throughout the country (DONRE, 2009). A booming economy and a growing population not only pollutes but also consumes water, depleting the underground reservoirs and causing the salinisation of aquifers in the coastal zones (Vietnam Environment Protection Agency, 2004, World Bank (WB), 2008). Environmental sanitation and health issues have made the news (Le Kien, 2011, Ha Van, 2010a), but, in legislative terms, they remain only partly addressed (Nguyen Thi Phuong Loan, 2010b, Nguyen Thi Phuong Loan, 2010a). Only 16% of the urban population in Vietnam is served by combined sewerage and drainage systems, with most of the untreated wastewater being directly discharged into water courses (ADB, 2007). By delaying action and not prioritising the adoption of integrated water management systems, the country's decision-makers are jeopardising the availability of water that is safe for human use (World Bank (WB), 2006). The government also appears weak in using the existing legal instruments to sanction and control the pollution stemming from industry, healthcare facilities and individual households (International Center for Environmental Management (ICEM), 2007: 197).

Tackling such pressing socio-environmental problems does not seem to be reflected in the overall priorities of the one-party government, which maintains the leading development vision of "urbanisation and modernisation to 2020" (Central Committee CPV and Communist Party of Vietnam, 2001). This vision has been materialising, with the growing share of urban population climbing to 21% nationally and increasing current at a rate of 5.18% (GSO, 2011b). The urban centres in the country have been marked by the expansion activity in the secondary and tertiary economic sectors, a rising number of employees working in industry and services[7] and a two-fold increase in the gross industrial output between the years 2005 and 2011 (GSO, 2011b). The Mekong Delta has largely followed this trend of urban agglomeration (Renaud and Kuenzer, 2012: 120), with the central province of Can Tho being upgraded to an urban City (level-I) in 2009 (Statistical Office of Can Tho City, 2009). However, the sort of development that is solely driven by economic growth and urbanisation tends to be blind to persisting inequalities and environmental consequences and, in many ways, runs contradictory to the core values projected by the Vietnamese Communist Party (VCP), namely those of progress and well-being for all.

Many authors contend that these contradictions owe to the fact that in Vietnam, political and bureaucratic elites have been appropriating the benefits of the open market and have been using the instruments and structures that operate under a one-party rule in order to safeguard their own powerful positions (Gainsborough, 2010b, Gillespie, 2001). This is seen to be taking place also through the technical and political exploitation of the country's water resources, particularly in the region of the Delta (Benedikter, 2014, Reis, 2012). As Beresdorf (2008) describes, the inflow of private funds since the renovation period came under the dominion of those who managed to associate and bond with the sources of those funds during the transition, thereby creating a new set of power dynamics in the country. Cheschier (2010) also speaks of how opening up to capitalism brought about unequally distributed financial gains and a so-called New Class[8], which was formed by those in close proximity to the state apparatus. These observations are in line with Gainsborough (2001) and King's (2008) discussions of an emerging socio-economic middle class that has been benefiting from much of what the new public-private mix in the economy has

[7] Rising from 32.2% of the population in 2005 to 51.3% in 2011 according to GSO (2011)

[8] By the term "New Class", Cheschier (2010) is here referring to Djilas (1957).

provided. In this constellation of events, Beresdorf (2008) sees that many have been excluded and that this exclusion owes to reasons connected to the absence of redistributive mechanisms in the country.

1.3.2 A blurry causality: water supply and sanitation and the control of diarrheal diseases

The sector of water supply and sanitation has gained significant attention during the last 20 years in Vietnam (GoV et al., 2006, MARD and MoC, 2000, The Prime Minister of Vietnam, 1994), accompanied by a noticeable decrease in the levels of cholera and typhoid (Kelly-Hope et al., 2008, MoH, 2012b). The rate of mortality for under-5 year-olds has also dropped during these last two decades (WHO, 2008, WHO, 2012c). Nevertheless, the results with regard to diarrheal disease appear on the whole neither clear nor sustainable. Firstly, cholera re-appeared with a big epidemic in 2007 and has not yet been eradicated in the country, with over 600 documented cases in 2010 (see also Fig 4.6). At the same time, there has been a significant increase in the incidence of dysentery throughout the 1990s, which is also still not tackled (Kelly-Hope et al., 2008, MoH, 2012a). Rotavirus appears to be the main cause for children being hospitalized (Van Man et al., 2005) while, in general, diarrhoea is still one of the leading causes of morbidity for people of all ages in the country (WHO, 2012c). Between 2001 and 2010, one in every hundred Vietnamese has been diagnosed with diarrhoea each year (MoH, 2012b). There is thus an emerging disparity between the increasing number of improved water facilities countrywide, on the one side, and the persistence of diarrheal diseases on the other.

Comparing national data separated by region, Soussan et al (2005) found that the Mekong Delta is a hotspot for diarrheal diseases. Regarding water and sanitation, the Delta was ranked fifth out of the six socio-economic regions for improved water supply (77.9%) and hygienic sanitation facilities (42.4%) (GSO, 2010a). The region thus combines comparatively poor WSS infrastructure and a high level of disease incidence. However, empirical findings provided by UNICEF (2012a) from the An Giang province of the Mekong Delta demonstrate why, despite this apparent correlation of facts, conclusions on the causal relationship between the two are hard to draw. Looking at the effects of seasonality on the incidence of diarrheal disease, the study showed that even during the dry period, when surface water quality (*E.coli* indicator) worsened and access to rainwater decreased, the incidence of the disease was not significantly different (UNICEF, 2012a). This means that the risk of disease did not seem to increase even when people were using water that was expected to be of lower quality than the improved sources. The authors suggest that this is probably because the changes in water quality were "masked by a complex mix of inter-household variations in water source and treatment methods, hygiene behaviour patterns and other risk factors that influence diarrhoeal disease risk" (Ibid., 2012:70). In other words, as earlier stressed (section 1.2.2), the complexity of behaviour and choices that characterizes the use, treatment and consumption of water within each household is what defines the water's quality at its point-of-use; this can (re-)shape the risk and the outcome of disease.

The effects of household behaviour on the spread of disease have been acknowledged in national policy and particularly in the National Rural Water Supply and Sanitation Strategy (MARD and MoC, 2000), which proclaims the target of health education as central. While the declared approach to WSS is to be "demand-responsive" and thus to cultivate demands through "Information Education and Communication activities and community participation" (MARD 2003: 12), the content and the orientation of those activities are not specified. Reis (2012) has discussed how WSS policy in the rural areas of the Delta is now pushing towards the construction of household-based sanitation and away from providing more centralised solutions or information for water that is safe for human consumption. As Cairncross et al (2010a) have warned, overshadowing the health education content with the promotion of construction (either of water supply or sanitation) might undermine the effectiveness of the health messages:

> "Hygiene promotion and sanitation promotion both suffer from the budgetary dominance of water supply, and from a loss of effectiveness when implemented too fast. Freeing sanitation promotion from its link with construction (of toilets or of water supplies) avoids these problems and makes it more suitable for implementation by the health sector." (Cairncross et al., 2010a)

The Vietnamese Ministry of Agriculture and Rural Development (MARD) has listed some of the problems that the demand-driven communicative approach faced during the first years of its implementation, acknowledging that "there were no regular in-depth surveys on people's knowledge, attitudes and practices, or any impact evaluations, which made it very hard to monitor change" (MARD, 2003). Ten years after these acknowledgments by the MARD, the question that arises now is whether it is informed demand that has raised the amount of WSS expansion and how well this reflects the public's awareness of hygiene and potential for improved health outcomes.

1.4 Study objectives and research approach

The aim of this study is to answer how cultural, social and political environments define and shape the spread of diarrheal disease in Can Tho City in Vietnam's Mekong Delta. In order to answer this question, data collection and analysis were based on the following four objectives: (i) To delineate the institutional structures behind the prevention and control of diarrheal disease and to question their contribution in limiting the disease's prevalence[9] in the country; (ii) to describe which environmental and socio-economic aspects create favourable conditions for the exacerbation of the disease in the Mekong Delta; (iii) to trace the existing perceptions and understandings around diarrhoea and around the practices that can drive its spread in both urban and rural settings in Can Tho City; (iv) to discover and discuss the socio-political factors guiding the discourse and underlying the implementation of public policy around diarrheal disease at both the national and local levels.

In order to address these objectives, this study draws greatly from the theoretical current of Political Ecology. The field provides a holistic approach as it demands the inseparability of ecological and social phenomena. Political ecology also poses questions of power. Here, power is understood as being distributed and negotiated in ways that inevitably affect the nature and the outcome of socio-ecological interactions. Tracing the roots of inequalities that have come together with the use of natural resources, apparent in the uneven distribution of risks and benefits, political ecologists have also sought to answer how knowledge around these risks is constructed. Through this questioning of socio-environmental problems, power emerges as the locomotive force which determines how policy turns into practice and whom this process benefits. Being able to locate 'the political' in disease, as in this study, is a similar sort of task, aiming to answer questions such as what guides the spread of disease physically, what hinders its control institutionally and what disempowers people from being able to be adequately protected from it.

Engaging with questions of how the risk of disease is constructed, communicated and understood, this study also calls for a better understanding of the agents who produce, receive and circulate that knowledge. Seeing how the issue of "behaviour" takes a central role in the control of diarrheal disease, it is important for the analysis to be able to capture and understand prevailing beliefs, habits and public perceptions. This turn to culture and agency has been commonly addressed in the methods and the concepts used in anthropology. Thus, in order to demonstrate the way the risk of disease is understood and experienced in the everyday life of the actors, this study also draws from the field of Critical Medical Anthropology. This field proved extremely useful in exploring

[9] Prevalence (of disease) = the proportion of the population that is infected at one time (Joralemon, 2010:32).

human health, as it lays bare issues of access to wealth and power, relating socio-political aspects to patterns of disease and the cultural meanings that are ascribed to disease.

In order to collect data that would support a critical and holistic analysis for the problem of disease from a social science perspective, the study followed an abductive research strategy, where "data and theoretical ideas are played off against one another in a developmental and creative process" (Blaikie, 2009: 156). In need of an approach that could accommodate interpretative and critical explanations on disease, a topic that is commonly understood through biomedical concepts of a technical and deterministic nature, the abductive approach was useful in its use of "both technical and lay concepts to link structure and agency" (Ibid., 2010:118). Without having a formulated hypothesis, the aim of the research was to understand problems with conceptual guidance from the fields of political ecology and critical medical anthropology. In order to better address the objectives of the research, the collection and analysis of data followed a mixed-method paradigm. Qualitative and quantitative data offered different kinds of information which, at different times, complemented and contradicted each other. The same series of data were seen under the light of statistical significance and interpretative meaning. Overall, qualitative analysis was emphasized, while quantitative analysis was seen as valuable to provide "an objective or observer's perspective that can then be supplemented (and reflexively contextualized) by an interpretive perspective integrating the views of the subjects themselves" (Harrits, 2011: 161). Using mainly semi-structured and in-depth interviewing (87 in total), qualitative results came mostly in the form of transcripts. However, these were complemented with observations of participants and the research context, documented daily in the form of field notes. A household survey was conducted in 131 households of urban and rural communities. The findings of the survey were meant to contrast with and complement unstructured discussions and observations. Material that is used for health communication purposes was examined both quantitatively and interpretively, placing it in the realm of discourse about disease that is formulated in an ongoing manner by state representatives and the interviewed household members. Secondary statistics were collected on the disease's prevalence, water supply and sanitation expansion, and water quality, but were mostly used as starting point for reflection and criticism rather than as a comprehensive and valid source of information. Scientific literature and media reports also contributed to framing the discussion of the findings, while photographic material helped in documenting snippets of information in visual form.

The findings of this work are discussed in the chapters that follow. Chapter 2 reviews how literature has approached the issues of environmental health and particularly of disease, tracing the parallels with approaches in development and pinpointing the gaps in critical scientific knowledge about health. To this end, the chapter draws connections between agency and structure. The chapter situates the study in the fields of political ecology of health and critical medical anthropology, delineating the analytical categories encompassing elements from both these fields. It also presents a framework of analysis that outlines the events involved in the course of the disease's prevention-infection-cure-control pathway, paying attention to the context of personal, social, environmental and political spheres, as well as to the issues that emerge from their interactions.

Chapter 3 elaborates more on the methodological approach, offering a detailed description of the steps followed during the data collection and analysis. The chapter also justifies the selection of the case-study areas and provides some background on their significant characteristics for this study. Furthermore, chapter 3 reflects upon the limitations posed by the "character" of the research field and discusses how those challenges were addressed.

The empirical analysis begins in chapter 4, which focuses on the health sector in the country and looks at how the changes following the renovation and decentralisation policies are reflected in the function of its services today, particularly in regard to public access to healthcare and its utilisation. The chapter offers a description of the sector's organisational structure, focusing on those aspects that are crucial in the management of diarrheal disease (primary healthcare, preventive health education and reporting of epidemics). Additionally, the status of some of the main infectious diseases is presented and critically discussed, focusing on how the incidence of diarrheal disease appears in statistics generated at national, regional and local levels.

Chapter 5 examines the expansion of water supply and sanitation in the region of the Delta and uses empirical and secondary data to question the actual contribution of WSS infrastructure in reducing the risks of diarrheal disease. Looking at the results of policy implementation, particularly in the region of Can Tho, the chapter questions the values that govern this sector, looking foremost at issues of equity, transparency and efficacy. Although advancements in WSS have been claimed to be a major component of health prevention, the findings presented in chapter 5 bring into question the capacity of those advancements to provide clean water and sanitary living environments in a sustainable manner.

Chapter 6 tries to look at the prevention of diarrheal disease holistically, moving beyond the technical measures of water supply and sanitation expansion. It traces the fragments of policy that exist in national legislation and examines their implementation within Can Tho City. The chapter particularly emphasizes the health education mechanisms that are employed to raise awareness about the issue of diarrheal disease. It analyses the means and methods used in the circulation of information, with a focus on the content of messages that are communicated to the public.

Chapter 7 focuses on the two selected case-study areas, the urban Cai Rang and the rural Phong Dien districts. Presenting and discussing the results of the household survey, the chapter portrays how the factors related to the spread of diarrheal disease are viewed and experienced by local actors. Complemented by qualitative information and analysis, the chapter presents a more informed understanding of household behaviour, placing people's documented practices in water supply, water treatment, hygiene and sanitation side by side with their perceptions on water safety and disease. People's preventive and curative attitudes are examined in relation to such perceptions to the structural constraints that they commonly face. Here, the statements of local residents often contradict much of the officially circulated discourse, and these help pinpoint gaps between policy and practice in public health.

Chapter 8 brings together the findings of the study and draws overall conclusions about the interplay of factors shaping the risk of diarrheal disease. It combines the insights drawn from institutional, anthropological and statistical analysis and traces two emerging phenomena: the "normalisation" of diarrheal disease and the construction of sick identities in poverty and rurality. These insights are then also discussed in relation to the two analytical categories that were chosen for the study, namely the epidemiology of health messages and the politics of risk communication. Chapter 8 also draws conclusions about how the principles of political ecology and critical medical anthropology proved to be a useful theoretical ground for this analysis. Ultimately, the chapter presents how the findings of this study can contribute to these theoretical fields and generally to the literature of interdisciplinary studies of health and disease.

A POLITICAL ECOLOGY OF DISEASE INFORMED BY CRITICAL MEDICAL ANTHROPOLOGY

CHAPTER 2

This chapter situates the research in the field of political ecology, justifying along the way why this theoretical approach is useful in the study of health and disease. First, some parallels are drawn between the modernist approaches to human development and the strictly biomedical approaches to human health. The limitations of such views in understanding problems holistically will be flagged (2.1). After discussing the potential for carrying out socially and culturally relevant studies in health and disease by merging the currents of political ecology and critical medical anthropology, the chapter traces the value of this pairing by drawing together analysis on human agency and institutional structure (2.2). Borrowing from the questions and the angles that have been traditionally examined in these two fields, the analytical fields that become the focus of this study are discussed in more detail (2.3). To conclude, the chapter offers a combined depiction of the study's analytical framework and conceptualisation of the problem. It does so by illustratively arranging factors that can determine the outcome of disease around the single incidence and conceptually situating these factors at the interpenetrating spheres of personal, social, environmental and political context.

2.1 Problematising health

Health problems have been usually viewed in development studies as an aftermath of socio-economic evils: a companion of insufficient growth, delayed progress or low institutional capacity. It is true that weaknesses of an economic and institutional nature often accompany major public health problems. However, the presumed trickle-down effects of economic and technological advancements have not been fully realised in relation to health and well-being, neither in the global North or South. This is because such presumptions often fail to consider the socio-ecological dynamics and the cultural landscapes that define the way economic and technological advancements are distributed and experienced in the wider population in the places in question (Gardner et al. 1996 cited in Chay Navuth, 2006: 24, Power 2008 cited in Potter et al., 2012: 66). Considering health as the aftermath, as a part, or as a goal of human development leads to the question: what kind of development is being pursued? Envisaging progress in health through a modernist lens would mean to pursue an overt technological and economic advancement of the sector led by western paradigms of advanced biomedical knowledge. This approach, however, would likely be blind to the inequalities and injustices that govern local institutions of health and, most importantly, it would exclude alternative visions and beliefs on health (and disease). It is for this reason that such visions need to be criticised, not as utopian or impossible to achieve, but as consciously apolitical.

2.1.1 Humanities in health and the link to development

There are many parallels between modernist views in human health and those in development. The conceptualisation of development as a desired "outcome" that human societies should pursue and which can be rigidly defined, has been heavily criticised and reframed by post-modern and deconstructionist theorists (Parfitt, 2002: 78ff). Scholars from these schools have argued that the modernist development approach disempowers, subordinates and controls nations, groups and individuals (Sachs 1992 cited in Schuurman, 2000). To contrast to the monolithic views of modernism, scholars have discussed different ways of discovering what are the desired outcomes in human societies, investigating concepts like "development from below", "people-centred development" or "another development" (Potter et al., 2012: 75ff).

Alongside the differing debates about development, approaches focused on human health and the risk of disease, have also been debated from different viewpoints. From the side of the social sciences, Deborah Lupton opines that a western-centred focus on health has used biomedical solutions as "the ultimate weapons against illness, disease and premature death" (Lupton, 2012a: vii), often overlooking cultural aspect of health. Western narratives about how to bring about or maintain good health, and of what constitutes disease, have influenced curative means across the globe. Such narratives have "all generated ideas and practices which tend to deny the fragility and mortality of the human body" (Ibid. 2012a). By discursively taking away the (cultural) meanings assigned to health, its social significance is also stripped away. Bambra et al (2005) argue similarly that this medicalisation of health explains, in part, why our scientific views of it have been largely depoliticised. The rendering of medicalised and depoliticised approaches in health as the dominant paradigm, has been an ongoing process globally. According to Nichter and Nichter (1996a) such processes are "constituting an agency of socialization where relations of power, dominance, and dependency take concrete form" and, in some respect, are reifying the capitalist ideology, with the latter "being swallowed along with the pills that embody it" (Ibid 1996a: 269).

Nevertheless, even in parts of the world where biomedicine has a long history and many successful narratives, human health is still facing major challenges. Many diseases have been eradicated as a result of advancements in science that have come hand-in-hand with socio-economic growth and the mortality rate for other diseases has seen a significant decline. But despite what the "modern world" has achieved, the affluent West is now being "plagued" by health problems such as obesity (Ohtsuka and Ulijaszek, 2007: 11ff) and has to face the increasing mortality of chronic diseases. The fact that, even in exemplary contexts of technological development and economic prosperity, people have not been freed from disease, indicates that good health is not simply a technical matter and it is not only guided by economic growth. For this reason, as social scientists argue, assessments of health cannot simply rely on statistical indicators which use narrowly defined categories (i.e. the rate of diseases mortality or the average rate of hospital bed availability). Instead, to better illustrate the sources of disease and the reasons of public health failures, observers need to take greater account of the social structures and the cultural meanings in each context. It is often the case, for example, that a decrease in disease mortality is not accompanied by a decrease in disease morbidity, suggesting that "there is an awareness of the availability of curative intervention, but the preventive intervention components have not been emphasized or have been unsuccessful" (Pollack 1983 cited in Nichter, 1996a: 400).

Problems of financial or know-how constraints might be part of the reason why advancements in medicine have not been able to reach everyone in need (Schlipköter and Flahault, 2010). But what the humanities emphasize with regard to health, as part and parcel of development, is that it needs to be more ethnographically informed. In the words of Leonard Syme:

> "We epidemiologists have suffered a whole series of very embarrassing failures. [...] Our model is to identify the risk factors and share that information with a waiting public so that they will then rush home and, in the interests of good health, change their behaviours to lower their risk. It is a reasonable model, but it hasn't worked. […] We in public health have important messages to give to people, but people have lives to lead. There often is a major gap between these two priorities. This is an issue that anthropologists think about, and it would be good to incorporate that thinking into the design of better interventions." (Leonard Syme in Trostle, 2005: xi)

2.1.2 Re-conceptualising health and disease

In the fields of anthropology, sociology and ethnography, the meanings that people assign to their experiences and actions are often interrogated, and the objectivity of "facts" is questioned. Nichter and Nichter (1996b) demonstrate the importance of metaphor and analogy in the communication of health messages, while Myrick (1996) argues that AIDS-related campaigns entail the construction of certain realities that place blame on the gay community.

But efforts to look at health holistically have expanded into more disciplines. A growing knowledge on the intrinsic connections and interactions between human societies and their surrounding ecologies has looked at human health in relation to natural environments and natural phenomena. Health Ecology for example, views health as a result of a constant dialogue between individuals and the environmental changes from local to global scales (Collins, 2001, Hunar□ et al., 1999). The discipline of Medical Geography (Jones and Moon, 1987, Jones and Moon, 1991) and the more socially influenced, Geography of Health (Kearns, 1993, Kearns and Moon, 2002, Gatrell, 2005), use space as an explanatory basis and a conceptual bridge that connects medical, natural and social explanations of health. These and other similar approaches, have provided the basis for looking together at systems previously seen mostly as separate and for understanding how the processes within and among these systems are shaping human health. The study of epidemics, in particular, can offer a fertile ground for opening the scientific discussion in this regard, as epidemics "offer a particularly vivid demonstration of the interconnections between biological, social and cultural components in the human experience of disease" (Joralemon, 2010: 29).

Many of the interdisciplinary attempts to conceptualise human health, however, fail to theorise enough outside their methodological traditions. Epidemiologists, for example, often relate statistical patterns of disease to other series of data that might be of an economic, social or cultural nature. Their claimed purpose is to illustrate the interplay between health and society through showing the statistical relationship between, for instance, the prevalence of certain pathologies and poverty (Weiss and Lonnquist, 2003: 57). However, such analysis rarely goes into examining and discussing why such relationships exist (Leatherman, 2005: 50) and, moreover, rarely reflects critically on the sources and the limitations of the quantitative data as such. Notwithstanding the interesting insights that can emerge from systematic large-scale statistical approaches, in isolation, they are limited in interdisciplinary depth and necessitate complementary explanations. Trying to approach the "cultural" side of biological expressions (reflected in health), some have instead focused on the genetic and evolutionary characteristics of human societies, coming up with biocultural explanations of disease. However, these routinely ignore the behavioural and social aspects, which in synergy with biology, define people's vulnerabilities and adaptive capacities regarding disease (Singer et al., 1992, Lock, 2001). As asserted in the work of Joralemon (2010: 42), only under a critical interpretive lens is the evolutionary/ecological approach able to answer the question of "who benefits and who suffers from the economic structures that provide [disease] the opportunity to take hold and spread".

In response to the limitations that the above approaches have presented, the works of critical and cultural disease ecologists and epidemiologists (such as: Brown, 2006, DiGiacomo, 1999, Trostle, 2005, Amsterdamska, 2005) have advanced toward a more comprehensive view of how social aspects affect health and, in doing so, broaden the boundaries of health studies. In the example of Kenya, Akala (2006) investigates the social and political ramifications of HIV, showing how the disease acts as "a sophisticated social condition responsible for unprecedented social injustices particularly against young uninfected and voiceless victims", thus pushing our conceptualisation of AIDS beyond "just a health condition requiring anti-retroviral treatment, a balanced diet and research focused on evolving a cure and/or vaccines".

Emerging from such problematisations, the field of Medical Sociology "places health and disease in a social, cultural and behavioural context" (ASA 2002 cited in Weiss and Lonnquist, 2003). Rudolf Virschow is considered the father of this discipline, as he was the first medical practitioner who traced the roots of an epidemic[10] in the prevailing socio-economic conditions of the time, arguing that "medicine is a social science, and politics nothing but medicine on a grand scale" (Virschow cited in Taylor and Rieger, 1984). Others have argued that a sociological approach of health is not really new, but a return to what was before holistically examined as people's well-being:

> "From a nineteenth-century perspective, when medicine was yet to throw its future in with the merging experimental laboratory sciences (and when sociological perspectives had not yet been purged of their psychological, organicist or physiological roots), health and disease were not clearly defined as biological and physiological processes but more commonly discussed in broader terms, better encapsulated within the concept of well-being." (Collyer, 2012: 5)

This blending of disciplines in the attempt to approach health socially, however, has often maintained strong ontological dividers between society and health. Falola and Healton (2006, my emphasis) for example, state that they seek to illustrate "the combination of real medical risks, with the social environment that often exacerbates them". While offering some powerful descriptive demonstrations of socially produced inequalities of health, the authors imply that there is an explanation of health which is objectively real (biological, medical, scientific) and thus not under question. In light of this "real" risk of disease, society is perceived as acting externally and not as an intrinsic player in defining risk. In contrast, cultural theories of risk see the important role of actors in constructing the meaning of a risk, recognising that "the fabric and texture of

---

[10] The author is referring to the typhus epidemic in Upper Silesia during the year 1847.

these constructions reflect both the interests/values of each group or institution in the various risk arenas and the shared meaning of terms, cultural artefacts, and natural phenomena among groups" (Aven and Renn, 2010: 39).

What the myriad conceptualisations of risk share is the collective recognition by various societies of an outcome as negative (Brooks, 2003). Despite the "realness" of a pathogen studied under a microscope, for example, its spread will not be treated as a health risk unless it is recognised as such within the affected society. Defining risks is heavily shaped by the available discourses, which in turn can be culturally, scientifically and politically driven. Though she is not using risk terminology, McIntosh (1996: 215) looks at food and nutrition as social problems and find similarly that "the sociological aspects of social problems concern the identification of groups that successfully define a situation as a social problem worthy of attention and the rhetorical tools these groups use to persuade others of the problem's existence and importance". Through the above scholarly problematisation of risk definitions, it becomes clearer why, despite the real, biological and tangible essence of nature and of human bodies, social workings need to be considered as a vital part in the shaping of risk understandings and thus, in the shaping of action taken to manage those risks. Twaddle (1994 cited in Hofmann, 2011: 21) for example, explains that while disease is seen as a tangible health problem "that consists of a physiological malfunction", illness is defined as an individual assessment of "an undesirable state of health", while sickness is understood as a socially-established condition concerning the relative ability of an ill person to carry out her social roles and duties.

Enriched by theories of cultural theory and social constructivism, sociologists of health and medicine have recognised that medical knowledge is "a series of relative constructions which are dependent upon the socio-historical settings in which they occur and are constantly renegotiated" (Lupton, 2012b: 8) and thus, that there is a need not only for more critical but also for more interpretive studies of health (Lupton, 2012b: 19). In her work, Mary Douglas has advanced the heuristic of questioning of disease as socially and culturally produced, proposing that physical and social bodies are not only co-dependent but also redefine and reconstitute each other (Douglas, 2002). Based upon Douglas' work, Gammeltoft (1999) explains this as a mutual struggle between these social and physical "bodies" of the same experiential and the cognitive self to understand and define each other:

> "The social body constraints the way the physical body is perceived. The physical experience of the body, always modified by the social categories in which it is known, sustains a particular view of society." (Gammeltoft, 1999: 132)

Along similar lines, Di Giacomo (1999) supports the idea that disciplines like cultural epidemiology should move away from naturalist approaches towards the body and from unproblematised views of society and, instead, should embrace interpretative analytical pathways. Gadamer has argued that if do not take the anthropological perspective into consideration, the concept of health can turn into a hardly definable 'enigma' (Gadamer 1993 cited in Hofmann, 2011). While agreeing on the essentiality of anthropological inquiries in health, some medical anthropologists like Margaret Lock also emphasize how dangerous it would be to treat the human body only as a social container and assume that biological factors play no role at all in the experience of disease (Lock, 2001, Lock, 1993):

> "There is no doubt that biological and genetic determinisms must be rejected outright. But it is also necessary to reject those equally deterministic arguments for the social and cultural construction of the body and related medical practices in which the material body is black-boxed. Truth claims about the body demand contextualization and critical appraisal, but to ignore the reality of biology entirely and its interdependence with history and culture is short-sighted in the extreme." (Lock 2001)

In line with the work of Douglas, a 'three bodies approach' is discussed by Scheper-Hughes and Lock (1987) who try to conceptually delineate the individual, the social and the political through an anthropology of the body. The individual body, then, depicts what people experience, both physically and mentally. The social body is understood as the medium through which bodily elements are turned into social categories and, conversely, social structures are transformed into health experiences. This is also related to the idea of the body politic, which refers to the use of health as an object of regulation, to be controlled and to effect control through various means. Michel Foucault (2003) elaborates how the political is inseparable to the individual and social body of health. According to him, both medical and sociological knowledge "began to operate, hand in hand to make the individual and social body and its diseases legible" and thus allow for the creation of a means to control it, and thereby determining how closely power is tied to assigning meanings of health.

Trumper and Phillips (1995) show how the construction of discourse regarding cholera was used to perpetuate social power structures in Ecuador and Chile. Similarly, Nations and Monte (1996) describe how entire favela communities in Brazil were stigmatised as carrying and spreading cholera, leading to an old favela resident to claim: "we are the disease", which suggests how state-generated discourse saw the problem as the people and not the disease. The authors go on to discuss how the members of these marginalised communities then refused any help from state-led prevention campaigns (Ibid. 1996) and effectively exacerbated their individual risk through their common reaction to a politically constructed socialisation of disease against them. In light of the theoretical review thus far, the 'three bodies approach' seems to serve as a useful entry towards a holistic view of health issues (Joralemon, 2010). This is not only because it can capture the many dimensions of disease through individual, social and political spheres, but also because it emphasizes the permeability of these spheres, an aspect rarely showcased in literature.

2.2 Theoretical grounds

This study draws greatly from the theoretical current of Political Ecology. A recent definition by Baer and Singer (2009) sees political ecology not only as a field examining the power exercised over natural resources, but as "an approach to understanding the factors that impact and result from environmental-society interaction that recognizes the fundamental importance of political economy, including capitalist production, market-driven distribution of resources, urbanization, and population growth". Before elaborating on the particular angles that will be examined in this study, it is necessary to explain why the framework of political ecology is particularly useful in the study of diarrheal disease. The answer is centred on the disease's main transmitter: water.

Water is a resource often scarce in good quality. It is no surprise that it has frequently been the focus of political ecology analysis, showing how natural resources do not "naturally" get exhausted, polluted or distributed and how the experienced scarcities are socially and politically constructed (Aguilera-Klink et al., 2000, Kallis and Coccossis, 2003, Bakker, 2000). As a carrier of intestinal pathogens and also a major determinant of hygiene, water undeniably takes a central part in the study of disease. Water pollution is an environmental issue with direct repercussions to human health, including diarrhoea. The mechanisms in place to control water pollution therefore determine the spread of disease, albeit indirectly but nonetheless to a great extent. Pathogens, and with them the risk of disease, are being transferred and concentrated along with untreated sewage and bad water supply networks in households, communities and public spaces, at the same time when the benefits of safe water and sanitation are not equally distributed.

The rules that govern access to water are also likely bound to reflect on other crucial determinants of disease, like access to healthcare, as the systems of governance for both water and health operate side by side in the same social and institutional context of a place. Therefore, a critical study of diarrheal disease must examine not only the sectors of water supply and sanitation, but also the sectors of health and healthcare. Political ecology offers a useful framework to trace the roots of inequalities that might exist in these sectors and to explain them, but also to help answer questions such as how and why knowledge around environmental health risks is being constructed and spread. Power is a central concept, as, of course, it underlines the political in political ecology. Power is seen as an implicit force which fills the gap between policy and practice, defining which discourse will be turned into what action. Thus, the "political" is highly relevant when seeking to answer questions like why diseases are spread (physically), why they are not addressed and controlled (by preventive environmental and health policy) and why people cannot adequately protect from them (behaviourally and socially).

2.2.1 Building on political ecologies of health

Political ecologists have often interrogated how the marginality and vulnerability of populations is produced and by what means it is maintained, relating these aspects to an unequal access to resources, to power and to knowledge claims, which in turn define the fate of environments, natural resources and again reflect on societies (Bryant, 1998b). Looking at water, Swyngendouw (2009) elaborates a political economy and political ecology of the "hydro-social cycle", stressing that "particular attention needs to be paid to social power relations (whether material, economic, political, or cultural) through which hydro-social transformations take place". These kind of questions are, also for Bryant, immensely important for studies of development (1991 cited in Mann, 2009). But even though water has gained increasing attention from political ecologists over the past two decades (e.g. Budds, 2013, Kaika, 2003, Loftus, 2005, Otero et al., 2010, Swyngedouw, 1997), such research has rarely been overtly coupled with issues of health.

However scarce, the political ecology of health and disease is not an entirely new field. Mayer traces the political ecology of disease back to Turshen (1977) and stresses how important it is to "understand the social, cultural and political factors which influence disease; the environmental characteristics which influence and frequently determine the nature of host-agent interaction; and the behavioural dimensions of individual or group susceptibility to disease" (Mayer, 1996b: 442). Mayer (1996b) sees the value of integrating human agency within specific spatial, cultural, political and social contexts, which would, according to him, reveal aspects that were never before directly linked to the spread of diseases or epidemics. However, the criticism of his work by King (2010), points to a deficit of theoretical and empirical links supporting his claims and to a mistaken interpretation of political ecology as "the integration of cultural ecology and political economy".

King (2010:40) offers an evaluation of the sporadic studies in the political ecology of health and argues that the discipline "offers a needed framework for understanding how social and environmental systems intersect to shape health across spatial and temporal scales" and thus "it would assist in illustrating how these relationships shape the transmission of disease and the ability of institutions to provide effective treatment". Using the example of the governmental reactions towards HIV in S. Africa, King (1996) recognises that politics penetrate discourse and policy around disease. However, he does not go into exactly why and how this happens, and as such his case is lacking in empirical depth. A better example comes from Richmond et al. (2005), who drew from Mayer (1996b), and applied his concept to the case of Aboriginal Canadian Peoples (First Nations). These authors describe how processes of globalisation affected aquaculture and caused local communities to lose their access to resources of land and water, leading eventually to their economic and social degeneration (Richmond et al., 2005). The impacts that environmental changes had on the population's health and well-being are detailed, and they way in which people understood and reacted to such changes is brought forward in order to merge global and local analytical scales and include human agency in the analysis (Ibid. 2005). An interesting study by Guénel (2004), that could be characterized as a political ecology of disease, even though it does not claim to be one, looks historically at the co-evolution of the French colonisation process and the spread of malaria in Vietnam. The author discusses how the surrounding ecology and the movements of migrating populations affected the epidemiology of malaria, at the same time underlining the effects of economic and political changes in determining the formulation and the success of certain control strategies against malaria in the country.

A more comprehensive political ecology of health approaches issues from a slightly different vantage, focusing additionally on the access to health services and not strictly on the patterns of disease. Blaikie and Brookfield (1987) have discussed the socially-produced unequal access to decision-making in health and have demonstrated how this consequently renders certain groups in society more vulnerable than others. Similar works to this direction have come from authors who do not identify themselves as political ecologist but incorporate questions, methodologies and analyses that are typical of the discipline. A study of the birth-control policy in S. Africa by Susanne (2006: 106), for example, reveals how the official decisions entailed elements of national pride, discrimination against "poor whites" and political pressures from groups "whose competing interests whether nationalist, politically moderate, feminist or eugenic".

The work of Farmer (2005) closely looks at how access to healthcare is intricately linked to people's struggles for social and economic rights and how the experienced inequalities in those fields "can indeed generate a kind of quiet brutality" (Amartya Sen in the Foreword of Farmer, 2005) against the health of the least powerful.

Studies such as those referenced above are not clearly addressing aspects of access to natural resources or environmental change, but are rather focused on the political economy and institutional analysis of health(care). Nevertheless, these studies are good examples of what is missing from the so nascent field of political ecology of health and disease. As Collins (2001) has noted, "studies that are able to identify the processes and perceptions that define a political ecology of healthcare, are rare" (Ibid 2001: 240). This additional focus would enable research to see health in its institutional complexity and to question it as a cultural and social category, as a subject of control and as a means of controlling. In other words, a political ecology of disease would have to deal with the idea and the concept of health, not only as an outcome, but more as part of the process that shapes health outcomes (Fig. 2.1).

Figure 2.1: From non-problematised views to an integrated and critical analysis of water-related disease

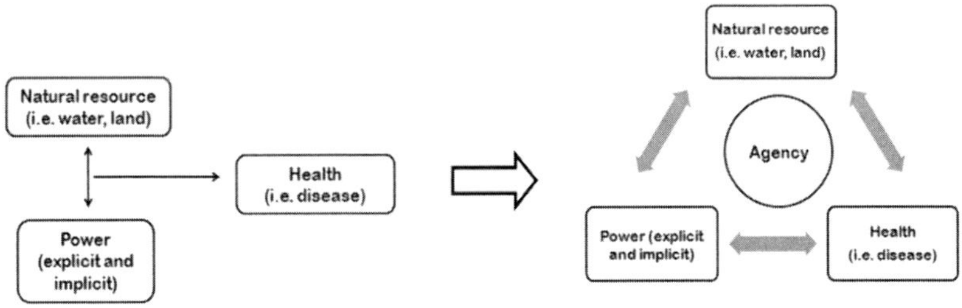

Author, 2014

As Roseberry (1988 cited in Leatherman, 2005) has pointed out, uniting structure and agency is exactly where the strength and unparalleled potential of political ecology lies. It is therefore crucial to involve agency when looking at how structures of health, water and power interact and what this interaction produces. In doing so, the conceptual and methodological tools used in critical medical anthropology become indispensable.

2.2.2 Borrowing from critical medical anthropology

In the first part of this chapter, I discussed why ethnographic and deconstructive approaches to disease are valuable. Although this study is not entirely anthropological, the field is considered the main conceptual and analytical resource for dealing with health risk perceptions and health-related behaviour. The latter aspects are considered important in understanding why certain preventive measures are successful in specific contexts and why others are not. Observing the connection between health behaviour and cultural norms, social structures and local beliefs can point to useful approaches for the control of health risks but can also reflect back to the society and illuminate important structures therein.

Previous studies from an anthropological vantage, particularly on diarrhoea, have illuminated its cultural aspects and how these shape people's attitudes and actions towards the disease, which eventually shapes its outcome:

> "Connotative aspects of a diarrheal episode might involve subtle cues which trigger the memory of a past illness experience, feelings of fear or vulnerability related to a particular season, celestial event, or environmental happenstance, or ideas about causality linked to humors, sexual behavior, the excessive consumption of sweet foods, witchcraft, or the evil eye. They might also index cultural notions of blame or responsibility, issues related to entitlement which influence health seeking behavior; or the need for secrecy associated with stigma." (Nichter, 1996b: 116)

Under the light of such studies, when seeking to adequately explain the disease's spread, and to provide recommendations about its control, questions of meaning, belief and culture gain in significance. Some medical anthropologists have further acknowledged how inextricably linked culture and behaviour is with the accumulation and the exercise of power. Young (1982 cited in Lock, 2001: 480) locates this political aspect of health in that "all medical knowledge and practice is historically and culturally constructed and embedded in political economies, and further, subject to continual transformation both locally and globally". When looking at the prominent or implicit forms of knowledge about disease or about health and the human body, one will inevitably come to question the scientific field of biomedicine. As Starr (1982 cited in Wolpe, 1985) comments that the medical profession has acquired through time a sort of "cultural authority" in society. According to Navarro (1984 cited in Weiss and Lonnquist, 2003), this is achieved through the use of coercive mechanisms that powerful groups possess and use in order to force this authority onto others. Thus, when anthropological accounts examine issues of health discourse and practice, they ought to also look at how struggles and claims around health connect to socio-economic spheres of national and international levels. Critical medical anthropology has advanced the study of health in this regard.

In the field of critical medical anthropology, health is explored by laying bare issues of access to wealth and power, relating them to patterns of disease and to the cultural meanings ascribed to it (Joralemon, 2010). Baer and Singer define the field as:

> "[...] an approach to understanding human health at the local, regional, national, and international levels, that emphasizes the central role of interaction between structural factors (like the distribution of power in society and the structuring of social inequality), biological factors (like human biological evolution and pathogenic adaptation to human hosts), and cultural patterns (like social beliefs systems, practices, and organization) on human health and health-related behaviours." (Baer and Singer, 2009)

Such an approach would not only offer explanations about how disease is experienced, but would also answer the question of *why* this happens. In this regard, the principles and themes that are considered in critical medical anthropology are very relevant for a wide range of fields. Looking at its typical fields of enquiry (Box 2.1), one observes the complementarities and overlaps between critical medical anthropology and a political ecology of health and disease, as discussed above.

Box 2.1: Lupton's fields of enquiry for critical medical anthropology, adopted by Lupton (2012a):

(i) The social production of medical knowledge; (ii) The functions of medicine and public health in social control; (iii) The importance of consciousness and agency in health-related behaviours and beliefs; (iv) The relation of health and medical language to power; (v) The identification and labelling of disease; (vi) The contestable nature of medicine and disease as biomedical realities; (vii) The meaning of the illness experience (here citing Singer, 1990)

Baer (1996) highlights the potential of uniting these approaches in that "critical medical anthropology shares with political ecology a commitment to merge theory and social action", while content-wise they address the coupling of socio-environmental and cultural aspects in the study of health. This merging however leaves room for criticism of the epistemological contradictions between these two fields. Although there are numerous exceptions, political analysis has tends to maintain a rather positivist and constructivist scientific view. Anthropology, on the other hand, has been predominantly deconstructivist in its approach. The importance of balancing the two analytical pathways (the critical and the interpretive) has been a main contention of critics who argue that critical medical anthropology can lose focus from the subjective personal experience of illness (Scheper-Hughes and Lock 1986 cited in Joralemon, 2010: 47). As Joralemon (2010) argues however, critical questions are inherent to cultural-anthropological enquiry and should not be seen as complementary or external to the lived reality of people. In accordance with him, Lupton (2012b) contends that "at their most political, social constructivist approaches are hard to differentiate from critical medical anthropological studies".

Whether to greater or lesser extent, the different orientations that characterize different studies is not to be seen as a daunting barrier, but as an indicative mark of where attention should be paid when attempting to merge theoretical approaches and follow a clear epistemology. Transcending the boundaries between these two fields is more of an opportunity than a constraint to research, one which has largely not been carried out. Even though medical anthropologists have considered engaging in a political economy type of analysis of health at least since the beginning of the 1980s (Morsy, 1979), the integration of views from political ecology is a more recent endeavour. Baer and Singer (2009) discuss and embrace the unity of the two currents, tracing their differences and their meeting points. The problems put forward by political ecology, critical medical anthropology and the political economy of health might stem from different orientations and might also describe phenomena using distinct concepts and methods, but they converge on the questioning of political, social and economic systems in relation to human health. Drawing from the meeting points of these disciplines, this thesis aims to elucidate what connects the sectors of water, healthcare and disease, in terms of policy, politics and practice, as well as how and why these sectors are connected.

2.3 Analytical fields

Within the theoretical fields discussed, the angles that this study seeks to analyse can be roughly divided between the politics of risk communication and the epidemiology of health messages. Information about diarrheal disease is risk-related information, which according to Bennett et al. (2010: 25) is continually and extensively "constructed, tested, communicated and validated". The politics behind the prevailing discourse and thus, behind the policies that follow, are situated at the core of this study's enquiries. The communicative process can be seen as "a tangled web of signs symbols and messages" (Krimsky and Plough cited in Bennett et al., 2010: 56); the perception of risk that is shaped through these processes is "a critical part of risk amplification and stigmatization" (Kasperson and Kasperson, 2005: 175). The 'infectiousness' of health messages and their potential to be internalised in the form of healthy behaviour depends on this communicative process, both on its content and its ability to include and involve the public. In turn, these elements can reflect aspects of the wider socio-political environments within which disease is encountered. In consideration these dimensions, the analysis in this thesis focuses on the processes of health education and health-related information circulation, questioning the levels of public participation and social empowerment that they involve.

2.3.1 The politics of risk communication

Discussing the politics of risk communication, one has to begin with the content of such communication. Risk discourses are shaped through processes that involve contestation about the origin and the nature of a risk, as well as about how to mitigate it. Bryant (1998b) wrote about how political the process of identifying problems in a society is, emphasizing that "the process of knowledge production reflects and in turn often reinforces social and economic inequalities in so far as knowledge claims may be used". Since problems are the negative outcomes of risk factors and risks often constitute social problems, any message that seeks to be informative or educative entails an assumption or a claim about the validity and relevance of some piece of knowledge over another. It is thus useful to examine which messages came to be prominent in health risk communication, through which processes this took place, and whose interests it reflected.

Apart from the content itself, the means and methods employed in risk communication can also be imbued with intentions of exercising authority and control. The use of language, the room allowed for questioning and altering the communicated messages, and the underlying discourse that accompanies them, can all emerge from and result in, a certain distribution of power. Looking, for instance, at how certain groups - or places - can be discursively stigmatised as the carriers of a health risk, Bennett et al. (2010: 34) stress how "language used to communicate complex scientific issues is important in helping to shape the nature of the debate and the attendant understanding that comes with it". Similar observations of how risk perceptions are built, emphasize that "as a place comes to be dominated by a single negative attribute, while other attributes characterizing the place recede into the background or insignificance, identity is altered and stigmatized" (Kasperson and Kasperson, 2005).

Seeing the centrality of political and social power in shaping the messages around risk and the means to communicate these messages gives rise to the question of where is, and what is, "the political". One should begin from the concept of power, which Paulson (2003) explains as not only an exogenous pressure exercised on individuals but also as "a social relation built on an asymmetrical distribution of resources and risks" (Hornborg 2001 cited in Paulson, 2003) and an internal characteristic that constitutes the subject: us and the others (Butler 1997 cited in Paulson et al., 2003). Based on these understandings, a definition can be prepared that looks at politics as "the practices and processes through which power, in its multiple forms, is wielded and negotiated" (Paulson et al., 2003). Politics, then, can be found not only in the official political and decision-making arenas but also in every day interactions, language expressions and people's practices. Politics in this form can often be silent, indirect or underlying.

Based on this definition of politics, risk communication processes and outcomes are worth examining in formal and informal spheres, through the officially circulated discourse but also through the discussions and meanings to be found in lay contexts. In line with Paulson's approach, Swyngendouw (2008) argues against the conceptual compromise of the political as simply a part of what politics involve. He defines the political as "the articulation of voice that demands its place" (Swyngedouw, 2008) and "the space for the arrangement of public encounter of heterogeneous groups and individuals" (Marchant 2007 cited in Swyngedouw 2008). Unlike Parfitt (2002), who holds that politics is (rather than should be) "about controlling power, stipulating rules and conventions to limit abuse of power", Swyngendow (2008) sees politics (of today) as being post-political. Nonetheless, Parfitt (2002: 101ff) does recognise that the space between indecisiveness and decision is where the political works; meaning that one decision necessarily excludes another and thus, in the process of decision-making "some will benefit while others not". When such inequalities are exacerbated, according to Farmer (Farmer, 2005: 16), some people's political rights become hollowed out - even if they are exercising them - as their voices are unable to translate into policy.

Being a one-party rule state, Vietnam is a particularly interesting field for examining the implicit and explicit demonstrations of power though direct and indirect political processes of risk definition and communication. The central government's authoritarian attitude in policy and decision-making has been seen as preventing the development of truly bottom-up processes (Brocheux, 2012). According to others, it is Vietnam's Leninist tradition that cannot allow for true participation and restricts to what was termed by Roeder as a process of coproduction; "an implementation of decisions already made" (Roeder, 1989 cited in Smith, 2002: 34). Nonetheless, many authors have recognised that the Vietnamese public has developed ways of acting politically, even if political rights are formally restricted (Gainsborough, 2010a, Smith, 2002). Beresford (2008) has noted, for example, that the □ổi mới' policy changes made information more accessible and allowed the rise of more critical opinions, coming both from the press and from within the government. Fforde (2013) has even come to question the sovereignty of the ruling Party, seeing the unprecedented criticism that it received in the aftermaths of recent economic policy mistakes. On the other hand, as Fforde (2012: 108) emphasizes, the local arms of the party-state remain faithful to state ideology and have managed to maintain their top-down authority, "often leading to striking results in terms of local development and order".

Through the process of communicating disease-related information, the Vietnamese state produces messages that shape public opinion around the causes of disease and around the ways to address them. In the context of direct control through party politics and the potent political expression that is found in socio-cultural processes, it is interesting to examine how interpretations and explanations of a water-related disease are worded and communicated. How much are the voices of people who suffer disease heard compared to others and with what means does the state control the formulation and the voicing of public concerns and demands? Who is given space to participate in shaping the discourse around disease? What shapes the ability of making health-related decisions and how can different groups in society get access to valuable resources and information that will empower them towards this direction?

2.3.2 The "epidemiology" of health messages

It was discussed in the beginning of this chapter how failures in public health continue to occur worldwide despite the ample knowledge developed in the field of disease prevention and treatment. One of the main challenges for public health has been to find ways to adapt information and expertise to the various contexts in which they are needed. An even greater challenge has been to do this with the participation of local people and with respect to local culture (Trostle, 2005: 26ff). Studies on the perception of risk have recognised that scientific knowledge can be very different from the public awareness of the same risk, stressing the importance of education and information processes "where both sender and recipient interact in order to develop a common frame for the understanding of the problem" (Hampel, 2006). Nichter (1996b: 125) asserts that "as important as an epidemiology of disease is an epidemiology of health communication". In other words, in order to understand which aspects determine effective public health measures, one needs to examine why certain health messages become "contagious" and useful, while others fail to gain traction in certain social and cultural contexts. Nichter (1996b: 140) further argues for an approach to health education that departs from "studying what a population does know, conceptually and experientially" and against an approach that tries to inject understandings about issues that the public is assumed to lack knowledge on.

Public participation is a crucial aspect in shaping and communicating health messages, as it informs policy-makers about the community's concerns, ideas, abilities and demands about health risks. Any approach that would treat such aspects of public knowledge and attitude towards risk as irrelevant, would "fail to understand the basis of public concerns and [would] provoke feelings of antagonism and rejection" (Bennett et al., 2010: 32). Moreover, the receptiveness of health messages depends greatly on the utility that the public sees in them. As Moore (2002 cited in Bennett et al., 2010) points out, "people do not need information for information's sake, but as a means of taking responsibility for personal choices, improving their own or their family's well-being or supporting their role in society". As more and more studies have come to show, a successful process of health communication needs to be informed about the understandings and the experiences of the people whose health is at stake. In the words of Nichter (1996a):

> "Lack of sensitivity to the health concerns of lay persons, and the introduction of educational messages that fail to take their health culture into consideration will result in misinterpretation, the compartmentalization of information, and desensitization to priority issues." (Nichter, 1996a: 399)

Given the position of academics like Nichter and Nichter (1996a), and in accord with wider efforts to combine epidemiological and anthropological undertakings[11], there is an urgent need to examine the "epidemiology of health messages" around diarrheal disease in the hotspots of its prevalence, in places like Vietnam's Mekong Delta region. This would require questioning whether the health education approach has been participatory and inclusive or not and seeing how this has affected the public's receptiveness to the message, as well as the utility and sustainability of health messages within local communities. It would also require engaging firsthand in exploration and analysis of those lay understandings and concerns that one might expect to find reflected in health education messages. In combining the above elements, a medical anthropology would look at the discourses and the practices around disease through a combination of cultural and institutional analysis. But in the spirit of making medical anthropology more critical, a critical aspect of risk communication connected to the "epidemiology of health messages" within the wider politics of risk

---

[11] For a historical review of how the disciplines of Anthropology and Epidemiology began to bridge their approaches during the last decades of the 19th centuries, see Trostle (2005: 21-41).

definition and communication (section 2.3.1) deserves particular attention: the potential of health education to empower.

The empowering potential of health education

When health education efforts are able to foster good understandings of how and why one can protect oneself from disease, they can achieve not only a change in disease-specific behavior but can also have "broad effects and benefits for prevention, disease management, and well-being across the life span" of a population (Fisher et al., 2011). Strengthening the sector of health education via widespread comprehensive information on various health topics is a process that promotes people's health literacy. Health literacy is a concept which, according to Nutbeam (1998 cited in Nutbeam, 2000), can be defined as "the cognitive and social skills which determine the motivation and ability of individuals to gain access to, understand and use information in ways which promote and maintain good health".

One of the key points of this definition is the necessity for health literacy to address three aspects of health-related information: access, understanding and use. With regard to the prevention of diarrheal disease, for example, health literacy is not achieved solely through increasing the availability of hand-washing promoting messaging if hand-washing benefits are not understood and/or if the practice of hand-washing is not meaningfully adopted by the public. Similarly, the benefits of health literacy cannot be really achieved when the emergent need and desire for ORS treatment against diarrhoea, cannot be satisfied when people lack the financial capacity to attain such treatment. The second key point in the above definition is that health literacy entails social skills. Thus, the ability of taking health-related action is socially shaped within society and goes beyond the individual's awareness of preventive health measures and their usefulness. As Nutbeam (1998 cited in Nutbeam, 2000) suggests, "[...] by improving people's access to health information and their capacity to use it effectively, health literacy is critical to empowerment".

Seen in this social light, health education is not only about individual understanding and participation, but also about involving the community, setting common goals and motivating each other through emergent health beliefs and social expectations of behaviour (Rosenstock et al., 1988). Bandura (2004) has elaborated on the 'social cognitive means' of health promotion, discussing how the effects of health education can be strengthened or hampered. Focusing on the importance of people trusting in their own capability to effect change in their health through their choices, Bandura (2004) stresses the notion of trust in one's self-efficacy. The author (Ibid., 2044) argues that people's health behaviours are shaped by a multitude of concerns, which include: what kind of outcomes people expect from their changed health behaviours; what reactions are those changes expected to receive in their social environments; how well do they think they can execute those changes; and how much are those behavioural changes attuned to wider goals that people value.

Through this approach, it becomes clear that an epidemiologically successful and socially empowering health education is not only a personal but a social matter, as "it requires changing the practices of social systems that impair health rather than just changing the habits of individuals" (Bandura, 2004). The views of Bandura are in line with what Nutbeam (2000) described as health literacy, which cannot be achieved without appropriately shaping the content and the methods used in health education programs and campaigns. Wallerstein and Bernstein (1988) inform us of Paulo Freire's empowerment approach to education and offer a model adapted to health, defining empowerment as "a social action process that promotes participation of people, organizations, and communities in gaining control over their lives in their community and larger society". In this regard, the goals of empowering health education is to bring structural change to individuals and groups through promoting community organisation and control over circumstances that people are aware that affect their health.

Health information, education and communication (IEC) activities have largely been used in the prevention of infectious epidemics, such as diarrhoea. Behavioural change is usually proclaimed to be one of the basic instruments for the eradication of disease (GTZ and Zimbabwe National Family Planning Council, 1994), but ideas of health literacy, self-efficacy and empowerment in health education have not seen much emphasis or application in public health approaches. In consideration of the Vietnamese socio-political context, it is interesting to question issues of inclusion and bottom-up representation with regard to health. Seeing how the political is to be found when voices try to be heard and groups strive to encounter (Swyngedouw, 2008), the spheres of access to health education and of empowered community action appear very relevant. Recognising people's uncertainty about the science of health and the professional authority that medicine has gained, it is easy to see how feelings of self-efficacy can be hampered and control over health can be lost, both at individual and social levels. Questioning why this is the case appears to be a lacuna in literature, which could be filled using a framework of political ecology and critical medical anthropology

2.3.3 A framework of analysis

Human health is a complex field and research on health needs to embrace the challenge of employing complexity in its empirical and analytical endeavours. Many of the reports addressing environmental health and proposing models for examining how the human-nature-society interaction results in the exacerbation or mitigation of health risks have largely failed to consider how inter-woven the socio-economic, environmental and cultural contexts really are. As a consequence, many of these approaches remain fundamentally restricted in their analytical approach. Briggs (2003), for example, offers a framework of examining children's health, looking particularly at health risks that are shaped by environmental phenomena. Although he elaborately develops a set of indicators, he provides no clear explanation of the connections between the "contexts" and the preventive or remedial actions (of individuals, communities or institutions), apart from recognising that both the contexts and the actions have an impact on risk exposure (Fig 1 in Annex). In a similar example, Morris et al. (2006) discuss environmental health by encapsulating context as one important, but rather non-problematised, determinant of people's exposure to health risks. The authors provide a framework which deals with health challenges in reference to environmental, behavioural, social and economic factors, but in a rather depoliticised context. Namely, the approach falls short of analysing contextual aspects of culture and politics and of relating those not only to the exposure and the effect of a risk, but also to its drivers and to the policies (actions) around it.

Despite the potential usefulness of the above models to fuel discussion on integrating approaches to health problems, they can hardly capture the complexity that human issues present in the different cultures and places where they are encountered. The concept of complexity has been a re-occurring theme of scholarly pursuit, especially in research that moves across disciplines (Urry, 2003). Gatrell (2005) has linked complexity with health studies and emphasized the analytical advantage of using complexity "as a vehicle for moving away from reductionist accounts [...] in research on health inequalities, spatial diffusion, emerging and resurgent infections, and risk". Complex systems, according to him, are basically composites that exhibit emerging characteristics and thus behave in ways that cannot be predicted using knowledge about their individual elements (Ibid. 2005). Conceptualising the incidence of diarrheal disease as it evolves in time and as it is affected by preventive, treatment, healing and curative strategies and experiences, the present work tries to organise its analytical sub-fields without drawing strict dividing lines between the sources and the outcomes of phenomena (Fig 2.2).

Figure 2.2: Conceptualisation of the analytical framework for the study of diarrheal disease

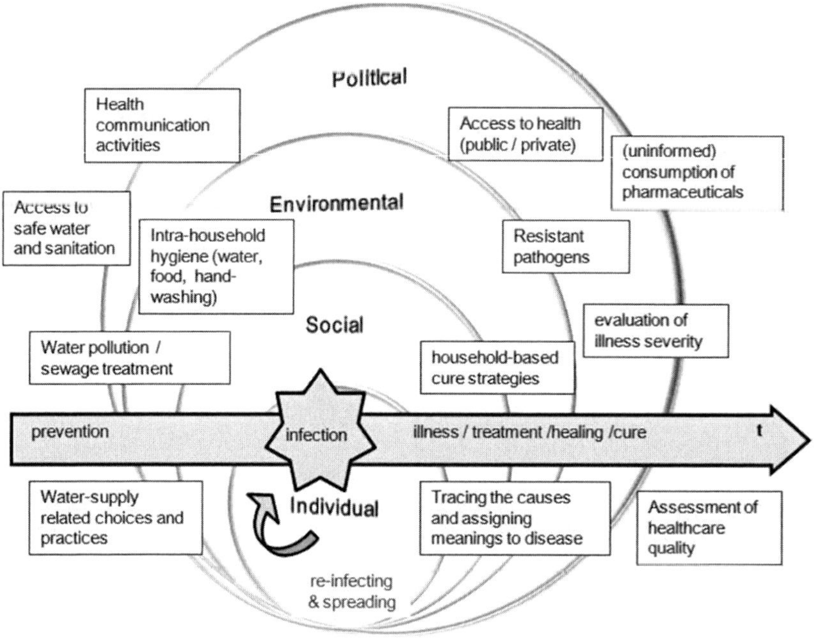

The placement of the different boxes (events, conditions and processes) is random in relation to the nested contextual spheres. As it is explained in the text, each of these boxes represents an expression and an outcome of the interplay between these spheres.

Embracing the concept of complexity, but also attempting a level of systematic analysis, this research traces some events and conditions that relate to the incidence of diarrheal disease and seeks to examine how these are shaped through the interaction of four contextual spheres: the individual, social, environmental and political. The above presented framework is meant to address the challenge that "both pathogens and ideas about pathogens are transmitted through populations" and thus that "the tools and theories to understand these phenomena must be able to move between the intracellular and the interpersonal, tracing causal relationships among pathogens, behaviour, power and disease" (Trostle, 2005: 41).

The temporal assortment of conditions and events that shape the vulnerability of individuals to disease is seen in relation to the interpenetrating spheres of environmental, social and political contexts. At the same time, it is acknowledged that individual experience, reaction and behaviour in relation to disease can impact on the other spheres as well. For example, the excessive use of antibiotics (individual), promoted by practitioners or pharmacists (institutional/socio-economic) can contribute to pathogens' resistance-building (biological/environmental) and make other individuals more vulnerable to disease (social). In contrast, an organised reaction of a community against an industrial source of water pollution (social/political) might have an effect on the adopted policies of water management (political/environmental) and, in turn, benefit the residents of the communities who were previously exposed to such waste (social/individual). It is therefore important to emphasize that the four contextual spheres are not meant as non-interacting boxes, but rather as being in constant interplay.

This conceptualisation was inspired by Scheper-Hughes and Lock's (1987) 'three bodies approach' to health, adapted particularly for the exploration of diarrheal disease in the Mekong Delta. The individual sphere resembles what the authors describe as "the individual body" of health, here referring to the physiological characteristics of individuals, such as their health record or their nutrition habits. Moreover, it refers to the different ideas that people have about how disease is caused and treated and their practices in relation to these beliefs. The individual sphere also captures the structural conditions that define the individual, regarding for example the access one has to healthcare of good quality or the ability to pay for medical treatment. The social sphere, following the idea of the "social body" (Douglas 1970 cited in Scheper-Hughes and Lock, 1987), consists of categories that are ascribed to certain social groups in relation to disease and the various ways in which the risk of the disease has been connected to social values, morals and behaviours.

The environmental sphere is something which Scheper-Hughes and Lock (1987) do not extensively question. The introduction of an environmental sphere in this case was considered important for two reasons. First, due to the inextricable connections between diarrheal disease and water, it was seen as useful to underline issues of water management and water pollution, as well as flooding events or experiences of clean water scarcity. Secondly, the environmental sphere was meant to represent the biological aspects of disease from the side of the pathogens' complex ecology, and not only from the side of the human body physiology, where the focus usually lies. This sphere therefore represents the biophysical conditions and phenomena, including pathogens, ecosystems and the climate, but also human population dynamics and their activities in using natural resources or causing the pollution and degradation. Finally, the political sphere includes more than the "body politic" of health as it is discussed in the three-body approach of Scheper-Hughes and Lock (1987). The political sphere is meant to capture the wider spaces and topics around which negotiation takes place and through which power is expressed. The result of such negotiations might not only act to directly control human bodies, but also to define the fate of natural environments, distribute the benefits from the use of resources, and define access to public goods and services. Therefore, the political sphere includes the processes through which certain knowledge claims come to dominate in the discursive practices of various actors around issues of health, water and disease.

FIELDWORK METHODOLOGY

CHAPTER 3

This chapter outlines and discusses the methodological approach that was followed for the collection and analysis of data. It describes in which ways research investigated aspects of individual, social, environmental and political spheres that relate to the spread and the control of diarrheal disease, as guided by the theoretical and conceptual framework described in the previous chapter (2). With the purpose of the research being to link the biophysical attributes of disease with the discursive practices around it, the analysis was meant to move from statistical to interpretative grounds and from obtained "factual" data to more critical views of their origins. The logic behind the combination of qualitative and quantitative methods is explained and the advantages discussed (3.1). After briefly justifying the research approach and the use of the case-studies, the chapter provides a listing and description of the data collection methods. This includes a discussion of the key characteristics of Can Tho City and the two case-study areas (3.2). Finally, the special characteristics of Vietnam as a field for social research are commented on with regard to how they affected the research methodology (3.3).

3.1 Understanding the social side of disease using a mixed-methods approach

Informed by the epistemology of medical anthropology, which "has so thoroughly grounded its contribution to the study of health and disease on a combination of qualitative (e.g. participant observation and open-ended interviews) and quantitative (e.g. surveys and questionnaires) methods of investigation" (Joralemon, 2010: 11), this research similarly embraced a mixed-methods approach. Each method that was used produced various types of information (e.g. interview transcripts, printed material of health communication, legal documents, health statistics and household survey results) that were analysed both quantitatively and interpretively, with primary and secondary data being reviewed critically with the goal of placing them in context with the circumstances and the motivations that guided their generation.

According to Blaikie (2009), "the use of single methods is usually associated with narrow and perhaps one-off research topics. Such research provides limited opportunities for advancing knowledge. The use of a variety of methods, however this is organized, should be seen as the norm". As this research follows a grounded theory and constructivist approach, it uses multiple methods in order to shed light on the various angles of the problem. Investigating the socio-political and cultural determinants of disease required a research orientation aimed at tracing policy, practice and the type of discourses that institutions and people generate. For this, critical analysis of printed documents, official reports and statistics was essential, but it was also necessarily accompanied by an analysis of the views and opinions that are circulating within the related formal and informal spheres. Although both qualitative and quantitative approaches were employed, the focus of data collection and analysis remained mainly on qualitative data, as this was considered to be most appropriate in the overall scope of this research. Having the flexibility to move between institutional, sociological and anthropological analysis was essential for exploring how the spread of diarrheal disease is affected both by the macro-level processes of policy and by the micro-level aspects of policy acceptance, transformation and implementation.

Using semi-structured interviews as the main qualitative research method, specific topics were discussed with a range of respondents, from state representatives and experts to residents of urban, rural, poor and non-poor households. Necessarily, some of the findings could be successfully confirmed through triangulation, while others would be contradictory or inconsistent. Complementary qualitative methods of observation and in-depth interviewing were also employed, in order to understanding conflicting information or to strengthen certain the findings. In order to obtain information on local people's current practices around water, disease prevention and healthcare, as well as to capture prevalent ideas and attitudes about these issues, a household survey was conducted. While carrying out the survey, an open-ended and in-depth manner of interviewing was attempted, allowing for discussions beyond the questionnaire's pre-defined formulations and categories. Secondary statistics provided by the government (for healthcare, disease, water supply, sanitation, water quality, and hygiene) were analysed and compared with survey results and secondary scientific literature about the region. In this regard, the research followed a rather praxeological knowledge approach, in which contradictions between quantitative and qualitative results were not seen as undermining various assumption about reality, but instead were critically examined and understood as "part of reality" (Harrits, 2011: 162). It is, however, important to stress that the combination of research methods that was employed for each institution and each respondent was limited to what was allowed by Vietnamese state authorities and local behavioural norms, which I respected as thoroughly as possible with the advice of a local research assistant (see also chapter 3.3).

3.1.1 *Abductive research strategy and the use of the case study*

The use of qualitative methods, particularly during the first stages of a study, allows for more nuanced research questions to crystallize (Maxwell, 2004a, 2004b cited in Harrits, 2011). In this case, a central research question was developed after a number of semi-structured interviews with local experts and state representatives, and taking account of information coming from the field. The research maintained a grounded theory approach by identifying and examining issues through an explorative and reflective process, rather than having clearly defined research hypotheses. Experiences from these initial encounters in the field led the decision of selecting and examining two areas: one distinctively rural and the other primarily urban.

This site selection arose because it was consistently argued by public office representatives that people living in urban and rural places get affected by diarrheal disease in different ways. Moreover, the studied literature and the collected secondary data were indeed pointing to the phenomenon of urbanisation as an on-going process strongly affecting the everyday lives of the local population. The drive for urbanisation was a consistent leitmotiv in nationally and locally proclaimed targets of development. For all these reasons, urbanisation was considered to be an important background against which to further the analysis of health risk. To this end, a comparison of urban and rural areas should allow "for a very intensive dialogue between theory and evidence" (Mahoney and Rueschemeyer 2003 in Mollinga, 2008) about the process of urbanisation itself and of how - or whether - urbanisation affects the incidence of disease.

Gerring (2004) defines a case study as "an intensive study of a single unit with an aim to generalize across a larger set of units". In this sense, the units of this study would be considered to be (i) the urban and (ii) the rural division of a district, representing accordingly both rural and urban parts of the Mekong Delta (or perhaps of the country, depending on the generalisation that one is willing to attempt). Urbanisation, however, is not considered as a static outcome; indeed, it can hardly be seen as completely absent from some places (that are mostly rural) or a finished product in others (primarily urban areas). In viewing urbanisation more as a process, it is then perhaps more useful to use Yin's definition of a case study as "an inquiry that investigates a contemporary phenomenon [like urbanisation] within its real-life context, especially when the boundaries between phenomenon and context are not clearly evident" (Yin, 2003: 40, my addition in bracket). Based on Yin's (2003) typology of case-studies, this study looks at the nexus of diarrheal disease determinants in the geographical context of the Mekong Delta. This two-case design involves embedded units of analysis that include the state, organisations within and beyond the control of the state, as well as individual citizens (for a visualisation of Yin's typology of designs, see Picture 1 in the Annex).

3.1.2 Methods of data collection and analysis

The qualitative methods of collecting data included semi-structured interviews, unstructured in-depth interviews and participant observation. In total, there were 87 interviews, of which most (78) were semi-structured interviews with local cadres who were involved in water and/or health issues. The remaining nine were in-depth interviews with selected households in the case-study areas. Additionally, there were eight informal discussions held with informants who prefer to remain anonymous; these are therefore not included in the listing of the interviews (Table 3.1).

Table 3.1: Number of interviews conducted by research phase and by administrative level

Research phase (chronologically)	Number of interviews				
	Commune	District	Province	Ministry	TOTAL
Phase 1: Contextualisation with the field	-	13	10	4	27
Phase 2: Selected districts	3	18	-	-	21
Phase 3: Household survey in the communes	131				131
Phase 4: Selected households in-depth	9	-	-	-	9
Phase 5: Targeted public offices*	8	10	6	6	30
TOTAL	151	41	16	10	218

*For details on the different research phases, see the section "Trajectory of Fieldwork" in the Annex

More informally, notes that were used to document observations from interviews were transformed daily into fieldwork diary entries. Photographic material was also collected on occasion to complement these observations. The quantitative method of collecting data centered on the household survey, in which in a total of 131 households participated. Nearly half of these households were located at the urban case study of Le Binh ward[12] (62 households) and the rest at the rural case-study communes of Truong Long and Giai Xuan (69 households)[13]. The findings of the survey were geo-referenced through the collection of GPS points (see Picture 3.2).

Secondary material was collected from governmental offices, libraries and from the internet. This included statistics, laws, policies, reports and maps. Data related to the presence of water supply connections, the use of other water sources, the types of sanitation, the quality of water in the households and the prevalence of diarrheal disease were analysed in Microsoft Excel. Local news articles were collected from online versions of provincial and national newspapers, amounting to 53 selected pieces, most of which were published during the research period (2011 – 2012). All the written works and documents that were not available in English were translated by a local research assistant. The overall duration of fieldwork was no more than ten months (from May 2011 to March 2012). Throughout this period, any interaction with governmental offices or local household members had to be pre-scheduled and approved by the Vietnamese state administration of the district and the provincial level. In order to comply with this process of 'official research permit' acquisition, the fieldwork was divided into five distinct chronological phases (Table 3.1).

The need for official approval was also often an obstacle to the intuitive flow of research activities, taking away opportunities for extended discussions, informal meetings and spontaneous interviews. However, it also allowed for the longer periods of reflection in-between data collection. As a consequence, each new research phase was not only guided by the original research objectives but also enriched by the field data already collected. Details about the methods followed during each of the above research phases, and about how these methods corresponded to each of the study's objectives, are provided in the section "Trajectory of fieldwork" of Annex).

---

[12] In Le Binh ward, interviews took place in two distinct areas: Yen Binh and Yen Hoa.

[13] In term of vertical administrative divisions, the urban *ward* is equivalent to the rural *commune* and, accordingly the urban *area* to the rural *hamlet*.

3.2 Location background: rural and urban case-studies

The research was situated in Can Tho City, the central province of the Mekong Delta (Picture 3.1). The selection of Can Tho versus other provinces of the Delta had been already established by the WISDOM project team and by the academic supervisors before the start of this study[14]. Can Tho used to be a primarily agricultural area but in recent years has begun to urbanise rapidly, including concurrent development of its infrastructure and industrial capacity. Much of the past agriculture and aquaculture is still present but these sectors are also experiencing their own transformations. At the same time, an evolving mesh of new socio-economic activities has been on the rise during the last 30 years. The trend to modernise and develop is being witnessed in the entire Delta region and experienced individually by the residents of Can Tho City.

The combination of traditional living habits and new emerging realities that one keenly encounters in the different parts of the province makes Can Tho a fertile ground for exploring how socio-economic changes affect health outcomes. The fact that Hau River, one of the main legs of the Mekong, constitutes the province's northeast border makes it ideal for studying a waterborne epidemic disease such as diarrhoea. After the first few months in the field, the study areas within Can Tho were specified. The collection of data in the district-and-below levels focused on the urban district of Cai Rang and the rural district of Phong Dien (Picture 3.2).

> Box 3.1: Rural and urban definitions in Vietnam
>
> It needs to be noted that the official administrative characterization of urban and rural areas in Vietnam is mostly made on the basis of population numbers, population density rates, prominent types of land use and economic activities. The law recognizes areas as "urban centres", as long as they fulfil the minimum numeric requirements of certain indicators, such as population, hectares of land, number of administrative subunits within the area, presence of ethnic minorities and other (GoV, 2001, GoV, 2009b). In summary, an area of any level (from district to city) can be characterized as urban if the majority of its population is occupied in economic sectors other than agricultural and if most of its infrastructure is "developed". The interesting consequences of this definition are described below:

[14] The fact that the project had already established collaboration with a network of local academic and administrational institutions in Can Tho City was an advantage which cannot be overlooked. Moreover, the project's previous and ongoing research provided for a knowledge pool, from where the researcher could continuingly draw on.

(i) Once an area is labelled as urban, the entire population within this area is counted as urban, even if a significant part of this population lives in predominantly rural circumstances and is occupied in agriculture.

(ii) This is not the case with rural characterizations, for which there exists no specific law. Namely, even if a district is characterized as rural, the centre of this district (town capital) can still be counted as an "urban centre" if the latter satisfies the criteria of the above law. As a consequence, the rural population in urban districts is not counted along with the rest of the rural population (of the province, or the country), but they are counted as urban.

(iii) Can Tho has been recently established as a "city", but it still contains rural parts. Some of this rural population is collectively reported as urban because the administrative unit within which they reside (district) satisfies the criteria of an urban area, as described above. Taking into consideration that urban provinces and districts are able to absorb funds easier (Han Sun Sheng and Vu Kim Trang, 2008) and also that urbanisation is a nationally proclaimed goal accompanying modernisation and industrialisation (Central Committee CPV and Communist Party of Vietnam, 2001), this legal particularity seems to intentionally push some districts and provinces towards the urban label, without them actually having an urban character.

Picture 3.1: Map of the Mekong Delta, Southern Vietnam

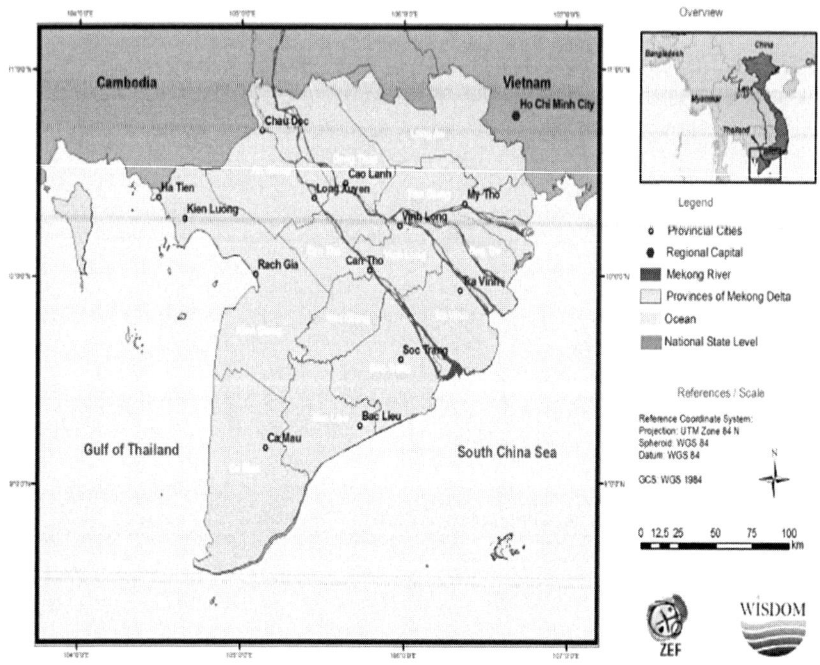

Scale: 1: 2.000.000. Original source: Sven Genschick, ZEF

Picture 3.2: Map of study area and location of surveyed households

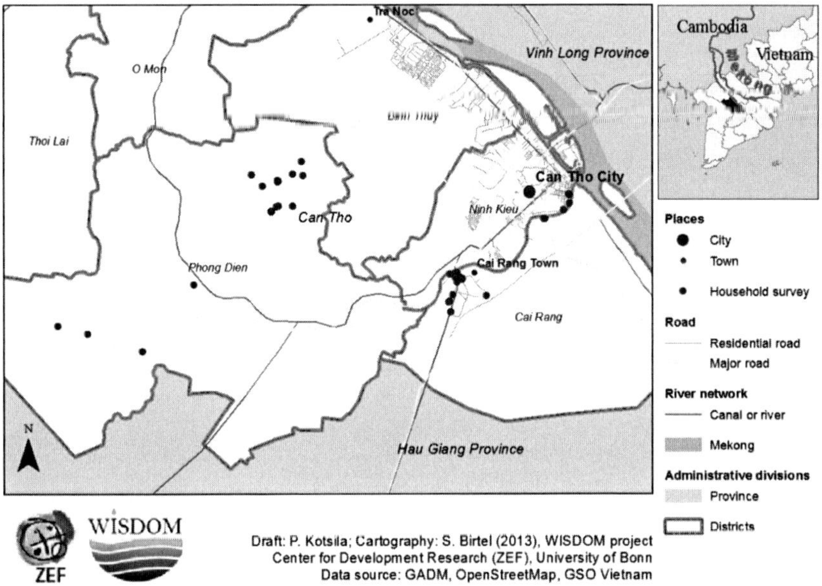

Note: The marked spots do not represent individual households but rather the different neighbourhoods where the households were located.

3.2.1 The rural communes of Phong Dien district

Neighbouring to urban as well as rural districts, Phong Dien is quite diverse but most of its communes are still sparsely populated and maintain an agricultural character. According to development plans, Phong Dien is on its way to urbanisation, but is still being officially reported as a rural district (Statistical Office of Can Tho City, 2011). Due to its proximity to the centre of Can Tho City and also due to the promotion of a tourism sector, not all of the communes within Phong Dien would be representative of the Mekong's Delta rural character (for a map of the district see Picture 2 in the Annex). To ascertain representative communes, interviewees from 15 offices and organisations were asked to assess and compare the socio-economic situation in each of the district's six communes, with particular reference to water supply and sanitation infrastructure.

This revealed that Truong Long and Giai Xuan communes are those that most closely represent the character of other rural areas commonly found in Can Tho City. These two communes were subsequently selected as the rural case-study areas. Other communes in the district were also agricultural (like Nhon Nghia and My Khan) but, on the contrary, have a micro-economy that is more versatile than simply rice agriculture, including big areas of fruit gardens and a "floating" river market. Attracting tourism and being supported additionally by the government constitute a different dynamism towards economic developments (Hoang Xuan Thanh et al., 2008) and thus make these communes slightly different from the typical rice-cultivating rural areas of Can Tho.

In the selected case-study communes, land-use was mostly dedicated to rice, with two thirds of the residents being rice farmers. Small-scale aquaculture also existed, though in much smaller numbers and following a rather declining trend in recent years (DSO Phong Dien, 2010). Aquaculture was claimed to be a significant source of water pollution in both these communes, affecting the quality of water in the canals that flow along the villages:

> "Aquaculture happens mainly in Giai Xuan and My Khanh communes with large-scale fishing activity, which causes the discharge of untreated wastewater in the channels." (Top official in the district branch of the YU, Phong Dien, 13.09.11; group interview)

It is along these same channels and canals that houses are traditionally built by residents in the area so as to have direct access to surface water sources. The scattered hamlets are nowadays interconnected with roads but many of the inner neighbourhoods, farms and houses are still often only accessible via canal bridges. These bridges are typically narrow and are thus only suitable for a bicycle or a moped. Despite the numerous other practical limitations that this entails, the remoteness of some households is also claimed to be an impediment to the expansion of the piped water network in those areas:

> "Truong Long is a rural area which lacks a transportation network, has a big size and some very spread out houses, which is not really suitable for water to be easily delivered to each household or establishment." (Official in the district Office of Education, Phong Dien, 08.09.11; personal interview)

> "Giai Xuan represents many faces of the district; it has a main street cutting through it but also has those areas in the borders that were only recently connected with roads, meaning that they still have remote characteristics and the people face difficulties in everyday life." (Official in a rural commune branch of the YU, Phong Dien, 13.09.11; group interview)

When looking at official statistics, Truong Long and Giai Xuan present a rather better rate of access to piped water when compared to the rest communes. On the other hand, these areas appear to have much higher percentages of poor households and also present the lowest rates of access to hygienic sanitation facilities (Table 3.2).

Table 3.2: Demographic, poverty and WSS characteristics of Phong Dien district, by commune

Comm.	Pop.	Pop. density (pop/ km²)	HH classif. poor	HH hygien. water access (%)	Pop. with piped water (%)	Pop. using treated river water	HH hygien. toilet (%)	Pop. using fishpond toilets
Phong Dien (central town)	10.760	1.425	134	74%	35%	-	12%	913
Giai Xuan	15.337	738	320	70%	33%	-	22%	2.493
Tan Thoi	13.692	782	166	77%	27%	1.124	35%	1.738
Truong Long	18.308	616	499	68%	48%	155	27%	3.125
My Khanh	10.451	893	179	74%	32%	2.427	44%	1.418
Nhon Nghia	17.139	825	188	66%	36%	-	29%	2.842
Nhon Ai	14.040	899	158	56%	25%	5.988	37%	2.034
Total	99.727	807	1.644	69%	35%	9.694	35%	14.563

HH= households. Data sources: The Phong Dien district statistics office (2010) for demographics, the OoH of Phong Dien (2011) for poverty and CERWASS (2011a) for water supply and sanitation data

Illustrating this dynamic, a doctor from the hospital of Phong Dien discussing people's access to hygienic water supply and sanitation in relation to the incidence of diarrheal disease, suggested that Truong Long commune was one of the most problematic in the whole district (Medical doctor in Phong Dien district hospital, 08.09.11; personal interview).

The data in Table 3.2 shows that the number of people using "hygienically treated" river water is much lower in Truong Long and Giai Xuan than in other communes. But how about those using river water that is not "hygienically treated"? And what are the definitions for this treatment? At the same time, the number of fishpond river toilets presents the highest rates in those two communes. But to which extent do these statistics reflect the real situation of clean water and sanitary facilities? Moreover, to what extent can this be linked with the spread of disease? The above data and questions are all fields of further inquiry but the selection of these communes as case-study areas was based on the premise that they were perceived by most of the interviewees in the local administration offices as the most rural and most problematic in terms of diarrheal disease risks.

3.2.2 The urban ward of Cai Rang district

Cai Rang district is a vibrant and rapidly urbanising district, despite its very small size of about 70 km^2. The share of the population that is occupied in agriculture shifted within the last ten years from 69% in 2000 to only 36% in 2009. This is particularly visible in the district's central ward of Le Binh, where only five people are documented as farmers in the latest statistics (DSO of Cai Rang, 2010). Although it is overall classified as an urban district (Statistical Office of Can Tho City, 2011), Cai Rang has not entirely lost its rural characteristics. Of all the wards within Cai Rang, it was only in Le Binh ward that one could clearly see a more modern and dense architecture, an extended and busy road network, a total shift to third-sector economy, and an evidently higher population density (Table 3.3).

Table 3.3: Demographics, poverty and WSS characteristics of Cai Rang district, by ward

Wards	Pop. density (pop/km²)	HH classif. poor	HH hygien. water (%)	Pop. with private tap[15] (%)	Pop. using treated river water	HH hygien. toilet (%)	Pop. using fishpond toilets
Le Binh	6.559	88	97%	73%	-	97%	212
Hung Phu	2.371	163	96%	72%	2.793	96%	278
Hung Thanh	1.007	139	61%	19%	512	61%	423
Ba Lang	1.129	91	66%	3%	202	66%	623
Thuong Thanh	927	172	87%	50%	142	87%	1.318
Phu Thu	874	392	64%	30%	2.625	64%	1.730
Tan Phu	653	186	34%	12%	587	34%	920
Total	1.249	1.231	78%	44%	6.861	65%	5.504

Data sources: Cai Rang District Statistics Office (2010) for demographics, Office of Labour, Invalids and Social Affairs of Cai Rang district (2011) for poverty data, and CERWASS (2011a) for water supply and sanitation data

The tendency to urbanise has of course affected many of the other wards, with at least half of their land being now non-agricultural (DSO of Cai Rang, 2010).

[15] The total population reported by CERWASS does not correspond to the total population reported by the Statistics Offices for each district within Can Tho. CERWASS reports on the population within the parts of districts that still have no access to centralised piped supply. In other words, what CERWASS reports as total population might correspond to the population in rural districts, but in urban districts this is not the case, as the tally does not include the central parts which are served by a private water company (see also chapter 4). To get an accurate number, the percentages in the table are based on the number of people CERWASS reports as having access to water and sanitation (2011) divided by the total population reported in the district's statistical yearbook (2009).

Nevertheless, the population density in those wards is much lower than in Le Binh, with the only exception being Hung Phu ward (Table 3.3). During the explorative research phase, Hung Phu ward was also visited. The developments there attested to the effort to radically re-organize the housing pattern to prevent exposure to flood episodes. In Hung Phu, as in a number of places in the Delta, development programs have suggested the relocation of people to newly constructed residential areas that are constructed inland and not near the flood-prone river (Stumpf, 2012). Hung Phu ward is one example where these residential areas have expanded and have, in many ways, dramatically changed the livelihoods of people:

> "People are being bought off their land and pushed to live elsewhere. Some cannot be farmers anymore; therefore they try to learn something else to do." (Top official in WU district branch, Cai Rang, 22.09.11; personal interview)

> "There are many different classes of people living there [residential areas]. There is a lot of movement. Some come as resettlers and the ones who were there before have to go. There is a lot of disorder in these areas." (Top official in the OLISA of Cai Rang district, 29.09.11; group interview)

The spectrum of socio-economic changes in wards like Hung Phu touches upon particular issues of resettlement, ownership, international intervention and the use of space, all of which go beyond the locus of this study. Therefore, despite its urban characteristics, the Hung Phu ward was not included as an urban case-study area.

The official statistics on the wards of Cai Rang show how the better coverage of clean water access and sanitary toilet facilities is correlated with the level urbanisation. Le Binh ward has an extended network for water supply, a high percentage of households with hygienic sanitation facilities, and the lowest number of fishpond toilets compared to the rest of the wards. Due to the high price of land in urban areas, occupying it with fishponds is a poor investment and this is probably part of the reason why fishponds are not so common in Le Binh. Moreover, houses are built close to each other and often have no direct access to surface waters; thus, open defecation in the river is rather restricted. Nevertheless, there are many households along the river that have access to surface water, one of which was included as a case-study area (Yen Binh area). Some of those households had the front door facing an asphalted road while the back of the house had direct access to the river (Picture 3.3). The part of the households with access to water would be usually where the kitchen is located and, in some cases, also a river toilet. It is not clear whether this housing model serves the purpose of collecting water or for disposing sewage, or whether it is just a tradition that has survived (Le Anh et al. 2007 cited in Herbst et al., 2009).

Picture 3.3: The back part of houses built along the river in Yen Binh Area of Le Binh ward

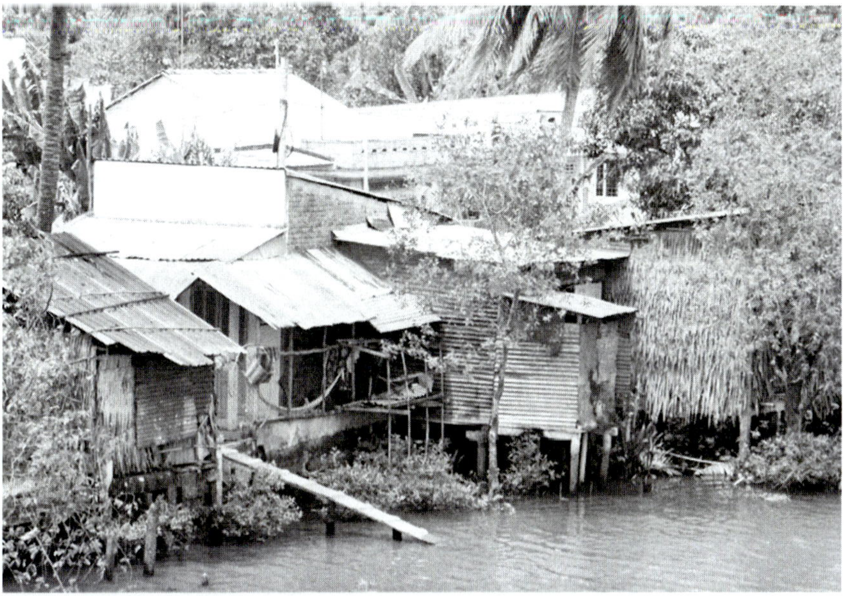

Picture by author, 2011

Despite the expanded network of water supply and the improved sanitation facilities, Le Binh ward faces increasing environmental sanitation problems as a consequence of its congested population, and the insufficient or non-integrated disposal and treatment system for sewage and solid waste. The busy floating market in the Hau River is one example of concentrated economic activity and to the production of waste, which, according to interviewees, is leading to increased health risks:

> "The floating market area is a place where one can easily get waterborne disease because all the garbage and wastewater is being discharged into the river." (Top official in WU district branch, Cai Rang, 22.09.11; personal interview)

Near where the floating market takes place, one finds the so-called "floating houses" of Yen Binh area. Their residents have very limited financial capacities and this is reflected in their housing infrastructure. Unable to afford buying land, they build their houses over the river. Interviewed families described their problems in water supply, sanitation and healthcare, which owe to their poverty and to their lack of bureaucratic recognition. As one interviewee claimed, "because we live in a floating house we are not registered, therefore, we cannot get free health insurance for our kid" (head of household N16, Cai Rang district; personal interview). The household survey included 13 of such households, constituting about half of the sample from the area of Yen Binh; one of the purposes of this sampling is to document this poorly recognised and understood reality that co-exists with the modernity and development of the surrounding urban environment.

3.3 The field's character: social research challenges in Vietnam

An important part of outlining the methodological limitations and decisions is to portray the distinctive character of Vietnam as a field for social research. Previous works have documented how the region is particularly challenging for researchers that aim for participatory and unbiased data collection (Reis, 2012, Scott et al., 2006, Howie, 2002, Ehlert, 2011). However, the entrance of foreign researchers in the country is now easier than in the past and the research process is more facilitated, even though it is still strictly controlled and overseen by state administration. The Vietnamese government has a long history of introversion and has a sceptical attitude towards any activity that involves intermingling with what the state does, let alone questioning it. Social science is inherently interrogative and critical, thus a researcher faces the additional challenge of framing her research so that it will not cause undesirable reactions by the government. Apart from the limits on the nature of questions one can ask, the research activities also have to be organized in ways that local authorities are familiar and comfortable with.

In the case of this study, the above constraints have moderately changed the way research methodology was chosen and carried out. Firstly, requirements for foreign researchers demand a research permit to be issued by provincial level authorities for every part of the research activity (i.e. visiting public offices and interviewing individuals). After central approval is obtained, the district authorities must also approve the planned research activities and each targeted office or organisation has to also confirm their consent and availability. If any of these steps is hindered, the whole process must be repeated. The limits placed on the researcher about directly contacting the offices of interest caused considerable delay and limited the overall flexibility of the research. Moreover, in order for the research permit to be issued, the researcher had to provide a detailed schedule of activities (i.e. which day and time) and present a sample of the interview topics. It was often the case that interviewees would not answer questions that had not been pre-stated in the research permit application and thus were not approved by the central authorities. It was also very common that the selected representatives of each office or organisation would come prepared with answers to the questions made available to them beforehand by the central authorities.

This very rigid idea of interviewing revealed not only the suspiciousness that the Vietnamese state showed towards the researcher (in some cases there would be a secret police officer to supervise a number of interviews), but also cast a feeling of state-supervision on representatives of offices in the lower administrative levels. Public office staff of the province and the district would be very wary of distributing state-produced information and of speaking openly on policy implementation matters. This reservation was not so much observed in the administrative extremes of the lower (hamlets, wards) and the higher level (national), where opinions were usually more freely expressed. Nevertheless, all cadres tried to project an image of a well-managed, well-informed and legally complying peasantry, community or nation. This was evident not only in their all-positive descriptions of party-policies with regard to local problems, but also in their behaviour when accompanying the researcher to interviews. For example, local cadres would be constantly prompting household members to give the "correct" answer; one that would correspond to the official guidelines and the social duties prescribed by the state (i.e. water treatment, hand-washing practices, sanitation facilities present in the household). This restricted the spontaneity and openness of the respondents who often hesitated to answer difficult questions in the fear of giving "wrong" answers. Notwithstanding the above challenges, these limitations were confronted as findings in and of themselves. The hesitation of the interviewees, the contradictory statements by representatives of the state, and the obvious effort of the Vietnamese government to hide part of the picture in water and health issues while projecting another, were all analysed as aspects of policy implementation and politics. Since the generation and communication of messages were central parts of this study, it was of great value to be able to observe the kinds of channels that information goes through and to gain insights on how official discourse is built. These aspects are further discussed in the empirical chapters of this thesis.

Not being able to speak Vietnamese was a further research obstacle, as the process of holding a conversation or an interview was naturally less spontaneous. Discussions were necessarily filtered through the research assistant's translations and thus, the resulting transcripts often lacked the richness of expression that can be found in everyday language and verbal mannerisms. In order for the instant oral translation during the interviews to be accurate, a significant amount of time and effort had to be invested in order to perfect the collaboration between the researcher and the research assistant. Moreover, getting more familiar with the context through time helped me transcend language barriers. As Farmer (2005) notes, understanding a place and its people "is not about linguistic competence. To get beyond the first (people's) silence, requires compassion and solidarity". In that sense, ultimately the fieldwork became enriched with interaction, collaboration, shared everyday life experiences and mutual appreciation between the researcher and the research subjects. This to some extent enabled the understanding of things that would otherwise go untold or untranslated.

HEALTH AMIDST CHANGE

CHAPTER 4

Vietnam has experienced a noteworthy economic progress of fast pace, after the opening of its markets to the global economy in 1986, when the renovation processes (□ ổi mới) began. These changes led to a system of market socialism which, under a one-party rule, allowed private investment to enter spheres previously entirely owned and administered by the state. One such domain has been healthcare. The transition of the Vietnamese health system has become an interesting subject of study, partly due to the changes it has gone through. From the socialist system in the 1960s, which included expanded basic healthcare provision and led to improved health indicators (Bryant, 1998a), it has now adopted a market-guided orientation which matches the economic policy directions of the last 20 years. Three of the most significant changes to the health sector after the initiation of the renovation policies are: the allowance of a private sector in health since 1987, the financial autonomy of health units - with the consequent introduction of fees - in 1989, and the obligatory contribution to health insurance schemes for the population (nevertheless, not including farmers and self-employed workers) in 1991 (Minh Nguyen Thang and Popkin, 2003, Nghiem Tran Dung, 2010). This chapter looks at how the health system is structured today (4.1) and at the repercussions of the recent changes to public healthcare accessibility, availability and usage (4.2). Additionally, the chapter reviews the health status of the population as this has been reflected in the morbidity and mortality rates of common infectious diseases, particularly looking at the frequency of reported diarrhoea episodes during the last decades (4.3).

4.1 Declared policy objectives and contradictory realities in healthcare

The government of Vietnam has been changing the legal framework of the health sector over the last 20 years, with a number of governmental decisions and directives that have accompanied policy strategies and plans. The most recent of these, the 10-year Plan on Vietnam's healthcare system (MoH, 2007b), addresses a spectrum of problematic issues like the need for the expansion and stronger implementation of preventive medicine, grassroots healthcare, healthcare services and drug regulation. As an example of what is often proclaimed as "socially relevant" health policy, the Plan projects an image of a welfare state, emphasizing the purpose "to achieve equality, effectiveness and development, to meet the increasing and diversified demands of the people for health protection, care and improvement, to reduce morbidity and mortality rates, increase life expectancy and improve the living quality of the population" (MoH, 2007b: 172). As this section will illustrate, the legal confluence of declarations can hardly be said to have translated into tangible improvements in the sector.

4.1.1 Past achievements and the challenges ahead

Vietnam has been improving its basic health indicators since the 1980s. Compared to neighbouring regions, Vietnam performs better in some selected indicators of healthcare services than the average of countries in South East Asia and falls slightly behind the average in West Pacific countries (Fig 4.1).

Figure 4.1: Selected health indicators for Vietnam and surrounding regions

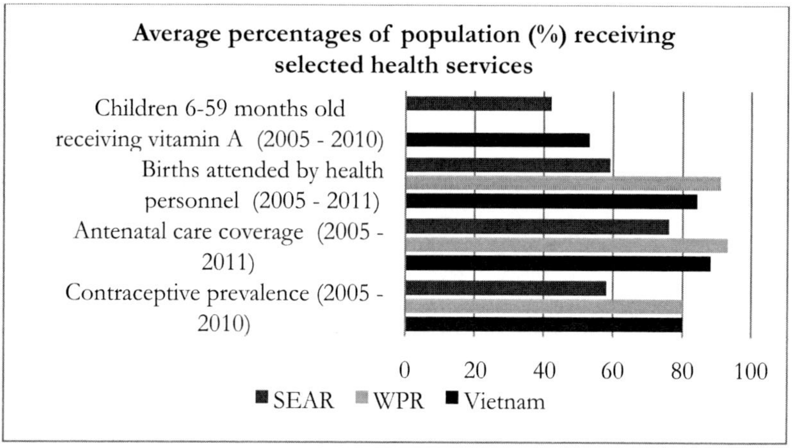

WPR= West Pacific Region, SEAR = South East Asian Region. Figures are given in percentages (%). Based on data by WHO (2012e). Design by the author.

Improvement in healthcare services are accompanied with better results in population health status indicators. This includes a crescent life expectancy that is now reaching 75 (World Bank (WB), 2011) and the significantly lower rates of infant and maternal mortality compared to 30 years ago (Fig 4.2). In fact, Vietnam managed to reduce by half the mortality rates of children under five years old, compared to the year 1990 (WHO, 2012c), showing progressive towards achieving the Millennium Development Goals[16]. That being said, some events took place in parallel during these three decades that have certainly assisted in raising life standards and in the general improvement of the population's health, including the exit of the country from extreme poverty, the recovery from war and the fast-paced economic growth (Gainsborough, 2010a: 265). It is, however, noteworthy that despite Vietnam's overall upward course, basic health indicators seem to have stagnated after the year 2006 (Fig 4.2).

Figure 4.2: Trends of infant and maternal mortality rates in Vietnam

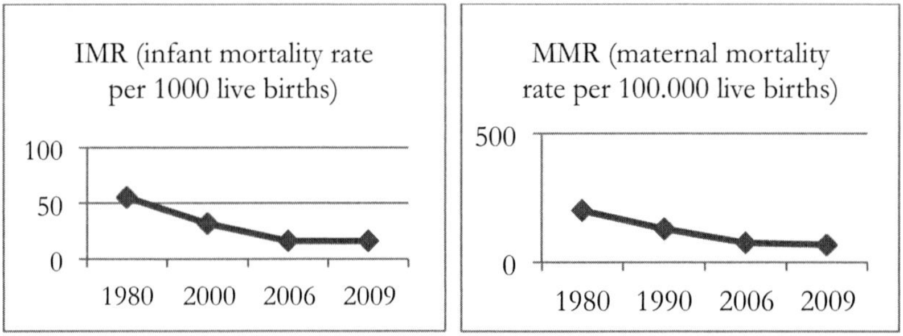

Based on WHO (2008, 2012c). Design by the author.

The World Health Organization (WHO, 2012e) has before recognized that in order to assess the health and healthcare conditions in a place, it is important to look beyond the reported incidence of disease and to include questions about the functioning of health institutions and how those functions are reflected in society. Specifically, the authors of the report have highlighted the need to examine health outcomes together with issues like health workforce, health inequities and public health expenditure[17] (Ibid 2012a). In particular, the WHO has recognised elsewhere how health systems inherently have the potential to improve the health of a population and that "a failure to achieve that potential is rather due to systemic failings than to technical limitations" (WHO, 2000: 2).

---

[16] In order to reach the MDG objective for MMR, the global community must reduce the rate by 5.5% each year. The fourth MDG is to reduce children mortality (infant and under-five) by two-thirds between the years 1990 and 2015 (WHO 2012: 58).

[17] The dimensions proposed as suitable for assessing health systems are: life expectancy and mortality of the population, cause-specific mortality and morbidity, status of selected infectious diseases, healthcare service coverage, health risk factors, health workforce, infrastructure and essential medicines, health expenditure, health inequities, demographic and socioeconomic statistics, health information systems and data availability.

In Vietnam, the post-reform period has been marked by a dramatic decrease of state investment in healthcare, which has largely impacted on the functioning of health institutions. As a number of authors note, the changes shook the grounds of a previously established system with universal access to healthcare (Fritzen, 2007, Minh Nguyen Thang and Popkin, 2003, Witter, 1996) and has come to the expense of the poor, who are actually now facing exacerbated health risks (Priwitzer, 2012: 185). Therefore, despite the noticeable progress in health indicators during the last decades, the extent to which this progress was brought forth due to the effective functioning of health institutions is as questionable as its current sustainability.

4.1.2 A pyramid with weak foundations

Following the wider administrative and political system in Vietnam, the organisation of the health sector has a pyramidal structure, with various subdivisions from the hamlets and the communes to the central-state level (Fig 4.3). Gradual decentralisation in the sector gave many health institutions which were previously under the control of the Ministry of Health (MoH), mainly at the provincial and district level, room to operate more freely and with a certain degree of autonomy. The MoH is still the overall governing body but does not maintain direct funding and reporting relationships with all of the health units in the levels below the Province. In fact, only a certain number of health research institutes, colleges and hospitals have remained under the immediate jurisdiction of the ministry (MoH, 2007b: 178, MoH, 2006).

This autonomy, however, has had serious economic impacts both in the curative and the preventive sector, with most of the assigned national health budget (80%) since the beginning of the reformation period going towards level-III[18] hospitals and away from local healthcare and prevention units (Fritzen, 2007). The responsibility for the economic survival and the functioning of these local units has been transferred from the central state to the local governments of the province and the district. At the same time, however, in spite of economic and functional "independence", the decision-making powers have remained

---

[18] All hospitals are graded according to a point system of evaluation that follows the criteria of location, mandate, number of beds, organizational structure, human resources, qualifications of staff, available expertise, technology, infrastructure, equipment and the number of specialization units (GoV, 2005). The administrative position of public hospitals under higher-level control "rewards" them with points, as does the possession of more resources and expertise proven through the above indicators. The grading system corresponds to the classification of hospitals as Level I, II or III (MoH, 2007a), a result of which is, for example, that most level-III hospitals, are usually directly under the administration of the MoH or the province.

concentrated in the Ministry. The importance of strengthening grassroots health units for the prevention of epidemics has been emphasized in the official national strategy (MoH, 2007b: 88ff), but the actual economic practices contradict these policy declarations.

Figure 4.3. Health institutions offering curative and preventive services in Vietnam

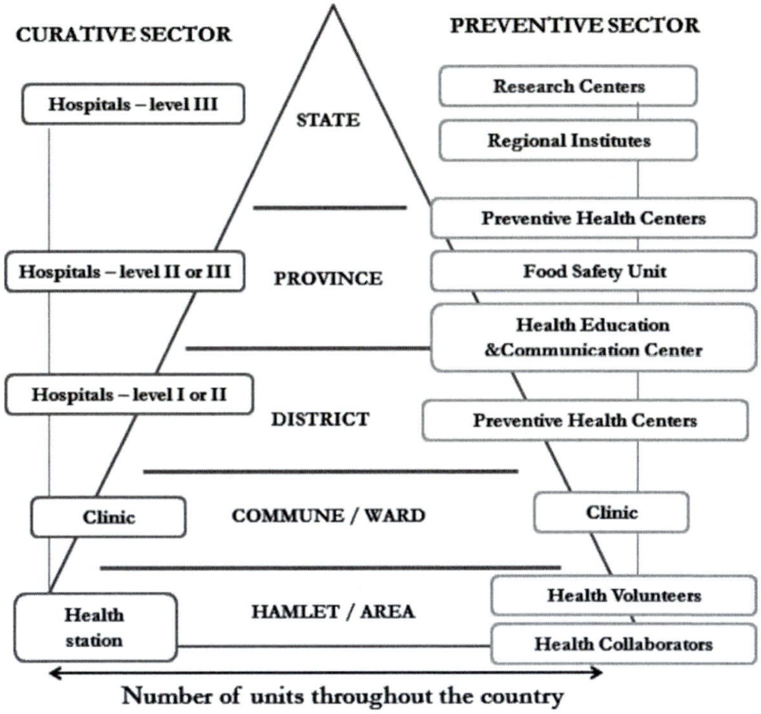

Based on fieldwork material and documents issued by the MoH (2007b, 2006). Design by the author, 2011.

Grassroots healthcare

The healthcare units in the rural hamlets and the urban areas are called health stations (Fig 4.3), which comprise the foundations of the health pyramid together with the health clinics of the communes and wards in the next level of administration (Fig. 4.3). Both of these types of establishments deliver curative and preventive services, but neither of the two is entirely supported by the state. Previous research by Bloom (1998) showed that, in practice, health stations operate purely on their own expenses. The current legal regulation states that the staff of stations and the clinics (which are collectively referred to as "local health workers") are entitled to monthly allowances by the state, as well as to additional funds from undefined "other" sources (GoV, 2010b). However, fieldwork confirms that Bloom's findings still stand valid, with respondents repeatedly pointing to the 'open' character of the above legislation, which does not define a salary nor specifies what the additional sources of funds could be and, thus, leaves room for very little actual economic support for these units[19].

Empirical observations from the five health stations in hamlets within Can Tho City showed that they are usually staffed by no more than two people and can only handle outpatient conditions. They are considered to be the first step of care in the local level, prescribing medicine and performing basic health examinations. However, availability of these units is not guaranteed in all the hamlets or at all times, because of the unpredictability of staff that are capable and willing to take charge. The financial viability of the health stations also depends on the income generated from the retail of medicine[20], but as informants said, running a health station is anything but a profitable occupation:

> "This is a place to treat simple, normal diseases so that the people don't have to go to the higher levels of healthcare. They just come here and get cheap medicine: only 10,000 for three doses of medicine for normal disease [....] and the people get well, they are satisfied with the treatment. We only get support from the state for the information material that we will distribute. The place or the equipment is our responsibility. Luckily we make enough from the medicine we sell. We only keep 5% of the price, so we can make some living. But if I was to ask for something, it would be some chairs for the people to sit and a new bed, because the one we have is rusty." (Top official of a Health Clinic in rural commune, Phong Dien district, 15.09.11; personal interview)

The requirements for the staffing of health stations are not demanding and they simply include: "(i) having a minimum level of health education, (ii) living and working permanently in the locality, (iii) having a sense of responsibility and enthusiasm for participating in social activities and (iv) being physically fit to perform the prescribed duties" (GoV, 2010b). The blending of professional and

---

19 Sources: NGO expert in Water Supply and Sanitation (11.12.11), top official in the district Office of Health (Co Do, 18.07.11), top official in the health station of a rural hamlet (Phong Dien district, 15.12.11) and a top official in central health station (Cai Rang district, 13.12.11); all personal interviews.

20 Health stations are only allowed to sell medicine that is manufactured within the country and mentioned in a list issued by the MoH (top official in the health station of a rural hamlet in Phong Dien district, 15.12.11; personal interview).

social attributes is worthy of notice in this regulation, since – as research findings have indicated - the required "social enthusiasm" can be translated as a willingness to work for very limited economic rewards. As a consequence of the limited professional demands and necessity of working in a nearly voluntary manner, one can find a wide spectrum of individuals in the health station post, from retired doctors to nurses and pharmacists, as well as simply people who have received a minimal three-month vocational training[21]. Thus, instead of the healthcare and consultation centres they are supposed to be, the limited quality of infrastructure and staff that they can recruit leaves local health clinics only able to provide cheap medicine.

Generally, allocating medical staff to rural and remote regions has become very difficult, especially in the case of doctors. Many chose to live in more central and urban areas, as the opportunities for work in the private sector there are increased (Fleßa, 2003). This difficulty is reflected not only in the staffing of health stations, but also in the rural commune clinics and district hospitals; it is pushing towards more lax controls on the requirements and the licensing of medical facilities, especially in the more remote areas (Nguyen Ha, 2011: 3). The national five-year plan for the health sector (MoH, 2010a), suggests that improving local healthcare quality, especially in the more remote areas, should be attempted by rotating some better-educated and experienced personnel to the health stations, in order to train health workers and enhance their capacities (Ibid. 2010). Nevertheless, this policy was not mentioned by any of the 45 interviewed health cadres and medical personnel in Can Tho City; indicating its limited implementation in the provinces thus far.

The commune (or ward) health clinics are more professional and better-equipped establishments. They are generally better able to deal with a wider variety of health issues and can offer examinations as well as some basic treatment services. According to reports, there is a health clinic in each of the 85 communes within Can Tho (Statistical Office of Can Tho City, 2011). Notwithstanding their expanded presence, the quality of healthcare offered in these clinics can vary a lot and depends on their space capacities, their infrastructure and their available personnel (London, 2008a: 122). According to national regulation, there should be one health clinic worker per 1000 – 1200 inhabitants (MoH, 2007b: 180). The reported figures from the two case-study districts of Cai Rang and Phong Dien noted the presence of an average of half what these

---

21 Sources: Top official in district Office of Health (Co Do, 18.07.11), top official in the health station of a rural hamlet (Phong Dien district, 15.12.11), top official in the central health station (Cai Rang district, 13.12.11); all personal interviews.

standards demand (Statistical Division of Cai Rang district, 2010, Statistical Division of Phong Dien district, 2010). This shortage of personnel, however, was not recognised as a problem by any of the interviewed state representatives, many of which insisted instead that the clinics are in good shape and are performing their duties very well. Some Vietnamese authors have argued that the quality of clinics has at least ameliorated in the last 15 years (Tuan Tran Van; Thi Mai Dung; Neu, 2005: 324), while others do not see any significant improvements (Minh Nguyen Thang and Popkin, 2003: 260). The poor capacity of clinics has been attributed to their funding dependency on local governments since the 1990s, a particular consequence of which is that the quality of basic healthcare in poor and usually rural areas is compromised (Tran Tuan 2004 cited in Fritzen, 2007: 1613).

Despite the present difficulties in meeting staffing criteria, the government promulgated a new and more demanding law for the clinics, according to which all clinics should have a medical doctor employed for at least three days of the week (GoV, 2011). Furthermore, each clinic is required to have an examination room and ten more types of specialised rooms[22], a pharmacy and available traditional medicine services (Ibid. 2011). Centrally-produced documents encourage local governments to invest and improve commune clinics, setting a high target that 80% of the clinics meet national standards by the year 2010. This target is, however, still far from being reached (MoH, 2007b). Despite the legislative provisions, the MoH indicates that only 69% of the communes in the country had any doctors at all during the reported year of 2009, while the nurse-to-doctor ratio remains among the lowest in the region of South East Asia (MoH, 2010a). Observations from the study sites within Can Tho confirm the lack of staff, space and equipment (Picture 4.1), confirming previous empirical findings from Fleßa (2003), who showed that only 5.8% of his study-communes in Cao Bang district had a medical doctor. More recent literature also suggests that legal requirements for health clinics are not commonly followed and especially not in the country's rural communes (DSW (German Foundation for World Population), 2011: 9).

[22] These consist of: a laboratory room, a sterilisation facility, a first aid room, an emergency room, a room for pregnant patients, a room for gynaecological exams, a delivery room, a vaccination room, a population and family planning counselling room and an administrative room.

Picture 4.1: Health clinic in Le Binh ward, Cai Rang district

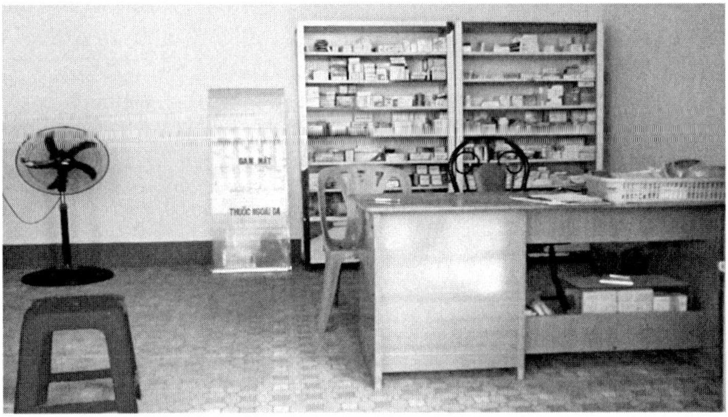

The picture shows the receiving area, where medicine is also being sold. The rest of the clinic consists of an examination room and a laboratory room. Photo by author, 2011

Being the first stop in public healthcare and the most accessible units for medical advice, the grassroots network of the health stations and clinics is crucial for the timely diagnosis, treatment and control of infectious diseases like diarrhoea. Not only is healthcare offered by these units supposed to be the closest and cheapest option for most of the rural and poor inhabitants (see also section 4.2), but is also meant to serve as a cushion for common episodes of easily treatable disease, thereby relieving hospitals of patient overload. Apart from recognising the above and praising the functions of primary healthcare, the central government has, however, not sufficiently implemented the supportive policies that could realize the potential of primary healthcare in safeguarding people's health. The financial dependency of health stations and clinics on the local office's budget is making their transition rather challenging, with repercussions not only in their ability to offer curative services but also on the prevention of disease and the control of epidemics.

4.1.3 The weaknesses reflected in preventive health

One of the national priorities regarding healthcare and prevention is to control big epidemics (MoH, 2007b). Some of the stubbornly prominent diseases, such as HIV, human influenza and children's malnutrition, are placed at the centre of attention (Ibid. 2007b: 123), emphasizing the need to raise public awareness about their prevention through health information and education activities.

Similarly to primary healthcare improvements, preventive health priorities are stressed but are not given a concrete framework of action upon which to create tangible outcomes. The National Strategy distributes preventive medicine responsibilities to ten different ministries, to all People's Committee divisions and to all the organisations under Vietnam's Fatherland Front (Ibid. 2007b: 130) and is, thus, making public health an issue for which everyone is responsible but no one is accountable.

Box 4.1. A summary of the priorities relevant to the prevention of diarrheal disease proclaimed in the "National Strategy on preventive medicine to 2010 and orientations towards 2020" (MoH, 2007b):

- Among the Strategy's future targets is to strengthen the functionality of the provincial and district Preventive Health Centres (PHCs) and to improve the surveillance system of disease (:126).

- Environmental sanitation and food safety are placed at the centre of attention, with the need for more enforcement and control in these sectors being underlined. Safe water supply is not considered a priority anymore, since good quality drinking water is considered to be "assured" for the majority of the population (:103).

- Intestinal diseases are recognised health risks that have the potential to become outbreaks (:106). Specific target-measures for the prevention and control of diarrheal diseases include: (i) to keep mortality rates of cholera less than 1/100,000 (deaths per population) and to contain the epidemic and (ii) to control the mortality rate of typhoid to less than 8/100,000 (deaths per population).

- The mitigation of diarrhoea, which is not classified under cholera or typhoid, is not mentioned as an overall health target, but rather only seen as part of protecting children's health (:122). Moreover, there is the aim of reducing child malnutrition rates to below 20% and to reduce the rates of Vitamin A insufficiency to below 5%, both of which would assist in the prevention of diarrhoea.

The national targets in the sector of preventive health need to be reflected in the priorities of the Preventive Health Centres and thus in the formulation of their "preventive health programs"[23] (MoH, 2007b: 89). The PHCs have two responsibilities with regard to these programs. One responsibility is to report on the incidence of each prioritised disease or health issue. The second is to keep the public informed about these health risks and to promote adequate preventive measures. The district PHCs are responsible for compiling and re-

[23] In Can Tho City, seventeen of such national programs were reported to be in operation, targeting: dengue fever, children's vaccination, food safety, malaria, tuberculosis, HIV-AIDS, eating disorders, diarrheal disease, sanitation expansion, malnutrition, medical education, occupational hygiene and maternal and neo-natal health (top official in PHC of Cai Rang district, 16.12.11; personal interview).

porting such health-related statistics, while the PHCs of the provinces are mostly coordinating and supervising these activities. The tedious collection of data from the communes and wards was seen to basically relegate the activity of the district PHCs to purely bureaucratic procedures. Empirical research in Can Tho showed that the health education activities performed by these units were limited to the occasional banners or posters within their jurisdictions. The MoH (2010a: 32) admits that the preventive health network remains weak "especially in the district level" and as a consequence, "the understanding and the awareness of the people and of some cadres, about health protection and promotion, is weak".

Contrary to the limited spectrum of activities that was observed at the district PHCs in Can Tho, the provincial PHC had multiple departments[24] apart from collecting data and producing reports and a wider range of responsibilities, including the organisation of public health educational and informational campaigns. However, as it will be discussed in detail in the following chapters (see chapter 5 and 6), these campaigns are scarce and do not manage to reach the majority of people in the localities. Many of the representatives from district and provincial PHCs claimed that the preventive health programs are implemented with great success. These claims were justified by the reported execution of certain activities and the relatively decreasing numbers of certain diseases (PHC Cai Rang, 2011a, PHC Cai Rang, 2011b, PHC Can Tho City, 2011a, PHC O Mon, 2011b, PHC O Mon, 2011a, PHC Phong Dien, 2011). The evaluation of public health success was thus based on quantifiable criteria, most of which describe what the local health bureaucracy does and not whether there is a positive impact on the population's health understandings and preventive practices.

Local communicators

While the provincial PHCs set the preventive health priorities and the district ones compile the reports, most of the communication in preventive health programs, and the most of the surveys for the collection of information, are undertaken by the health staff in the commune and hamlet levels. The health

---

[24] In the PHC in Can Tho City there were claimed to be departments of: (1) public health, (2) infectious disease management and vaccinations, (3) malaria and internal disease (covers lesions of lungs, heart, gastrointestinal tract, rheumatic lesions), (4) public nutrition, (5) laboratory – for the chemical and physical analysis of samples which includes water quality samples and blood samples suspected of carrying epidemic diseases (Top official in PHC Can Tho City, 14.07.11; personal interview).

clinics are the units of reference for the collection of statistics in these lower administrative levels and are assigned the responsibility to mobilise and train the health workers at the health stations in issues of public health (GoV, 2011):

> "Commune health clinics will deploy communication and health education activities, population and family planning, through mass media and through communication in the community when visiting families and when people come to have examination and treatment in the commune clinic and in the schools" (GoV, 2011).

The public health duties of the clinics expand to areas of food hygiene, malnutrition, maternal health and many more (GoV, 2011). Considering their shortage of qualified staff, their infrastructural limitations (see section 4.1.2) and the fact that commune clinics principally offer curative services, the requirement of successfully executing preventive activities appears to be a real challenge. Results from the field revealed that there exists a complementary network of health "volunteers" and health "collaborators", who help in the execution of these activities and are unique to the region of the Delta[25].

Uncovering the actual legal rights and responsibilities of the health volunteers and collaborators is a truly confusing issue. Representatives from health-related offices and organisations across Can Tho have all referred to them as being the communicators of preventive information to the public. They are selected and trained by the commune clinic's staff[26] and their main method of public health education was said to be visiting households and remaining in direct contact with local people at the same time collecting survey data. Their financial compensation, however, do not reflect their important and demanding responsibilities. To begin with, as their title already insinuates, health volunteers do not receive any payment for their services. Interviewees vehemently claimed that health volunteers and collaborators do not do this job for money, but to help their communities:

> "In this commune there are 13 health volunteers, some of them are also health collaborators, and some of them are the same people who run the health stations in the hamlets. They don't get paid; they do it from their hearts. They will go around and talk to people, telling them how to prevent accidents [...] Also regarding diarrhoea, they will talk about keeping a clean house environment and being hygienic when eating and drinking." (Top official of a Health Clinic in rural commune, Phong Dien district, 15.09.11; personal interview)

> "Most of them [health volunteers/collaborators] are living in the commune and are somehow related to the health sector. They are either the ones who run the

---

25 Source: Official in the National HSPI, Hanoi, 09.02.12; personal interview.

26 Source: Top official in the central ward clinic, Cai Rang, 13.12.11; personal interview.

commune or hamlet clinic, or retired doctors or people that have been trained on health in the army." (Official in the National HSPI, Hanoi, 09.02.12; personal interview)

The health collaborators were said to be specifically trained for carrying out the family-planning health program[27], reporting the number of kids in each family and keeping track of new births. Despite their thematic focus, health collaborators were found to outnumber the volunteers in the case study areas by a proportion of up to three or four to one. Their work was compensated with a monthly salary of an amount that is not defined by law, is unstable and depends on the locality (usually 100,000 VND[28]), in what seems to be a symbolic gesture to create incentive. As UNICEF (2011) reports, the majority of health collaborators in An Giang province were not getting any financial support and many were abandoning their posts every year.

In the case of these local public health communicators, it becomes again obvious how the proclaimed priorities in health do not translate into actual support for the sectors that need it. Whereas the issue of limited access to preventive information is acknowledged openly (MoH, 2007b: 96) and the importance of an effective network for health education in the hamlet level is stressed (MoH, 2010a), the role of health communicators is not mentioned. The legal absence of these posts was justified by the claim that they only operate in a rather informal fashion and only in the South of the country[29]. The lack of clarity concerning their duties was, nevertheless, also evident within the Mekong Delta, with health representatives unable to give clear definitions:

> "There are the health care units who are basically retired doctors or nurses that offer health care services in return to a very small payment. They don't get paid from the government, they are somehow volunteers. They have a sign outside their doors, so that people know who they are and where they are. They also have the right to sell some normal, over-the-counter medicine." (Top official in the district Medical Centre, Co Do, 18.07.11; personal interview)

> "The health volunteers or collaborators are people that talk to people and work on family planning and HIV prevention. These people are trained on these and more topics, like malaria, malnutrition, and prevention of disease, by the district

[27] Source: Top official in the health station of a rural hamlet in Phong Dien district (15.12.11), top official in the central health station (Cai Rang district, 13.12.11); personal interviews.

[28] This is equal to about 3.5 Euros.

[29] Source: representative of the National Health Strategy and Policy Institute (HSPI) in Hanoi 09.02.12

> or the city's Preventive Health Centre. Some of them have specialisations, but many don't and they just get the training afterwards." (Top official in the district PHC, Phong Dien, 15.09.11; personal interview)

Overall it seems that health workers, health volunteers and health collaborators are usually the same people revolving between the same interchangeable posts. They constitute the vestiges of what Bloom (1998) refers to as the Vietnamese brigade nurses of the 1980s who were part-time health personnel at the hamlet level and who had received training in order to offer basic preventive and curative services. They also have been mentioned as being very knowledgeable about each household's situation, particularly regarding their practice and awareness of preventive health measures. They are, for example, supposed to be good evaluators of households that are in need of water supply or sanitation (WSS) improvements. The results of their assessments affect the execution of support policies in the sectors of WSS (see chapter 5.2.2) but their work is, however, not adequately documented anywhere. Moreover, it was common in the case-study areas that their duties would be taken over by local cadres, such as the head of the hamlet, the head of the Farmer's Union or - as mentioned above - the health workers from the commune/ward clinics. In consideration of this fact, the validity of their assessments with regard to the distribution of support funding demands further investigation (see chapter 5.3.2).

Most of the interviewed local cadres have praised the work of local communicators as honourable, appreciated and very successful. However, the efficacy and impact of their work with regard to its quality and its coverage, is also frequently upbraided as being purely bureaucratic and not motivated or engaging for the public:

> "The problem in the execution of information and education activities in practice is not only that people at the local levels do not have the capacity or the education to understand everything that is involved in a health issue, it is also that the [health workers/communicators] do not care whether the population understands or not; they only care to fulfil the objective of visiting a specific number of households, ticking that box and filling in their reports that they did it." (NGO expert in Water Supply and Sanitation, 11.12.11; personal interview)

Whether due to the poor compensation, their undefined legal status and their unclear responsibilities, or due to their limited educational backgrounds and insufficient training, it seems that what these posts actually serve is again the bureaucratic gathering of statistics and not the targets of health education and promotion. Ironically, the resulting collected statistics (on water safety, hygienic toilets, environmental sanitation) are viewed by higher-level experts as unreliable[30]. However, it is on the basis of these reports that local and district authorities compile their short-term assessments on how successful the preventive health programs have been. This focus on numerical, rather than quality-based, results stems from the objectives that higher-level offices set and which they expect the local levels to realise. A pattern emerges from this brief analysis of the institutional function of the health sector, one in which the state - at least on paper - declares its support for the fundamental units of primary healthcare and preventive health action, while in practice neglects the local health curative and preventive networks. As will be further analysed, this is paralleled with a shift in people's health-seeking behaviours, as well with the - yet unmitigated - prevalence of preventable diseases, such as diarrhoea.

4.2 Reshaping access to public health

In 2008, the government allocated 7.3%[31] of the overall national GDP to public health, amounting to only 38.5% of the total health expenditures in the country (WHO, 2012a). The national health budget has overall been shrinking ever since the reformations of the 1990s and is nowadays unequally distributed among administrative levels, with most of the health funds being directed towards higher-level and centrally-managed hospitals and research units. This has been putting pressure both on health professionals who are unsatisfied with the compensation levels in the sector (HSPI, 2012a), and on patients, many of whom have to pay out-of-pocket for health services. The limited central support and the high rates of people without health insurance are far from facilitating a financial upswing of the public healthcare system; in contrast, this is hampering basic conditions such as staffing, internal organisation and functionality (London, 2008a: 125). In combination with the concurrent privatisation in the sector, the shift in public support has significantly altered public access to health.

4.2.1 New rules and new players in the "game" of healthcare: the private sector

It was mentioned above how the higher-level and specialised healthcare units of the country (hospitals) have, since the launch of decentralisation policies, been allowed to operate on a cost-recovery basis (GoV, 2002, GoV, 2006b). This has radically changed the landscape of specialised health examinations and treat-

[30] Sources: Top official in HIPH of Ho Chi Minh City (20.07.11), UNICEF representative (Ho Chi Minh City, 29.07.11); personal interviews.
[31] This is equal to about 7 billion USD.

ments that are offered in these units. The introduction of fees was expected to improve the financial situation of the hospitals and to boost their performance, but beyond the question of how far this has been achieved, it has also had a profound impact on re-shaping healthcare access opportunities (London, 2008a, Minh Nguyen Thang and Popkin, 2003). With hospital services being no longer offered for free and with the allocation of patients to hospitals at the different levels being subject to their residential registration, many of the poor, uninsured and rural residents face a multitude of obstacles in accessing the healthcare that they need.

Decentralisation came together with privatisation of healthcare. The number of private hospitals, pharmacies and medical practitioners has been on the rise during the last three decades. More than 137 private hospitals exist today in the country and a vast number of physicians are operating for private patients only. Most private hospitals are found in urban centres (Kieu Linh, 2012) and yet, despite their expansion, they are outnumbered by the public ones[32] (GSO, 2011b, Nghiem Tran Dung, 2010). Their further expansion is said to be checked by the legal complexity that surrounds opening institutes of health, as well as by the continuingly low demand for highly-priced healthcare from the country's poor and middle-income population (Kieu Linh, 2012). In fact, only 65% of the private hospitals in major urban hubs[33] have accepted to contract with the public health insurance program (HSPI, 2012c) and are thus making their services accessible only to individuals who can afford to pay the entire fees.

Unlike the elite character of the private hospitals, the charges for individual private doctors are not as high and thus not so exclusive. The numerous independent doctors that work on a private or "semi-public"[34] basis have the liberty of basing their clinics anywhere they chose. As mentioned before, this is seen as the reason why doctors have accumulated in the urban areas (see also section 4.1.2). However, the clustering of better health facilities (and health professionals) in urban areas has been, according to Bloom (1998), a trend in Vietnam since even before the renovation policies. According to Forsberg (2011), the private sector has given doctors the opportunity to improve their incomes relative to the low and apparently unsatisfactory salaries that they are paid in the public sector. Many of the publically employed doctors who were interviewed

[32] There are more than one thousand public hospitals in Vietnam, according to the GSO (2010).

[33] These are the cities of Hanoi, Ho Chi Minh City and Da Nang.

[34] This refers to the practice of moonlighting as a private clinician while employed in the public sector, as described by Priwitzer (2012).

admitted that they also work privately in the evenings. In fact, one of them claimed that, although his family lives in Ho Chi Minh, where he works privately, he also works in a rural district hospital in Can Tho by choice, and in order to contribute to the hospital's capacity. According to him, if he leaves his public health position, "the hospital will be left without a properly trained medical doctor" (Medical doctor in Phong Dien district Hospital, 21.07.11; personal interview).

Another problem that emerges from extending usage of private instead of public healthcare is that the activities of the former remain largely undocumented. Many of the clinics are unregistered and thus the services they offer are not standardized and thus remain unregulated. The Health Strategy and Policy Institute found that most of the private clinics in fact lack the equipment that is necessary to provide the healthcare services covered by the basic insurance program (HSPI, 2012a, HSPI, 2012c). Other authors have found that indeed many of the private clinics that are operating in rural areas were technically of much lower standards than the public ones (Tuan Tran Van; Thi Mai Dung; Neu, 2005). However, what makes private clinics generally more preferable for primary healthcare is the perception that they are more attentive to the patient's needs and they have availability at more convenient times when compared to the public ones (Dat V. Duong et al., 2004, Gaudine et al., 2009). As the next section discusses, the evaluations of the public with regard to their options for healthcare is not only shaping everyday health-seeking decisions but also has repercussions on longer term strategies followed in health policy, particularly in regard to people's participation in the public health insurance scheme.

4.2.2 Loopholes in the health insurance scheme

The approach to insurance policies has changed since the advent of the 'Health Care Fund for the Poor' (HCFP) policy in 2003, which ensured free basic healthcare for the members of households categorised as poor, as well as for those living in disadvantaged areas and communes, as well as for ethnic minorities residing mainly in the country's mountainous regions (International Labour Organization, 2012). The law also provides free healthcare for all children below six years old (Decree 63), while pupils and university students need to pay a reduced health insurance premium of three percent of the minimum monthly salary in the country[35]. For all the rest, the basic health insurance premium amounts to 4.5%[36].

When the public health insurance scheme was first introduced in 1992, the rate of insured individuals was below 10%. In 2006, the rate had climbed to 40% and has been increasing ever since. The government has been continuing its efforts by enacting a Law which foresees the insurance of all employed individuals and students, apart from those who are self-employed and farmers, under the 'Compulsory Insurance Scheme' (GoV, 2008). As a result, the rate of the population that was insured under the public scheme, either through their employment or by being beneficiaries of social policies, reached 60% (Nghiem Tran Dung, 2010). Notwithstanding these improvements, it is apparent that the number of self-employed individuals who voluntarily choose to join the insurance scheme has hardly increased throughout these years (HSPI, 2012b). With the goal of propping up the health system's finances, the government publically committed to make health insurance obligatory for all Vietnamese by the year 2014 (Vietnews, 2012).

Beyond the question of whether there will be a further rise in the rate of insured people in the country, is the question of why the finances of the health insurance scheme are not improving. With 60% of the population already signed up, the scheme should be viable. Instead, it has been continuously facing a financial squeeze since 2005 (Nghiem Tran Dung, 2010). This indicates that there exist some loopholes in the system. Literature suggests that one of the missteps in the system lies in the adverse selection of beneficiaries with free healthcare rights. Namely, local authorities which have the power to allocate free healthcare insurance cards according to the criteria mentioned above, often distribute them to people with increased health risks, even if the latter do not belong in categories of poverty or disadvantage (Lieberman and Wagstaff, 2009, Hien et al., 1995).

Considering the limited number of free health cards that the HCFP can provide, the local practice of adverse selection and moral hazard not only jeopardise the longevity of the insurance scheme (Lieberman and Wagstaff, 2009), but also take away health benefits from those who do belong in the socially sensitive categories that the law aims to support. A survey conducted in over two thousand households revealed that 20 – 30% of the poor were still not insured (Dam Viet Cuong, 2009). The national General Statistics Office provides simi-

---

35 Source: Top official in the district Office of Health, Phong Dien, 12.09.11; personal interview.

36 The minimum salary in 2011 was 830,000 VND, equal to about 40 USD.

lar percentages of poor people visiting public healthcare units but having no healthcare insurance (GSO, 2008). It is not specified whether the uninsured status of people in these studies was due to their non-classification as poor (or other categories), or because they were not yet reached by the HCFP program. Looking at the processes of formulating poverty inventories, however, it becomes clear that, similar to the distribution of free healthcare cards, the inclusion or not in these inventories often comes down to the personal judgments of local cadres. The pliable nature of these processes is worth taking into account not only when assessing the equity and the efficiency of the health insurance scheme but also a wide range of pro-poor policy implementation.

Box 4.2. A summary of how official inventories of poor and non-poor households are created:

1. Large-scale surveys take place every five years in order to define the poor and nearly-poor families. These surveys include questions and inventories regarding the family's income levels, their other revenue sources and an inventory of the household's belongings (see table 1 in the Annex).

2. Due to the possibility of a household changing status (i.e. shifting from poor to non-poor), there is an annual evaluation and re-examination of these five-year survey results. This is done by local authorities or more specifically, the district offices of Labour, Invalids and Social affairs (LISA). These offices produce updated inventories in consultation with local governments, as well as the health workers and health communicators of each commune/ward (Department of Labour Invalids and Social Affairs, 2010).

3. The results from these LISA surveys are discussed and assessed in commune level meetings, where cadres, citizens and health representatives confirm or deny their validity according to their personal knowledge on the status of each household under question[37] .

4. The responsibility for the final stamp of approval for the annual inventories of poor households lies in the hands of the 'Steering committee for the alleviation of poverty' at the district and provincial levels. These committees, however, have no other source of information at hand to help them question what is being presented to them by the local enumerators.

[37] Sources: Top officials in OLISA of Phong Dien district, 26.09.2011 & Cai Rang 29.09.12; personal interviews.

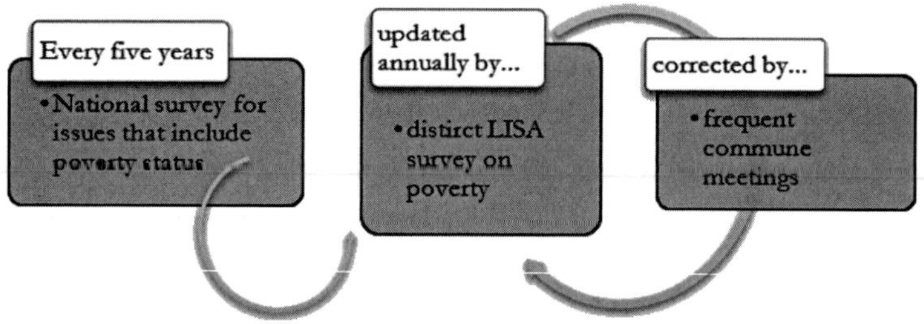

(Department of Labour Invalids and Social Affairs, 2010).

Looking at the performance of the health insurance mechanism and particularly at the persisting unwillingness of people to voluntarily join the schemes, suggests that there is public mistrust towards the benefits that the scheme can provide in return to the investments it requires. For those who sign up to the basic premium of public health insurance, the first step of care-seeking is to visit the health stations and clinics, where basic outpatient care is offered. If patients need to be hospitalised, they will normally be referred to the district hospital of their locality, based on their officially registered residency. If need be, the staff of the district hospitals can decide to refer patients further to specialised hospital units at a higher administrative level. Throughout this care-seeking path, the insured individuals have to contribute 20% of the treatment expenses if those surpass the amount of 120,000 VND[38]. People also have the option of directly visiting a public hospital of their own choice, but in that case they would have to pay 70% of the expenses. It is worth mentioning that these rules of access do not apply for medical staff and government cadres, whose special health insurance schemes provide for entrance to any public hospital with their contribution not surpassing 5% of the total expenses[39].

Even though the insurance scheme takes administrative divisions as the basis of assigning patients to hospitals, not every district or provincial hospital is of the same quality. Hospitals are classified in grades according to a system of evaluation that follows criteria of capacity (number of beds, human resources), administrational location (district, province, central), levels of expertise and avail-

---

[38] This amount is equal to about 7 Euros.
Sources: Top official in the district Office of Health, Phong Dien, 12.09.11 and top official in the Red Cross branch of Phong Dien district, 07.09.2011; personal interviews.

[39] Sources: Top official in the Central General Hospital of Can Tho, 21.06.11 and household representative, Yen Hoa area of Cai Rang district 18.10.11; personal interviews.

able infrastructure, technology and specialised equipment, among others (GoV, 2005). Interestingly, if a hospital is under central administration (level-III), it is granted more points in the evaluation system and thus gets a higher grade; even though the connection between healthcare quality and administrative position is not legally prescribed.

Following the pyramid model (Fig 4.3), there is one hospital (of level-II or level-III) in each district, which according to the above criteria could theoretically be evaluated highly or not (MoH, 2007b). Considering that funding for healthcare depends primarily on the socio-economic status of the localities, the quality of each hospital is also a function of how financially successful a district or a province is. As Priwitzer (2012) points out, district hospitals are less utilised than the ones at the province or in the city, and people have generally expressed their dissatisfaction with the quality of health services in local healthcare units (Phan 2006 cited in London, 2008b). This came up during a household interview in a rural district, in which the member of a better-off family explained why, since insurance only provided access to the district hospital that they considered lower quality, they preferred to quit the scheme and pay 'out-of-pocket' treatment in the central hospital of their own choice[40].

Specialised provincial hospitals have a reputation of offering the best quality of services. However, even though they usually have five times the bed-capacity of district hospitals, they are always overloaded with patients. Their specialised expertise is rare and thus they get assigned the treatment of many patients from around their region. Their good reputation brings in also many patients who chose to circumvent the official care-seeking path, even if their health problems do not demand for specialised care (Vian et al., 2012). The Paediatrics Hospital of Can Tho City, for example, attracts hundreds of visitors from around the Delta, as it is considered to offer the best healthcare for children. However, the hospital's capacities are not enough to support such huge numbers of visitors. The congestion of children patients in combination with a lack of nursing staff and somewhat poor organisation often results in the severe deterioration of inpatient care (Picture 4.2). Dramatic patient overflows are noted in many of the central high-level hospitals of the country, which are increasingly encountering difficulties in delivering consistently good healthcare services (MoH,

[40] Source: Household representative, Thoi Giai hamlet of Phong Dien district 05.10.11; personal interview.

2010a, Priwitzer, 2012), a reality that many administrative staff readily admit[41]. As Lieberman (2009) shows, this overcrowded status is to an important extent exacerbated by the hospitals' own policy to keep inpatients for prolonged stays. Following a "per diem" instead of "per case" system of charge, not releasing patients on time gives the hospitals much better economic returns, which works against the public benefit and compromises the overall quality of their services.

Picture 4.2: The department of diarrheal disease in the Paediatrics Hospital of Can Tho City

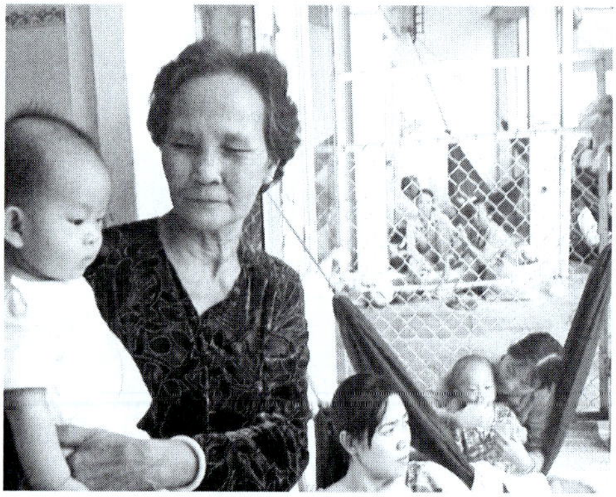

Children are held in hammocks outside of overcrowded rooms. The role of nurses is taken up by relatives and friends, as is the case in many overcrowded hospitals, presenting the risk of secondary infections and further spread of disease (Luxemburger et al., 2001). Picture by the author, 2011

The function of the public health insurance scheme must, therefore, be looked at in combination with the function of healthcare units and in relation to the policies that surround both. Regardless of where the best quality of healthcare is offered, the final decisions people make are largely dependent on their financial capacities. The health insurance scheme does not always guarantee the health access one might aspire for, either because public grassroots healthcare is too unprofessional or hasty, or because the specialised units are overcrowded, messy or not accessible. Most self-employed individuals seem to prefer to pay out-of-pocket for their "everyday" or "normal" health expenses and do not account for possible future "serious" problems in need of specialised and ex-

[41] Sources: Top official in Paediatric Hospital of Can Tho, 27.06.11 & nurse in Paediatric Hospital of Can Tho, 11.07.11 & Top official in the Central General Hospital of Can Tho, 21.06.11; personal interviews.

pensive healthcare, for which they will not be in the position to pay. As a result of taking such risks in their care-seeking strategy, many families are ultimately saddled with unbearable health expenses and fall into heavy debts. As the next section discusses, health access inequalities persist and are mostly acutely experienced by the country's poor and remote populations.

Combined impacts of inequality in health access

The picture of health access is not homogeneous, with the rural and the poor being the most underserved with regard to healthcare. It was mentioned above how, regardless of their vast number, local public healthcare establishments consistently fall behind in terms of technical and professional capacities (Axelson et al., 2009). Considering also the increased availability of private medical consultation (Nguyen Ha, 2011: 10), the decline in public clinic utilisation for outpatient cases does not come as a big surprise for either urban or rural areas (Bloom, 1998). Rural areas, however, have significantly fewer units of primary healthcare, most of which also have limited capacities (MoH, 2010a: 6). A recent survey by the GSO (2008) showed, the access to central hospitals is also conditioned by location. People from rural areas appeared to have fewer opportunities to receive examination and treatment in central hospitals, in comparison to their urban counterparts (Ibid. 2008). These observations cannot be viewed in isolation from factors such as health insurance and poverty, especially consideration that rural areas are mostly inhabited by farmers, who in turn are usually both uninsured and lower income.

Most of Vietnam's poor are indeed living in rural areas (General Statistics Office, 2009) and poverty is intensifying the difficulties in accessing health insurance schemes and healthcare services. Most of the rural inhabitants that could get inpatient treatment in high-level hospitals belonged to the rich quintile of the population; this disparity was even greater when considering the use of outpatient services (GSO, 2008). In general, the health spending of the poor is on average 3 times lower than that of the rich (GSO, 2008), while outlaws for health of the poor constitute 40.5% of their overall household incomes (London, 2008a). High out-of-pocket spending is one of the most persistent problems in the country, with many people finding themselves in need of unbearably expensive treatment due to their lack of health insurance coverage. It was reported that catastrophic health expenses are forcing three million people to go below the poverty line annually in Vietnam (Vian et al., 2012: 3). Even small unexpected health expenses might amount to more than is manageable for the uninsured, especially for those households with irregular income (Fleßa, 2003).

Apart from structural factors that define disparities in healthcare access, there are also institutional reasons why some people cannot get the same quality of healthcare as others. In hospitals, the offered services are seemingly different for those who are insured and for those who pay 'out-of-pocket', with the latter being more welcome and more attended to:

> "There are two different sections in the hospitals: one where people get medicine if they have insurance or a health card and they don't pay anything, and one special 'services' section, where people have to pay for treatment and medicine. The 'health insurance' section is slower than the 'services' and not as effective" (Household representative, Yen Hoa area, Cai Rang district, 18.10.11).

London (2008a: 125) has already written about this informal, but nevertheless strongly institutionalized, division of service delivery in the hospitals. Similar observations are made by Forsberg (2011: 4) regarding the better reception and treatment of governmental officials, in contrast to lay citizens with basic healthcare insurance. Noticing this type of double standards that are in play in public hospitals, Priwitzer (2012: 175) further describes how if patients are willing to pay doctors more money they will get better inpatient conditions, thus creating an overt "two-tier system" where public and private boundaries are blurred. The issue of corruption through "under the table" payments is a commonly discussed as a "plague" on the health system in Vietnam and especially in the healthcare units of high-demand (Than Tung, 2012, Dao et al., 2008, Hien et al., 1995, Vian et al., 2012, Thanh Nien news, 2012). The practice of additional illegal payments has become so common as to be considered necessary by a public desperate for good quality healthcare services (Ha Mi, 2013) and has contributed to the creation of high institutional boundaries to healthcare access for the poor. Other issues of mismanagement and corruption have been continually on the rise since the hospitals became autonomous, including the practice of unnecessarily prolonged bed occupancies, which has been described above (Lieberman and Wagstaff, 2009). This strongly suggests the need for the increased supervision, monitoring and inspection in the sector (Nguyen Khanh Phuong et al., 2009, Ha Mi, 2013). Although there was an attempt by the government to establish an independent auditing body for issues of health governance during the formulation of the Law on Examination and Treatment (GoV, 2009a), this idea was abandoned.

Having so far described the institutional structures and functions that underlie healthcare provision, it is understandable why people's attitudes towards the health system are governed more by fear rather than trust. Many prefer to visit a pharmacy and self-medicate rather than interacting with medical facilities (Khe et al., 2002), especially for sickness which they consider familiar or less serious. The majority of national health expenditures in Vietnam comes from people's out-of-pocket payments (Axelson et al., 2009, Ha Nguyen Thi Hong et al., 2002, Dao et al., 2008), a quarter of which is towards the purchase of medicine sold in the private sector (Lieberman and Wagstaff, 2009: 6). In a country of 88 million people, this has engendered a huge pharmaceutical sector. The prices of medicine, nevertheless, remain largely uncontrolled (Le Thanh Ha, 2010), despite regulations issued by the MoH (2007). What was apparent in the numerous pharmacies across the country is the promotion of certain medicaments over others and the inducing of patients to over-consume drugs (Ha Nguyen Thi Hong et al., 2002). The same has been noticed in the practices of doctors, who promote and illegally sell medication from their private clinics (MoH cited in Ha Nguyen Thi Hong et al., 2002: 2).

The uninformed consumption of medicine has been exacerbated by the poor enforcement in private pharmacies of the requirement for medical prescriptions. Many drug peddlers are not even licensed pharmacists (Lieberman and Wagstaff, 2009, Okumura et al., 2002: 1876, Vian et al., 2012, Bloom, 1998), yet they are deciding the medical treatment for millions of people in the country. A meta-analysis and review of studies on the issue (Van Nguyen et al., 2013) revealed that more than 90% of the doctors in hospitals overprescribed antibiotics in post-surgery cases due to their "lack of confidence in laboratory reporting and infection control policy". This type of irresponsibly prescribed medication can have serious repercussions on the health of those individuals and the wider community. Diseases that remain untreated, or are treated with the wrong medicine, can worsen and spread. Over-use of antibiotics causes pathogens to mutate and become resistant, constituting a serious threat to public health. A study conducted by Okumura et al. (2002) revealed that one third of their interviewed individuals (505 in total) were keeping medicine which they would take in case of future illness. Among these medicaments were various types of antibiotics, carelessly used for casual treatment of coughs and diarrhoea.

The line that connects institutional decentralisation and privatisation in the health sector to the illegal practices of bribing or unadvised retail of medicine is not visible at first site. The analysis shows that people's health access is defined by the organisational aspects that govern the sector of health and the mechanisms that exist to control and regulate its function. When seeking medical advice and attention, the poor and the rural population is usually faced with unqualified health workers and pharmacists or are compelled to take on significant economic losses in their efforts to access private and higher-level specialised units. Even though this might be easier for the urban and/or better off inhabitants, they are still subject to the challenges described above, namely internal hospital corruption, over-promotion of drugs and a poorly regulated private sector. When also considering the crippled system of preventive health education, people become extremely vulnerable to diseases and epidemics about which they are not informed and against which they do not know how to protect. The next section examines the current status of some major infectious diseases in the country, drawing parallels with what has been so far highlighted in the health system.

4.3 Controlling epidemics in Vietnam

4.3.1 The status of infectious diseases and the distribution of diarrhoea

The incidence and the mortality rates of certain highly infectious diseases are some of the main indicators for assessing the success of preventive health policy in the country (see also section 3.2.3). The WHO (2012a) reports that, in Vietnam, the morbidity of infectious diseases has decreased by 34.6% and mortality correspondingly by 5% from 2007 to 2010. One successful example is the control of malaria, the morbidity and mortality rates of which have come down significantly (Fig 4.4).

Figure 4.4: Reported malaria rates in Vietnam, surrounding regions and the world, during 2009

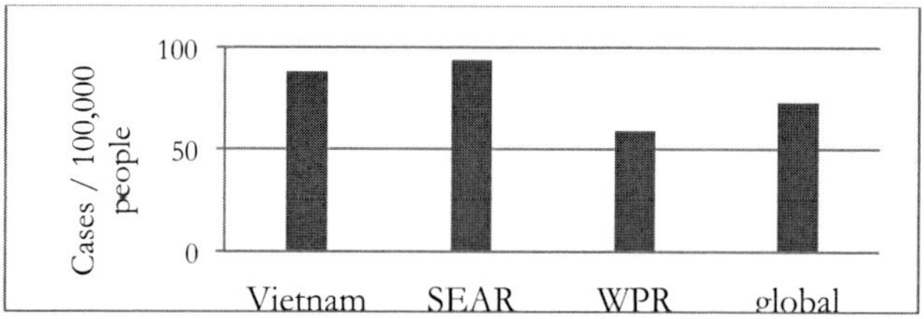

Based on data by WHO (2012e). Design by the author.

Considering that an outbreak of over one million cases was experienced in 1995, the progress made on this front is indeed noteworthy. Current research, however, detects some trends of resistance-building to anti-malaria drugs in the region, seen partly as a result of the manufacturing and usage of counterfeit medical products (WHO, 2012f). Despite the success in malaria control, some other infectious diseases like dengue fever, pneumonia, and tuberculosis continue to afflict much of the country's population (WHO, 2012a). Additionally, the HIV epidemic is particularly worrying, as the morbidity rates have been escalating during the last 10 years (Fig 4.5). Apart from these rather known diseases, new health threats are also on the rise and are proving extremely complex to control, including severe acute respiratory syndrome (SARS) and the influenza A (H5N1) virus (WHO, 2012a). Due to the social, epidemiological and environmental particularities of each the above mentioned diseases, it is hard to comment on what it is exactly that stands in the way of their effective management. Nevertheless, their persisting incidence does indicate that their prevention is facing institutional headwinds.

Figure 4.5: Morbidity rates for tuberculosis and HIV/AIDS in Vietnam and in surrounding regions

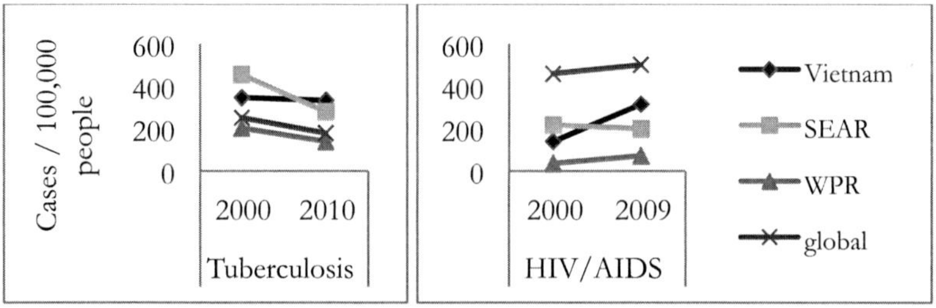

Note: WPR= West Pacific Region, SEAR = South East Asian Region. Based on data by WHO (2012e). Design by the author.

With regard to diarrheal diseases, the WHO reports that even though most outbreaks are being successfully detected and controlled (WHO, 2012a), it remains one of the leading causes of morbidity in the country. The more severe expressions of diarrhoea, seen in the infections of cholera and typhoid fever, have reduced dramatically since 1997, but they keep re-appearing as short-term epidemics (WHO, 2012a). The latest and most severe cholera epidemic took place in 2007 (Fig 4.6).

Figure 4.6: Annual numbers of cholera cases in Vietnam for the years 2001 to 2010

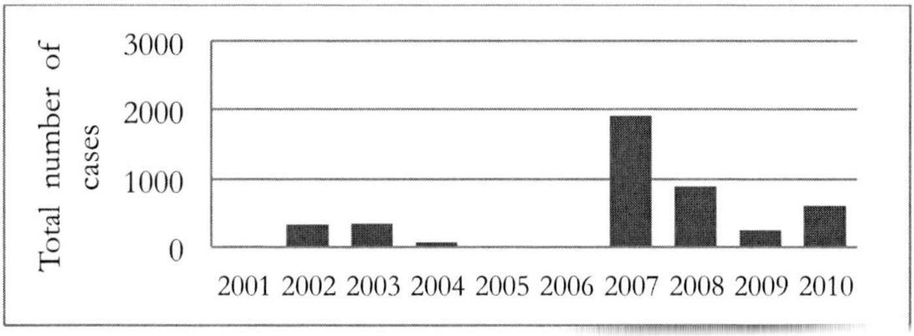

Data source (MoH, 2012b). Design by the author.

One of the diarrhoea types, Shigellosis dysentery, has been maintained consistently high incidence in the country (Kelly-Hope et al., 2008). Other types of diarrhoea that are caused by protozoa, helminths or worms, have been largely under-studied and unreported, both in Vietnam and worldwide. Acute diarrhoea that is neither dysentery nor typhoid is the most prevalent diagnosed type of diarrhoea reported in the country (Fig 4.7), with an average of over 1.5 million documented cases annually from the years 2005 to 2011. The Northern and Highland regions are comparatively more prone to the disease, presenting the highest morbidity rates for the same period (Fig 4.8). These provinces are characterized by high rates of poverty (Nguyen Thang et al., 2006) and high ethnic diversity. This already suggests some co-evolution of socio-economic and health phenomena. When looking particularly at the provinces of the Southern Mekong Delta, it is readily observable how the city of Can Tho is among the six provinces that are most affected by diarrhoeal diseases (Fig 4.9).

Most of the above reported southern provinces (Fig 4.9) are officially characterized as rural, apart from Can Tho City and Ho Chi Minh City, which are classified as urban (GSO, 2012b). The province of Ba Rau is the only one of the 18 rural provinces where the number of urban and rural residents is almost equal (Ibid. 2012); thus, Ba Rau could be seen as the "urbanising" case at the provincial level. Ho Chi Minh City aside, Can Tho is considered to be one of the most developed provinces in the Mekong Delta, from both an economic and an infrastructural standpoint. The health data shows that whereas the overall number of diarrheal disease cases has decreased in the South over the reported years, the urbanising province of Ba Rau is facing an increase and was actually the most affected province for the year 2010. Considering that Can Tho City is also facing more cases than many of the rural provinces, it seems that urbanisation does not necessarily coincide with public health improvements, at least in terms of diarrheal disease. To contrast, however, the least hit province is Ho Chi Minh City, which is indeed the most urbanised and developed in the South (Fig 4.9).

Figure 4.7: Reported morbidity rates of diarrheal diseases in Vietnam, by diagnostic type

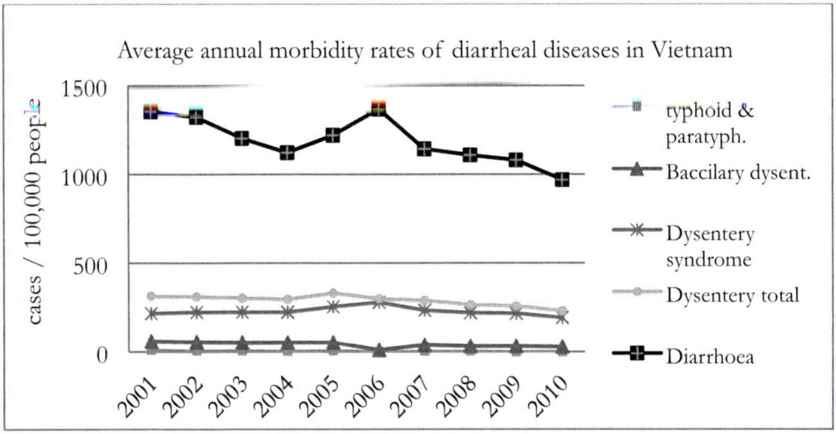

Data source: (MoH, 2012b). Design by the author.

Figure 4.8: Reported morbidity rates of diarrheal diseases in Vietnam by region, averages for 2001 to 2010

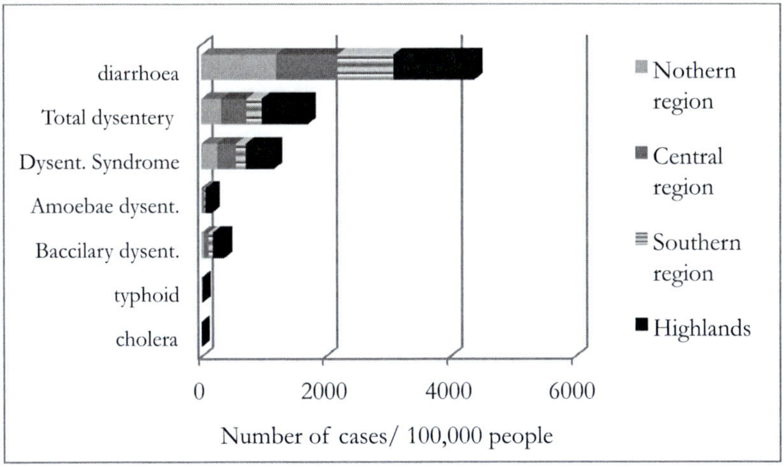

Based on data by MoH (2012b); design by the author.

Figure 4.9: Reported morbidity rates of all types of diarrheal diseases for the Southern provinces

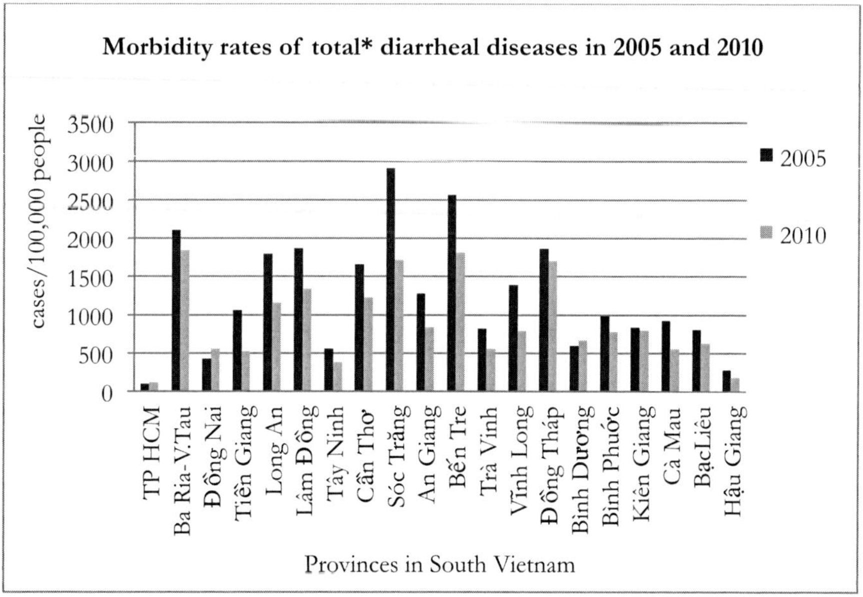

* Including acute diarrhoea, dysenteries, typhoid and cholera. Data source: IHPH (2012); design by the author.

Zooming in the nine districts of Can Tho City and focusing on what is being reported as acute diarrhoea, a rural or urban characterization does not seem to be a factor in the distribution of the disease's morbidity (Fig 4.10). To illustrate, the most affected districts of Cai Rang and Binh Thuy are officially classified as urban districts, while the most central and developed district of Ninh Kieu actually reports higher morbidity rates than the wholly rural district of Thoi Lai.

Figure 4.10: Reported morbidity rates of diarrheal disease in the districts of Can Tho City

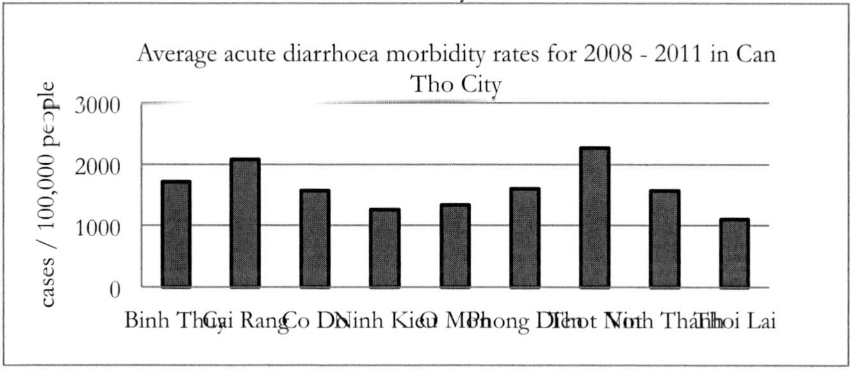

* Data for the population is from 2011 (Statistical Office of Can Tho City, 2011). Based on data by the PHC of Can Tho City (2011b). Design by the author.

What can be extracted from the health data above is that urban and rural categorisations cannot fully describe what shapes the spread of disease. Even if the process of urbanisation does impact on the risk of diarrheal disease, this impact is not to be understood as clearly positive or negative. More importantly, before rushing to conclusions about what the spatial distribution of disease incidence indicates, one needs to interrogate the credibility of health statistics and look at how this data is being produced from the local to the national level.

4.3.2 The disease reporting mechanism and the case of diarrhoea

The information on the occurrence of infectious disease is aggregated in a bottom-up manner from the communes up to the MoH, in a process that is coordinated by the PHCs (Fig 4.11). Reports on the status of disease are produced daily, monthly and annually, with the statistics continually being aggregated as the reports move up levels[42].

---

[42] For example, the district PHCs collect daily statistics of the number of diarrhoea cases per commune. The regional institutes of the South, to compare, only have aggregated data per province and in most cases they only keep monthly or annual statistics.

Figure 4.11: The reporting of infectious diseases within the health system in Vietnam

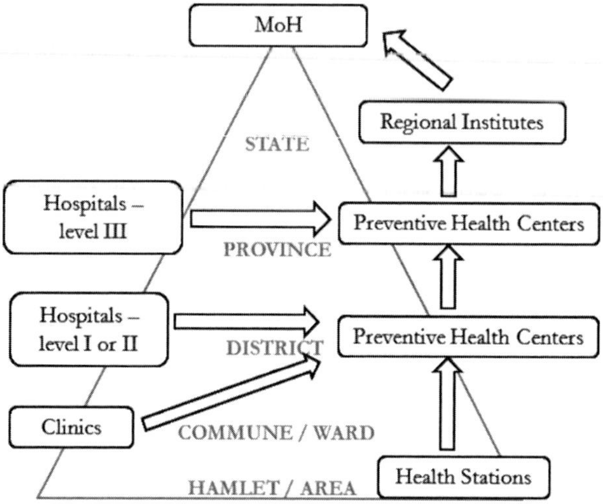

Based on descriptions of health representatives, collected health reports and Decree 48 of the Government of Vietnam (2010a)

If a case of highly infectious disease appears in one of the units of health reporting, the unit must immediately report it to the provincial authority (PHC), which in turn has the duty to initiate a "case management plan" and take measures to hinder the spread of the epidemic (Article 47 in GoV, 2007). The management plan for cholera, for example, includes the transfer of the patient to a district or provincial hospital, where a 'disease control strategy' is employed, according to the instructions issued by the MoH (2007a). The national guidelines for the management of children's diarrhoea define diarrhoea generally as "the passing of watery stool three or more times within 24 hours" (MoH, 2009c) but also classify it according to the different aetiologies and lay out the recommend treatments (see also chapter 6.2.2). Generally, health professionals claimed to base their treatments of diarrhoea on the diagnostic characteristics and not on laboratory analyses, prescribing antibiotics for the feverish type of bloody dysentery and oral or intra-venus re-hydration therapy for the acute watery diarrhoea[43]. From the overall answers of the interviewees it seems that

[43] Source: Top official in the Paediatric Hospital of Can Tho; 27.06.11; personal interview.

only specialised hospitals are in the position to diagnose and treat diarrhoea in detail and thus the cases that are not administered in the hospitals fall under the more general category of diarrhoea and are thereby reported and treated accordingly. Interestingly, there is no "case management plan" for diarrhoea that is not classified as cholera or does not concern children.

Citizens and health professionals usually referred to adult diarrhoea as a "light", "common" or "everyday" disease, characterized by mild episodes that do not reach severe de-hydration stages and thus do not receive special medication or inpatient care. According to informants, only when a case of acute ("serious") diarrhoea is detected in a health unit, the PHCs in the central, provincial and district level will coordinate to control its spread[44]. The preventive mechanism against diarrheal disease in the country is kept active by the frequent circulation of directives and decisions from the MoH to the localities, especially during periods of increased risk for foodborne or waterborne epidemics (see also chapter 6.2.1 and 6.2.2). The electronic Disease Surveillance System in the country is based on the reporting of infectious diseases (Fig 4.11) and is used for the early detection and control of the outbreaks of epidemics. However, the system will only recognise the morbidity rate of an infectious disease as an outbreak when this rate surpasses a set threshold. The thresholds are defined based on the average rate of each disease during the previous five years[45]. As a result, the constantly high numbers of a disease, like acute diarrhoea, are not considered to be outbreaks unless the incidence rises particularly abruptly.

To summarise, the detection and the confinement of a possible outbreak depend on the reporting that takes place in the healthcare units and on the fast communication and coordination between the preventive organisations involved. Although diarrhoea is the second most prevalent disease in the country, its spread seems to be considered rather expected and normal by the reporting and curative health institutions in the country. In terms of medical attention, the millions of episodes of diarrhoea that are noted annually are not considered alarming unless they are of a deadly type (like cholera). In terms of preventive action, diarrhoea episodes do not initiate further examination and control unless they spread at rates that exceed the established 5-year threshold. Further-

[44] This only takes place if the symptoms indicate the presence of infectious cholera or typhoid, or a group food poisoning case, but not for the case of the milder individual diarrhoea episodes.
Source: Top official in PHC Can Tho City, 14.07.11; personal interview.

[45] Source: Official of the WHO in IHPH, Ho Chi Minh City, 29.07.11; personal interview.

more, the reported statistics only show the tip of the iceberg of the actual cases of disease in the population and often prove untrustworthy, as there are inconsistencies in their reporting methodology.

Inconsistencies and "escaped" numbers in the case of diarrhoea

It is particularly difficult to judge the extent to which reported statistics on diarrheal disease reflect the reality of aggregate personal experience. The problems already begin when different reporting categories are used in the various health units[46], which are not well clarified in the produced reports and thus can easily lead to the comparison between "apples and oranges" (Table 2 in Annex). Many of the health clinics and hospitals in Can Tho City only report about patients that are under-five years old. And many of the reports from the district PHCs only report one number of total patients with diarrheal disease. The provincial department of health, on the contrary, separate statistics between children patients and the total number of patients (Department of Health, 2009), but the source of data for this separation is unknown. The Paediatric Hospital in Can Tho, however, which reports 1,500 annual acute diarrhoea cases on average for the years 2009 to 2011 (Can Tho Regional Paediatrics Hospital, 2011), does not specify that these numbers actually only represent inpatient and not outpatient cases. A closer look into the detailed records from the hospital's archive was able to show that, in fact, there were up to 12,000 check-in visits of children with diarrhoea, most of which were simply not diagnosed as "severe" cases and thus were sent home as outpatients.

When comparing the data from the different authorities within Can Tho, many discrepancies arise (Table 2 in Annex). The district PHC of Binh Thuy, for example, reported 140 cases of children patients for the first semester of 2011. This number did not appear in the report of "children's infectious diseases" compiled and provided by the PHC of Can Tho City for the same year, which only reported 10 cases of children's diarrhoea. As a result of this confusion and the unclear methodology for collecting data on diarrhoea, health statistics from the various organisations in the country can provide for various interpretations on its spread, depending on how much of the "meta-data" is available and to what extent triangulation can confirm the validity of the data. The problems of health reporting go beyond the issue of diarrheal disease, seeing how even the vital registration system in Vietnam has been proved flawed and regularly fails to provide accurate numbers for mortality and causes of death (WHO, 2012a). While the WHO and other international organisations have assisted some prov-

---

[46] For example, some units report only on children patients, some only on inpatients and some report all the patients with diarrhoea.

inces with equipment and technical training for properly reporting diseases, most provinces still rely on governmental support or hospital revenues, which so far, are not said to be sufficient (MoH, 2006). While reporting is a core activity for numerous health offices, it has proven to be a rather poorly synchronized and incomplete system of information exchange. In the words of a medical doctor from a rural district hospital in Can Tho City, "the real disease in Vietnam is the reporting system" (21.07.11, personal interview). In the case of diarrhoea, this also owes to the fact that both policy and action for its control are rather compartmentalised and de-prioritised (see also section 6.2.2).

Another issue that hampers the accurate representation of the spread of diarrheal disease involves cases that completely escape the reporting system. As earlier explained (section 4.2.3), many patients do not turn to the public healthcare system, either because they seek advice elsewhere (private healthcare, pharmacy) or because they do not consider their illness as requiring medical attention and treatment. Based on the findings by Nguyen et al. (1997) and on the reported rates of disease by IHPH (2012), the disparity between statistics and empirical findings is conspicuous (Box 4.3). Notwithstanding the significant drop in the disease's morbidity rates since the publication of the above study (Nguyen Thi Kim Tien et al., 1997), there appears to be a significant gap between what is captured by the reporting mechanism and what is revealed by in-depth empirical studies. As the representative of the IHPH concluded for the case of diarrhoea, "the numbers of reported patients are only the tip of iceberg that is visible on top of the ocean. What happens underneath, we cannot really know, but it certainly exists" (top official in IHPH of Ho Chi Minh City, 28.07.11; group interview).

Box 4.3: Comparing data from empirical collection with official statistics of diarrheal episodes

Empirical findings of Nguyen et al. (1997): A study from the Pasteur Institute in Southern Vietnam documented that in Cai Be district of Tien Giang province, the incidence of diarrhoea was high for infants (71.2 episodes per 100 children annually) and for the age-group of 6-12 months (60 episodes per 100 children annually); constituting a serious health problem in all of the 24 studied communes (Nguyen Thi Kim Tien et al., 1997). Considering that about 25% of the country's population are children under-five years old (CIA, 2012) and assuming that this applies also for the population in Cai Be district, a simple extrapolation of the study's data would give an incidence rate of about 50,000 annual cases of diarrhoea in children for Cai Be district. This figure is five times higher than what was reported for the whole province of Tien Giang during the years 2005 to 2010 (IHPH, 2012).

The confusing and only unrepresentative reporting compounded by the drop in utilisation of public healthcare, it is questionable whether the broadly declining numbers of diarrheal diseases in the country are of practical use. Taking into account the institutional normalisation of the "everyday" diarrheal episode, there is the risk of discounting a potentially very high incidence. Firstly, this explains to the failure of preventive mechanisms to take the necessary measures to eliminate the risk of its spread. Secondly, this indicates that many adults and children are disregarding the seriousness of the disease's frequency. If not treated on time and with proper medication, diarrheal episodes can transform into persistent diarrhoea (Nguyen Thi Kim Tien et al., 1997) with adverse effects on a person's nutritional status, their susceptibility to other diseases and their general development and well being.

4.4 Conclusions

As this chapter has portrayed, the changes in economic policy that Vietnam embraced after 1986 have deeply affected the functioning of the healthcare system and the health behavior of Vietnamese people, as well as the way they experience disease. The implementation of decentralisation and privatisation policies in the sector has not managed to balance pre-existing disparities, which have instead been actually growing since. The responsibility to strengthen healthcare services has been transferred from the central to the local state. Inequalities of access persist horizontally, with rural and the poorer areas finding it harder to cover their healthcare needs, as well as vertically, with the health units in the lower administrative levels (communes and wards) facing major hurdles in fulfilling the healthcare and preventive responsibilities that the law - subtly but consistently - has been transferring to them. The insufficient financial support that reaches the sector of primary healthcare does not allow these grassroots units to upgrade the quality of services they can offer. This is primarily felt by the poor, who cannot get access to more central public healthcare of better quality unless they pay additional fees. People who consistently encounter a low level of services seem to be losing their trust in them more and more throughout the years and therefore utilising them less.

As Roberts et al. (2003) suggest, assessing the performance of public healthcare systems needs to accomplish three goals, namely to determine: "the health status of the population, the satisfaction that citizens derive from the system, and the degree to which citizens are protected from the financial risks of ill health". The combined phenomenon of lack of trust and lack of access to healthcare often leads to individuals remaining uninsured and seeking out unadvised medication. As a result, many over-consume drugs, follow treatments incorrectly or are not being properly diagnosed in a timely manner by a physician. The practices of many medical practitioners is at the core of many problems in healthcare service provision, as they demand under-the-table payments, maintain a double status in care giving (both in the private and the public sector) and they are illegally selling medicine from within their private clinics. Overall, health status, satisfaction and the protection of citizens is currently guaranteed through the health system in Vietnam. By transforming healthcare from a state duty to a commercialised good and an individual responsibility, the Vietnamese government has put many of the country's citizens at risk of ill health and unbearable expenses. Instead, people are left alone to try to balance between what they think is best for their health and the financial burden that this would involve.

The impacts that the current set-up and functioning of the health system has on the spread of infectious diseases, like diarrhoea, are manifold. Firstly, the "everyday" or "normal" incidence often goes unreported and perhaps untreated until it reaches a stage of severe dehydration and thereafter becomes a risk to the individual's life. In the context of limited access to medical facilities and wide-ranging self-medication, timely examinations of diarrhoea are rare. Due to the circumvention of public healthcare, many cases of disease go unreported and thus the assessment of their spread is under-estimated. As the next chapters discuss, the weaknesses that have been evidenced in the foundations of primary healthcare and preventive action are bound to reflect negatively on the stability of the whole construction of public health, particularly with regard to the control of epidemics.

QUESTIONING THE PANACEA OF WATER SUPPLY AND SANITATION

CHAPTER 5

Having examined the context of health institutions and health-seeking behaviours within which disease is encountered, treated, prevented and controlled, some main weaknesses of the sector have been outlined. Institutions of health are, however, not alone in the shaping of disease risks. The sectors of water, sanitation and food safety come in as major determinants in the prevention and control of infectious diseases such as diarrhoea. Having seen that the rates of diarrheal disease episodes remain high in the country and particularly in the region of the Delta, this chapter will begin to question the way that the Vietnamese state addresses this problem from the preventive side. Focusing on the sector of water supply and sanitation (WSS), this chapter looks into how policy is implemented and what are the impacts on water-related household practices and, ultimately, on people's access to safe water and sanitary environments. Trying to clarify the factors that govern this access, multi-sourced information is used to compare and contrast the official discourse with local opinions on the subject and with secondary findings of water quality and environmental hygiene from the region. The long-disputed issue of whether and how much improved facilities of water supply and sanitation contribute to the elimination or lessening of the risk of (diarrheal) disease is brought to the table through a close examination of the case of Can Tho City.

5.1 A discursive jump: from infrastructure to health benefits

The fact that clean water and better sanitation are main players in the fight against waterborne disease is supported by numerous scientific works worldwide. In Vietnam, a study from the An Giang Province of the Mekong Delta found indeed that children with access to improved water sources suffer 75% fewer episodes of diarrhoea than children whose drinking source is the canal or river water (UNICEF, 2012a). Statistical findings of this sort are impressive and provoke enthusiasm for the potential of WSS facilities in solving persistent health problems. However, a focus on technical improvements might distract from the corollary issue of the use and maintenance of these facilities by individuals, which is truly crucial in defining the hygiene of people's water, food and living environment. Furthermore, the presence of improved WSS at the household level is not enough to provide for environmentally sustainable sanitation if the systems of wastewater collection, treatment and use are not integrated (Saravanan and Gondhalekar, 2013). Ultimately, the improvements found among the statistics do not imply anything about their distribution. Pre-existing and persisting social, ethnic or gender inequalities are not visible in the mainstream indicators and leave open the questions of who is benefiting from the investments in the sector and why. For all the above reasons, the contribution of WSS to the prevention of disease needs to be questioned on the basis of microbiological, social, cultural and institutional inquiry.

5.1.1 Water supply and sanitation vis-à-vis disease prevention

There have been a large number of studies about the benefits that improved WSS bring to communities around the world. Many of them emphasize how the positive impacts in relation to health mostly accrue when the technical improvements are combined with the promotion of hygienic practices, such as hand-washing with soap, proper treatment and storage of water and good kitchen hygiene (Cairncross et al., 2010b, Clasen et al., 2006, Fewtrell et al., 2005, Sugita, 2004, WaterAid Australia & International Water Centre, 2008, UNICEF and WHO, 2009). The question of whether positive health impacts would be of the same extent without the accompanying promotion of hygienic practices remains open due to the difficulty in drawing causal lines between these issues. Nevertheless, the importance of hygiene awareness is proving central in the sector of water-related improvements of well-being.

Ignoring this importance has been a recurring pitfall in Vietnam, despite the strong focus on expanding piped water supply networks and modern sanitation systems throughout the country. This has been carried out largely in the context of the fight against waterborne and water-related diseases. This goal is evident both in national documents which declare the fight against disease as a primary goal of WSS expansion (MARD and MoC, 2000), as well as in the content of health campaigns which promote WSS as the answer to disease[47]. The strong relationships between water quality, sanitation and the risk of diarrheal disease are indeed part of the discourse reproduced by many citizens and state cadres. Their descriptions and experiences, however, tell somewhat different stories:

> "The problem of waterborne diarrheal disease is intensified in the rural areas because of the lack of water access and sanitation and because of the inadequate hygienic behaviour of the people." (Top official in IHPH of Ho Chi Minh City, 28.07.11; group interview)

> "The awareness of people around issues of disease is on the rise continuously in Ninh Kieu district, judging from the declining statistics of diarrhoea incidence […] Households now use modern toilets and no longer the fishpond ones. I don't know of any programs for improving sanitation in Ninh Kieu, as the situa-

[47] This is discussed in detail in chapter 6.

tion is already improved, but I know in [rural] Ca Mau for example." (Official in PHC Ninh Kieu district, 23.06.2011; group interview)

"When I was using river water I would get a lot of diarrhoea. One time I was suffering for days, I turned purple and my neighbours took me to the hospital, I almost died. Now with tap water, diarrhoea only happens to me two or three times a month. The state said they would give us a subsidy to build a toilet last year, but they still haven't yet" (Head of household in Truong Long commune, Phong Dien district 11.10.2011, in-depth interview).

As the director of the IHPH underlines, it is not only the lack of facilities that results in the disease's spread but also the poor hygienic behaviour of people, which he particularly points to in rural areas. However, the difference between the two is blurred in the words of the PHC representative, who sees the declining rates of diarrhoea disease and the increasing rates of WSS facilities as the main indicators for people's hygienic awareness and behaviours. These assessments and assumptions take on a more social orientation in the descriptions of the female head of household quoted above, who describes her experiences with disease and with access to water and sanitation. Despite having less episodes of diarrhoea now that access to tap water is possible, the health problem persists, even if at a lower frequency. Moreover, continued improvement to sanitation is not possible for her due to financial constraints and lack of support from the state.

The issues presented above point, firstly, to the diversity of factors that create the problem of diarrhoea, which are found in the nexus of people's own hygienic behaviours, the quality of water that they have access to, and their ability to exercise safe sanitation without imposing health risks on themselves and their community. Secondly, it becomes obvious through these short excerpts how different the discourse is when reproduced by lay citizens, high-level representatives of health policy, or local cadres, and this reflects the different interests at play. The household interviewee states her experience and points to her problems and needs, while the local cadre portrays the result of a successful policy implementation without mentioning any of the problematic aspects in the sector. The director of the IHPH, on the other hand, gives a less involved and more technocratic view of the situation, describing the problem but not questioning its causes.

As this chapter discusses in detail, the claims of the PHC representative above contain a faulty argument and a false assumption. What he falsely assumes is that people's increased awareness about the issue of waterborne diarrheal disease is defined by the presence of WSS facilities. As literature has highlighted, these two issues constitute separate challenges and, even though related, are not equivalent to each other. The respondent is also rushing to argue that his point is proven by the health statistics concerning diarrhoea in the district of Ninh Kieu. However, this district actually reports much higher rates of disease than its rural counterparts which are significantly less developed in terms of WSS (see Figure 4.10 in chapter 4.3.1).

The same line of argument was provided by many other state representatives, who gave misleading evaluations of the diarrhoeal disease risk, by solely looking at the expansion of "hardware" solutions while not directly examining the success of "software" measures, assuming that the former well represent the latter. Moreover, the case of the interviewed woman points to the fact that even if the statistics of WSS coverage were to tell us something about the risk of disease and the levels of hygienic awareness, they fail to adequately portray the inequalities that persist in the sector, as they focus on the macro level and they do not usually distinguish between categories of poverty, gender, ethnicity, etc. As many observers have underlined, notwithstanding the potential benefits of Water, Sanitation and Hygiene (WASH) improvements, a disregard of the structural and social inequalities can even counteract the impact of such improvements in fighting disease (Cairncross, 2003, Carter et al., 1999, Elmendorf and Isely, 1983). One of the few interviewees that acknowledged this aspect of diarrheal disease was the representative of the WHO in Ho Chi Minh City. In his words, the study of diarrhoea in the region is representative of a deeper social problem which needs to be looked at beyond one-dimensional indicators:

> "One third of the population in the South of Vietnam will get waterborne diseases; especially the kids under five years old. The poor, those with no access to water supply, no ability to construct and maintain sanitation facilities, those with unequal access to health services and treatment, they are the most vulnerable." (Official of the WHO in IHPH, Ho Chi Minh City, 29.07.11; personal interview)

5.1.2 Seeing beyond "improved" indicators

In Vietnam, the promotion of water supply and sanitation gained momentum with the new millennium, when developments in the sector were boosted mainly in the urban areas (ADB, 2007). At that time, the National Strategy on Rural Water Supply and Sanitation (NRWSSS) was adopted as part of the National Target Plan (MARD and MoC, 2000) and signified the expansion of WSS into rural areas as well. These efforts were realised with the financial assistance of international donors (ADB, 2007: 124) and under the coordination and administration of the provincial Centres for Rural Water Supply and Environmental Sanitation (CERWASS) of the Ministry of Agriculture and Rural Development

(Reis, 2012: 56). This fast-paced development is now presenting results of remarkable progress in the country, with 95% coverage of improved water sources and 60% having improved sanitation in the year 2010 (Fig 5.1 and 5.2). However positive the overall change may be, the globally observed trend of disparity in WSS coverage between urban and rural areas (Graham and Selendy, 2011b, Graham and Selendy, 2011a) persists overtly in Vietnam (Fig 5.1 and 5.2).

Figure 5.1: The evolution of improved water supply access in Vietnam between 1990 and 2010, for rural and urban areas

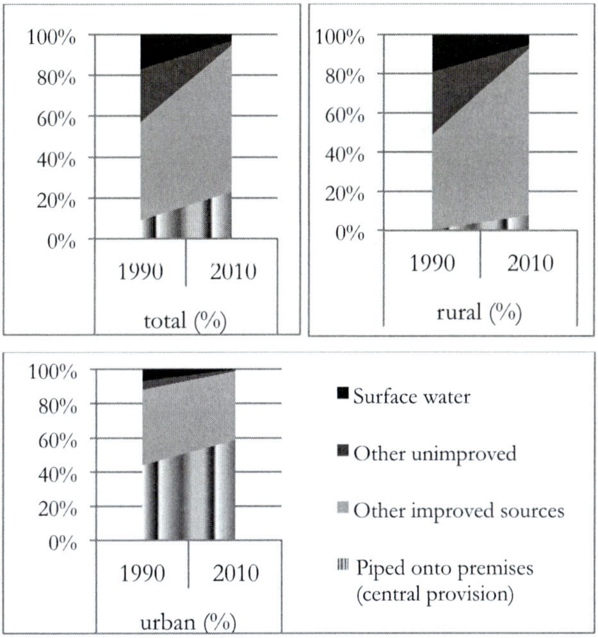

* The category of "other improved sources" includes: public taps or standpipes, tube-wells or boreholes, protected dug wells, protected springs, or rainwater collection. In the case of Vietnam, this category also includes mini-supply water stations that deliver treated groundwater in the rural areas. Data based on the Joint Monitoring Program (JMP Vietnam, 2012a). Design by the author, 2012.

Figure 5.2: The evolution of improved sanitation access in Vietnam between 1990 and 2010, for rural and urban areas

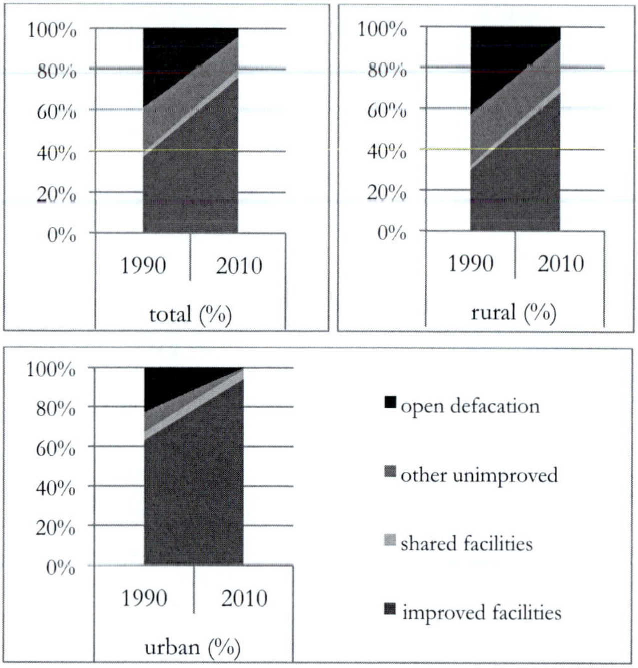

Data based on JMP of WHO and UNICEF (2012b). Design by the author.

Rural areas are still behind the targets of 70% hygienic sanitation coverage and 85% clean water access that was set for the year 2010 (GoV, 2006a, MARD and MoC, 2000). According to reports from the MARD, only 40% of rural residents had access to water that complies with national standards of safety[48] and only 43% had access to toilets that officially qualify as hygienic[49] by the target year of 2010 (MARD and MoC, 2000). Noticing the significant difference between what being reported by MARD and what is presented by the Joint Monitoring Program of WHO and UNICEF (Fig. 5.1 and 5.2), the differences be-

[48] Standards of domestic and drinking water are defined in Decision 09 of the Minister of Health, "on Issuing the Sector Standards-Hygiene Standards for Clean Water" (09/2005/QD-BYT. Hanoi).

[49] According to Decision 08 of the MoH, "on the Hygiene Standards for Various Types of Latrines" (08/2005/QD-BYT Hanoi).

tween "improved", "hygienic"[50] and "safe" also demands attention. Thus, interpreting statistics in order to understand the reality of the actual experience of water supply and sanitation is an important and challenging venture. Apart from questioning the trustworthiness of any produced data, it is the interpretation of what is reported as "improved", "safe" or "clean" with regard to health that needs to be carried through with caution.

Bain et al. (2012) elaborate why the availability of an "improved" water source does not guarantee health risk avoidance. Firstly, the source of water does not necessarily guarantee its safety. The quality of one type of water (i.e. groundwater) can vary significantly with location, even within the same village. Moreover, the quality of water at the point-of-use depends greatly on the treatment, the handling and the storage to which the water is subjected after its collection (Jensen et al., 2002). In most cases, these handling practices, which usually take place at the micro-level (the household) are assumed to be homogeneous and ideal, when in reality they are not so. Speaking of "improved" sanitation implies assumptions of a similar nature with regard to the hygienic benefits of a certain latrine type in personal and in community levels. The promoted toilet models are designed to safely dispose and treat sewage so that they remove much of the health risk factors related to bad sanitation. However, the details of their construction and, more importantly, the manner of their usage and maintenance are issues that depend on the individual households and can hardly be captured by the produced reports, due to their false underlying assumptions. Relatedly, but less important, safer household sanitation does not necessarily mean safer community or environmental sanitation unless systems of wastewater collection are integrated with systems of wastewater treatment (Saravanan and Gondhalekar, 2013). In a water-rich and water-complex environment such as the Delta, the disposal of sewage that has not been treated can increase spread of water-related disease and is interwoven with issues of safe water supply and usage.

In sum, "improved" models of water supply and sanitation might not agree with local definitions of cleanliness, safety or complacence, despite their scientifically proven hygienic virtues or practical usefulness. On the one hand, this might be because such models do not conform to the context in which they are introduced. The idea of having a toilet inside the house, or of reusing treated

[50] The use of quotation marks for the word 'hygienic' (or 'clean' and 'safe') is when the word stands for a category that is defined and reported by Vietnamese state authorities. It does not indicate any particular evaluation or standard of water quality that the author has conducted or agrees with.

wastewater, has often been rejected due to cultural sanitary taboos (Jewitt, 2011). In the example of Southern Vietnam, it is not acceptable to use plant fertiliser that originates from human waste compost and thus, the composting pit latrine is not an option. On the other hand, Reis and Mollinga (2012) have found that the idea of the modern and "beautiful" septic tank latrine is based more on its perceived social and aesthetic benefits than on a recognition of its hygienic and health performance. It is, therefore, important to emphasize the social and cultural aspects of preventive solutions like safer water supply and sanitation when attempting to understand whether and why these solutions are successfully adopted.

Recent global monitoring targets on WASH urge a step towards more in-depth and more finely disaggregated indicators, which would go beyond the typically reported "improved" facilities. The newly formulated indicators of improved WSS evaluate *quality* differently from *accessibility* and *availability* and recognise that non-discrimination should be a cross-cutting evaluation criterion for project success (JMP, 2012a). In addition, issues unique to urban poor minorities are also given more attention by asking for poverty-specific data that include urban areas (Ibid. 2012). Moreover, the need to address the "gap in access" between different income groups and other sensitive social categories is integrated into the organisation's future targets. In terms of sanitation, criteria do not only cover the number of types of latrines but also their durability and their ability to effectively contain excreta, setting also high priorities for safe treatment and possible re-use of sewage. Last but not least, the practices of hygiene (hand-washing, food hygiene, menstrual hygiene management) are emphasized "as fundamental to good health, dignity, and quality of life" (Ibid. 2012: A21). Based on international demands for a more socially and environmentally sensitive focus in the sector, the chapter continues to examine how effective the policy and the discourse around WSS in the region of the Delta has been, in particular regarding the prevention of diarrheal disease.

5.2 Safe water access in the Delta: whose reality and whose delusion?

The term 'safe water' is rather blurred in practice, and cannot adequately be described unless investigated in detail. In biochemical terms, water can carry different concentrations of many kinds of substances and microorganisms, some of which can be potentially dangerous to human health. These concentrations are not usually stable over time, nor do they lend themselves to monitor ing in full detail, especially for vast amount of water such as the flows in the Delta. Moreover, interpreting concentrations in relation to human health is a complicated and contested issue. Therefore, when talking of safe water, one needs to specify which water, at which instance, for what type of usage and in which amounts. International and country-specific regulations of water quality define the parameters for water that is safe to drink or adequate for daily use. It is not within the scope of this thesis to question the basis of these limits and thus, the analysis that follows refers to the established Vietnamese standards of water quality (MoH, 2009b) that defines allowable levels of bacterial/microbial pollution. This section examines whether various reports on "hygienic" water coverage reflect the reality of safe water access in terms of waterborne disease or whether they constitute more of a popular delusion.

5.2.1 Rural supply schemes, urban water companies and the hampered alternatives

The establishment of water supply mini-stations which use groundwater and can serve up to 100-200 households each (Reis, 2012: 73) has been promoted as the solution for the delivery of treated water in the rural areas of the Delta. There are about 428 of these stations today in Can Tho City[51] but not all of the rural households have managed to get access to the network. The morphology of the Delta region, it is claimed, makes water developments a challenge; "there is a complicated system of canals and channels so it is hard also for the water supply network to reach every household or every area in the communes" (top official in the Red Cross branch of Phong Dien district, 07.09.2011; personal interview). Essentially, it is a financial problem, as the expansion of the network to remote areas would demand increased outlays that CERWASS does not cover and the residents are not willing to pay for. Indeed, even when the demand is present, the local authorities will often continue to neglect the network:

> "Because the river flows along this commune [Nhon Ai], people seem to use river water and one third of them do not have access to tap water. There is the demand, but for some reason the government does not build the infrastructure. There is a road and it is close to the centre of the district so I don't understand why they don't take care of it. My family also takes water from the river." (Top official in the district branch of the Women's Union, Phong Dien, 08.09.11; personal interview)

The alternatives to piped water supply include collecting rainwater, drilling or digging private wells, using river water or purchasing bottled water. Among these, the use of untreated surface water is the most popular cost-free alternative and part of the local culture, as "most people traditionally live along the river in Vietnam and they follow the habit of using river water" (top official in

[51] Source: Top official in PHC of Can Tho, 12.12.11; group interview.

the Red Cross branch of Phong Dien district, 07.09.2011; personal interview). However, it is also this practice that exposes people to the risk of waterborne disease. It is often the case that even when households are connected to piped supply, they will continue making use of the many other alternatives and supplement their water needs for drinking or for daily usage (Herbst et al., 2009).

As it has been argued by Reis (2012: 96), a sustainable year-long access to clean water for rural households in the Delta presents a complicated dilemma that is, in the end, primarily a question of a household's financial capacity[52]. Discussions with local residents and state representatives from rural areas in Can Tho City confirmed Reis's findings:

> "Well, those who have money buy bottled water, or a purifier and their kids know when they get thirsty they can drink this water." (Household representative HH3, Phong Dien district, 21.12.11; personal interview)

> "Those who still cannot have access to mini-water stations will drill their own wells. The poor, who cannot afford to do that, collect rainwater." (Top official in district PHC, Phong Dien, 21.07.11; personal interview)

> "A lot of people don't want to connect to the water supply system because they don't want to pay for it and they don't care that much about their health. The government cannot force them, but they could support them financially to do so. Hopefully the policies will change towards this direction and the situation will improve." (Top official in district PHC, Binh Thuy, 12.07.11; personal interview)

> "It is really difficult for the government to give water to all the hamlets that want it. It is hard to satisfy all the people's demands. Some rich people cannot stand to wait, so they use their own money to drill a well." (Official in the district branch of the Farmers Union, Phong Dien, 09.09.11; personal interview)

In the urban areas, piped water supply is centralised, organised and managed by water companies. These are Joint Stock Companies (GoV, 2004), meaning that the every local People's Committee holds part of the shares (28%) and private individuals hold the rest (72%). In contrast to the sluggish growth of the CERWASS network (a rise of 0.6% annually from 2010 to 2011), the central water projects are very successful, with twelve operating stations in Can Tho and with the aim of reaching a consumption of 150 litres per capita by the year 2015[53]. The Water Supply Company of Can Tho City (CTWSC) is supposed to

---

[52] By classifying households into categories, Reis (2012) estimates that 30 - 50% of the rural population in Can Tho has poor water access in terms of availability, quality and/or reliability.

[53] Source: Top official in the DPI of Can Tho, 14.12.11; group interview.

only serve urban areas[54] but the definition of "urban"[55] can go beyond the administrative definitions of a district (Reis, 2012: 90). This means that water companies might deliver water to "urban" centres of rural districts if it makes financial sense. Working as private entities with a for-profit ethos, they do not include social considerations in their water provision plans:

> "The water companies in the urban areas are businesses that necessarily have to make profit. They have many shareholders and they manage their viability by themselves, getting loans from the bank. The households pay money to them and they have to balance their expenses with their profits, so that they survive and grow. It is hard to reach remote areas; it costs a lot for them, so they don't do it" (HELVETAS local representative 15.12.11, personal interview).

Having access to centrally provided tap water does not necessarily mean that households will use exclusively this source for their daily use and drinking needs. Groundwater exploitation is a popular alternative in both urban and rural areas as groundwater is considered a reliable (throughout the year) and improved water source. The issue of licensing water extraction remains under-regulated (KBR (Kellogg Brown & Root Pty Ltd.), 2009: 136) and problems of over-extraction are seriously threatening the sustainability of the resource. The expenses of drilling a well, which will be able to provide water for more than two years, vary from 800,000 to 1,700,000 VND[56]; this is equivalent to the monthly salary of a well-paid state cadre of the region. This is slightly higher than the cost of connecting to the rural piped supply network[57]. Considering the price of CERWASS-provided water (3,000 VND/m^3 in rural areas)[58], when comparing the free private extraction of groundwater, the investment in a well makes more financial sense in the long-run:

> "If the households have financial constraints, they are not willing to pay to get connected, they would rather drill a borehole and get groundwater. After they drill the hole, they don't have to pay for anything else, it is for free" (Vice-head of the district Office of Agriculture, Phong Dien 06.09.11, personal interview).

---

54 Source: Top official in PHC Can Tho City 12.12.11, group interview.

55 For rural and urban characterizations, see also chapter 3.2.

56 Source: Official in district branch of the FF, Phong Dien, 13.09.11; personal interview. The amount is equal to about 28 to 60 Euros accordingly.

57 This amounts to 700,000 VND (25 Euros) not including additional pipe-extension costs in cases where the household is located more than 20 meters away from the station.

58 Source: Official in primary school of remote commune, Phong Dien district, 16.09.11; personal interview.

Nevertheless, contrary to private groundwater which requires home-based treatment, CERWASS-provides water that has already undergone filtration and chlorination. Overall, it seems that many people choose not to connect to a water supply network or to keep a multitude of water sources available in order to strike a balance between the cost and quality of water.

In order to address the difficulties faced by some sensitive groups in accessing piped water supply, the Vietnamese government, with the support of numerous international donors (MONRE and UNDP, 2008: 34), has been offering free or subsidised water connections[59]. Providing subsidies for improvements has been generally discussed as a provisional strategy of development, one which cannot not foster sustainable change on its own (Pattanayak et al., 2006). Moreover, the process of becoming eligible for these beneficial programs is, according to many, not very transparent[60] and thereby does not reach or benefit the very poor in Vietnam. Previous literature discusses how the implementation of programs that provide financial support for household WSS improvements is subject to corruption (Reis, 2012: 81, SNV, 2010: 28). Apart from subsidies, this problem also faces micro-finance programs for households, which are meant to encourage people to invest in WSS. Micro-financing is an idea that has been put forward ever since the 1980s in development policies but its potential for alleviating poverty, empowering women and providing more opportunities, has been questioned (Karim, 2008, Rogaly, 1996, Elahi and Danopoulos, 2004). In Vietnam, the loans are provided with a low interest rate by the Vietnamese Bank for Social Policy (VBSP) and are administered locally through the formulation of credit groups, which also involve organisations like the Women's Union (Sakata, 2006, SNV, 2010).

In the study region of Can Tho, the promotion and administration of micro-credit has been presented as the strongest, if not the only, tool used by local cadres to enhance water supply and sanitation expansion in rural areas. More precisely, the microcredit loans seem to be primarily directed to the development of sanitation and not so much to provide for clean water solutions. Almost all of the interviewees from district and provincial authorities referred only to the construction of toilets when describing the usefulness of micro-credit programs. The only informant who mentioned the use of loans in the context of water supply improvements was hesitant to further discuss how the distribution between the two sectors is regulated, saying that "this is a sensitive

---

59 Source: Top official in the OLISA of Cai Rang district, 29.09.11; group interview. The implementation of microcredit and subsidizing policies is described in detail in chapter 5.3 for the sector of sanitation.

60 See Box 4.2 in chapter 4.2.2 on the example of official classifications of poverty.

matter and we can't talk about it" (Official in CERWASS, 30.06.11; personal interview). The official national statistics show a better coverage of "improved" water sources and a lower coverage of "hygienic" sanitation (Fig 5.1 and 5.2), thus the focus on sanitation can somehow be justified. Nevertheless, 60% of rural inhabitants still lack access to water that is safe to drink (MARD and MoC, 2000).

Investments in clean water provision are not only de-prioritised, the options that the state officially proposed and promotes are restricted. In Can Tho, the only solution provided to rural residents was a connection to the network of CERWASS mini-supply stations. However, the groundwater aquifers that CERWASS uses to supply water are being exhausted and suffering from salination (Thang, 2002, NUBER and STOLPE 2008 cited in Fortier, 2012). It is thus for both social and environmental reasons that more and better clean water alternatives need to be prioritised and developed 4in the region. Informants spoke of other alternatives that provide access to clean water and which have been implemented in several provinces of the Delta in a fragmentary manner[61]. These include SODIS (Solar water Disinfection) technology, which uses sun radiation and can disinfect rainwater, groundwater or surface water that has been filtered or flocculated (HELVETAS and NCERWASS, 2010). Sand-filter constructions have also been designed by the same NGO (HELVETAS), to be used in combination with SODIS in an integrated system for treatment of river or well water. Using plastic containers and sand of a certain diameter, these filters are able to yield up to 100 litres of water per day per household - a volume significantly higher than what a rural mini-supply station in Can Tho can provide in the same period of time (CERWASS, 2011a). Even though it requires the use of empty plastic bottles, the SODIS method was adopted by 40% of the households where it was introduced and was considered to be a cheaper and more convenient treatment method than boiling or buying bottled water[62]. In his explanation of a similar technology for community-based water treatment using UV disinfection, a water and sanitation expert discussed why these solutions are not scaled up:

> "Each installation costs only 500,000 VND and yields up to 0.6 litres of treated water per minute. It works well but the government did not want to continue its expansion, although it proved beneficial for the poor of the rural areas. I don't know why. Things are complicated with the authorities, the law is strange [...] the standards are very strict for water quality and the government keeps them

[61] These are the provinces of Ninh Thuan, Dong Thap, Tay Ninh and Long An.
[62] Source: NGO representative/WSS expert, 15.12.11; personal interview.

high so they can keep receiving money from violations. Even if the water is proven to be good enough - at least for people who do not have another better option - the government refuses to drop the standards or to somehow 'bend' the legislation around it" (NGO expert in Water Supply and Sanitation, 18.06.11; personal interview).

Another water treatment alternative to boiling, which can be used in the household-level, is disinfection through the use of chemical purifying tablets. In Can Tho City, these tablets were found under the commercial name 'Aquatab' and were only popular in the districts of Vinh Than and Co Do which are prone to flooding[63]. The positive aspects of Aquatab were elaborated by a local health representative who believes that "the promoted disinfecting tablets are an excellent solution for poor households, as their use is easy, fast, affordable and successfully creates safe drinking water" (Director of the medical centre Co Do district 18.07.11, personal interview). However, secondary results (Abt Associates Inc., 2011) show that this type of treatment was not a widely known practice in the above districts (Table 4 in the Annex), which is due mostly to the limited distribution and the poor quality of the promotion activities that health workers employed (Abt Associates Inc., 2011). A similar case of a poorly known alternative is that of chloramine-b, a disinfectant which is only distributed in flooding areas or during cholera epidemics (MoH, 2009a)[64]. When asked to answer why these solutions are not promoted, a top official from the PHC in Can Tho claimed that "people often mistakenly use it in water that has not been before treated (filtered)" and that "it is a rather expensive solution" (12.12.11, group interview).

These claims, however, do not clearly reflect the reality and do not explain why chemical disinfection is not included in the recommended preventive mechanisms. This has to do with the fact that, firstly, the possibility of people not filtering the water before using disinfecting tablets is just as likely to take place with boiling, and both lead to equally risky outcomes. Secondly, when the director talks about the cost of the tablets, he is referring to the rather moderate

---

[63] The PATH project, in collaboration with the Bill and Melinda Gates Foundation and Zuellig Pharma Co Ltd (the official exporter of Aquatab), has launched and has been promoting the product in these districts since 2010. According to the project's report, the tablets were available in Can Tho also before the initiation of the program, but were only sold by some limited number of pharmacies, mostly in the centre of the City (Abt Associates Inc. 2011).

[64] Sources: Top official in PHC of Can Tho (12.12.11), Official in CERWASS Can Tho (12.12.11); group interviews.

price of 0.15 USD for 10 units, which could treat 200 litres of water[65]. Based on Gleick (1996 cited in Inocencio et al., 1999), the maximum consumption per day and per individual is five litres of water and thus, for a household of four members, the monthly cost for treating the drinking water with Aquatab would not be higher than 0.50 USD. If the family chooses instead to treat drinking water through boiling it and thereby using wood to do so, the monthly cost could reach 1.60 USD (Clasen et al., 2008). The use of Aquatab compared to boiling is therefore fairly competitive both financially and practically. The hesitance of local governments to embrace and promote alternative water treatments has been described as a result of the adherence to central guidelines, which only prescribe rural CERWASS-connections and boiling water. The potential of local governments to make independent decisions and to affect policy was seen as weak by one informant, who claimed that the communication or the feedback from bottom to top is governed by fear:

> "In water supply and sanitation, there is not a lot of communication and collaboration between the authorities at the provincial and the local levels and there is no feedback from bottom to top. In the district and the commune level, there isn't much capacity for making innovative decisions; they just implement the guidelines. People are afraid to try something new because they don't know if it would be approved or not by the higher levels; they are afraid of being judged for not controlling things well enough or for taking too much initiative" (NGO representative/WSS expert, 15.12.11; personal interview).

Reis (2012) however, maintains that policy and implementation is a double-sided coin and that it is often the interests of local cadres, rather than simple obedience, that are secured through policy-making and implementation in rural water supply (Ibid. 2012: 199). CERWASS water-schemes are administered by state-designated cadres, while the above described water alternatives (SODIS filters and UV-disinfection or chemical disinfection) provide household-based water treatment without the need for state-administration. Officials might claim that most people today are well-served by CERWASS, that they follow treatment practices that ensure water safety and that, therefore, there is no need to complicate things by offering more alternatives. The next section demonstrates that, despite these claims, the waterborne health risks seem to be actually quite high for a large part of the population. The question of why sanitation is prioritised over water supply solutions will be taken up in the following sections.

5.2.2 Reporting water supply: "hygienic" labels and data discrepancies

---

[65] Source: Top official in the district Medical Centre, Co Do, 18.07.11; personal interview.

Many of the reports on water supply coverage produced by different authorities in Vietnam were found to contradict each other. For one, the terminology and the definitions differ and can easily create confusion. The terms "safe" (AN TOÀN), "clean" (NƯỚC SẠCH) and "hygienic" (NƯỚC HỢP VỆ SINH) have been interchangeably used in many official written documents and during discussions with state cadres of the water sector. A state representative claimed for example, that 63% of the total population in Can Tho City use "clean" water, but only 38% in the rural areas[66]. The latter figure coincides, more or less, with what CERWASS reports as the percentage of people with access to CERWASS-water (CERWASS, 2011a), but according to the definitions provided by MARD (2008a), tap water is not the only source that is considered as "clean" or "hygienic". One could assume that the state representative did not consider the other sources as clean, or that "clean" is defined differently for him and his organisation. The above terms appear also to be used differently, depending on location:

> "Clean water is water appropriate for everyday household activities and 95% of the population in the district has access to it. It can include tap water from the water supply network [...], drilled water from the wells and river water that has been treated. Safe water is the water one can drink without adverse health effects and for clean water to become safe, it has to be treated with a chemical like Aquatab" (top official in the district Medical Centre, Co Do, 18.07.11; personal interview).

> "The central part of the district gets piped water from the water company, but the rural areas either get served by CERWASS or people dig their own well. The percentage of people that have access to such clean water reaches 93.5% but that is not safe water; it does not comply with the 22 criteria that the regulation sets for water to be safe to drink" (Top official in the Office of Economy, Cai Rang district, 20.09.11; personal interview).

The above intuitive definitions of clean and safe follow the different realities of water use in each of the localities. In the district of Co Do, where many people use the chemical treatment promoted locally (Aquatab), the director does not mention boiling as a disinfection method. In Cai Rang district, where piped supply and well-water coverage prevails (see Table 4 in the Annex), the interviewee does not mention any other water sources as potentially clean. This is also reflected in the words of a citizen from the central ward of Le Binh in Cai Rang, who claimed: "I don't know what people who live near the river do, but here we have tap water" (representative of household classified as poor, Yen Hoa area 17.10.11, personal interview).

---

[66] Source: Top official in the DPI of Can Tho, 14.12.11; group interview.

Discrepancies of water quality definitions and categorisations are not only verbal, but appear also when comparing the reports of district and provincial authorities. The district-level reports usually show higher coverage than what is reported for the same districts by CERWASS (Table 5.1). When this issue was brought forth during an interview with CERWASS cadres, the answers were as conflicting as the data:

> "Respondent: The Preventive Health Centres in the districts report on the total population of the district, including the central towns. But we don't report on that, we only report on the rural areas. That's why their numbers are higher.
>
> PK: Looking at the datasets, I see that CERWASS also reports on the towns of each district. The data should coincide.
>
> Respondent: The data produced by CERWASS is more accurate, because we conduct surveys with questionnaires and we know exactly what the situation is." (Official in CERWASS Can Tho, 12.12.11; personal interview)

The problem of conflicting data is best demonstrated by the case of Phong Dien district. The figures provided by the PHC of the district for "hygienic" water access exceed by 10% what is reported by CERWASS for the same district (Table 5.1).

Additionally, the head of a local office of health claimed that "80.6% of the population has access to piped-water schemes" (top official in district Office of Health, Phong Dien, 12.09.11; personal interview), contradicting the CERWASS reports by 45%. The vice-head of another office in the same district spoke of 75% of households as being serviced with piped water and also claimed that "the other 30% harvest rainwater or river water, but they treat it with alum[67] and filters; thus, altogether 90% of the district's population has access to hygienic water" (top official in the OARD of Cai Rang district, 06.09.11; personal interview). To confuse things even more, the head of a third district office commented that 70% of people having access to "clean" water and more than 80% having "hygienic" water from either CERWASS stations or their own drilled wells (Top official in the district branch of the YU, Phong Dien, 13.09.11; group interview).

---

[67] Alum is a chemical compound used to clean the water. It causes the flocculation of fine suspended particles. This process of flocculation can significantly reduce the concentrations of pathogenic agents in the water, as the latter bond to the formed floccules and settle with them at the bottom of the container.

Table 5.1: Reported access to tap and "hygienic" water in rural parts of Can Tho City

		Access to "hygienic" water (CERWASS)	Access to tap water (CERWASS)	Access to "hygienic" /"clean" water (other agencies)
Vinh Thanh	104,867	59.15 %	29.8 %	-
Co Do	114,138	82.23 %	41.8 %	82.18% [68], 90% [69]
Thoi Lai	116,909	72.67 %	28.0 %	-
Binh Thuy	40,380	68.02 %	44.0 %	90.40% [70]
Thot Not	126,828	68.33 %	54.2 %	-
Phong Dien	98,450	68.75 %	34.9 %	79.52% [71]
O Mon	100,269	73.84 %	33.3 %	85,72% [72]
Cai Rang	76.711	77.76 %	50.2 %	91.04% [73]
Total (2011)	778,552	71.46 %	39.1 %	
Total (2010)	778,552	69.21 %	36.9 %	

Date based on CERWASS (2011a) and local authorities (as indicated). Design by the author.

The phenomenon of arbitrary reporting in the sector of water supply is not new (Reis, 2012: 129). One interviewee from the district level admitted that "the latest collected data are from the national survey of 2002 and the recently used

68 Medical Centre of Co Do 2011. Water Supply, Sanitation and Hygiene Statistics. *In:* Department of Health (ed.). Can Tho.

69 Medical Centre Co Do 18.07.11, oral communication.

70 OoH Binh Thuy 08.07.11, oral communication.

71 PHC Phong Dien 2011. Summary of the Preventive Health Activities for 2009 and 2010. Can Tho.

72 PHC O Mon 2011b. Report of Preventive Health Activities for 2011 and Future Plans *In:* Department of Health (ed.). Can Tho.

73 PHC Cai Rang 2011a. Annual General Reports of Preventive Health Programs for 2008 - 2011. *In:* Department of Health (ed.). Can Tho .

data are extrapolations of the old, thus they might not be really representative" (Top official in the district PHC, Binh Thuy, 12.07.11; personal interview). Whether a matter of having different information at hand, or of interpreting the same information differently, reporting water supply types and coverage is characterized by perplexity and confusion, even though (or perhaps, exactly because) it has been emphasized as a sector of national priority (GoV, 2006a, MARD and MoC, 2000).

The portrayed access to clean water in Can Tho City

Statistics from the provincial level (CERWASS) present a somewhat more realistic picture, usually with lower rates of access that consider both improved water supply and the hygiene sanitation. Looking at aggregation of statistics from the local to the higher levels, one might argue that the stricter reporting of CERWASS is balancing the eagerness of the district authorities to report better coverage. Nevertheless, a more conservative reporting does not guarantee accuracy. The surveys conducted by CERWASS follow specific guidelines and definitions (Box 2 in Annex), but the actual data collection rests in the hands of health staff and local cadres (described earlier in chapter 4.1.3). When asked about their sources of information, CERWASS officials confirmed that data is produced "by the health staff in the local levels", but they also claimed that additional independent surveys are conducted from time to time.

Based on CERWASS reports, more than 70% of the rural residents in Can Tho City have access to "hygienic" water (Table 5.1). CERWASS-supplied water is the dominant source of "hygienic" supply in the rural areas and is followed by groundwater (Fig 5.3). These data, however, only capture the main water source that is used in each household and fails to inform about the parallel use of other sources. Even so, it appears that nearly 19,000 individuals seem to be dependent on rain water and 29,000 on river water, accounting together for a not insignificant percentage of the rural population (6%) who lack access to a piped network as well as their own drilled well. The reports also note a 2.25% increase of the number of "hygienic" water users for the period between 2010 and 2011 (Table 4 in Annex). This increase corresponds exactly to the number of new CERWASS users during that period (17,507 people). It seems that the increase in CERWASS-users came solely from those who previously had no access to "hygienic" water whatsoever, which suggests that no household switched from another type of "hygienic" water source to piped water. According to the official classifications, water can be unhygienic due to a polluted water source or due to the poor conditions for water collection and water storage in the household (Box 2 in Annex). The CERWASS reports show that only

10% of water collected from deep-drilled wells and only 9% of rainwater collected in jugs did not classify as "hygienic". Therefore, the results show that most of the 222,221 individuals without access to "hygienic" water were river-water users[74].

Figure 5.3: Number of people using different water sources in the areas without access to the central water supply in Can Tho City, for the year 2011

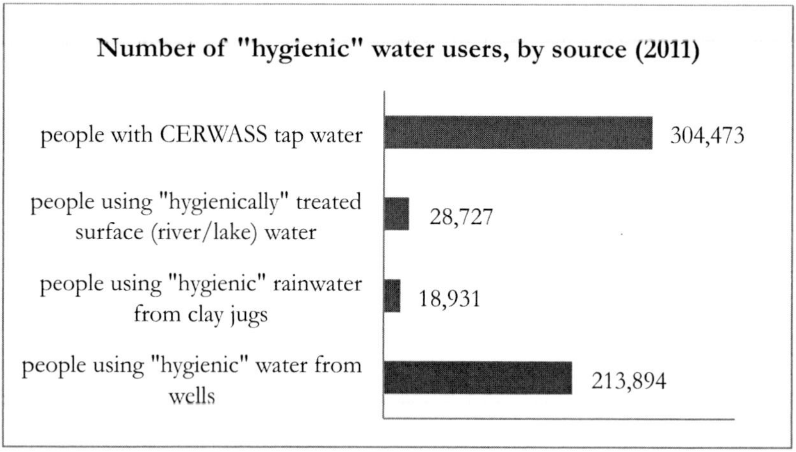

Source: CERWASS Can Tho City (2011a). Design by the author.

Considering the above, CERWASS statistics essentially suggest that none of the families with problematic (unhygienic) water access decided to alter some aspects of their existing strategies (i.e. to improve their wells, to store rainwater in cleaner jugs or to improve their water treatment methods), but instead chose to connect to the CERWASS water network, even though doing so was the most costly of options. If some of these newly hygienic – and the remaining 222,221 unhygienic – water users would be able to marginally improve their household practices of water storage and treatment, access to water of a better quality would not depend entirely on how fast CERWASS expands its network. As discussed above on the subject of water treatment alternatives, hygienic behaviour and household strategies are significant determinants of water quality for those with no access to piped water; unfortunately the public awareness around these issues seems to be limited.

---

[74] Unlike in other categories, CERWASS does not report the total number of surface water users, but only the number using "hygienic" surface water (Table 3 in Annex).

The fact that CERWASS does not report areas covered by water companies (Table 5 in Annex), does not mean that these areas are free of water access problems. Water supply was not reported by CERWASS for Ninh Kieu district because the central water network covers all its territory. However, not every household in Ninh Kieu has access to tap water. The reports from the PHC of the district indicate almost universal coverage (96.28%), but the remaining percentage consists of 572 households which are still using water from wells drilled by themselves as a primary source and 371 households which depend on river water for their "hygienic" water supply (PHC Ninh Kieu, 2011). This number of river-water users is comparable with the numbers reported for rural districts[75], where the problem of surface water usage is usually exclusively found. The fact that an almost equal number of people face water access problems in Ninh Kieu as in other districts is known to local cadres, but it is not mentioned as a particular problem since the majority of people have access to piped-supply:

> "The numbers [of piped supply access] are high on the reports; this shows we are doing well. This is a place where the 'social' aspect is very developed. Almost 80% are connected to central water supply in this district and the rest 20% are still getting water from the river [...]. Such are the areas along the river like Cai Khe and An Lac ward, where people get water from the river for washing clothes and bathing themselves. The people there will use chemical treatment, will buy bottled water for drinking, or if they are poor, they will boil the river water before drinking it." (Official in PHC Ninh Kieu district, 23.06.2011; group interview)

The phenomenon of small "pockets" of population that are living in an urban context and are facing complex problems of poverty, has often been detected in Vietnam (Harms, 2011), as well as elsewhere in Asia and the world (Allen et al., 2006, Simon, 2008). In relation to water supply, this comes into view when observing urban minorities with no access to "improved" water sources. These people also rarely benefit from support programs that exist for the development of WSS (subsidies or microcredit) because such programs are strictly designed for rural areas (see also chapter 5.3.2). The reported access to WSS by the majority creates a picture of disease-invulnerable modern urban communities, which provides a convenient pretext for leaving out urban areas from health education activities. Ironically, it is the urban poor who have the greatest need for improved hygiene which are often excluded from useful preventive

[75] These are the districts of Thoi Lai and Co Do, with, respectively, 452 and 868 people who depending on surface water (for details see Table 4 in the Annex)

health information. The showcased success in urban areas with regard to WSS might indeed be supported by statistics of consistently increasing piped-supply coverage, but it tends to overlook the reality of a considerable number of people who either lack access to safe water provision, or whose practices vary a lot more than what single answer surveys can capture. The complexity and the inequality of access that characterizes water access needs to be emphasized more.

5.2.3 Water quality fluctuations from source to consumption

So far, the issue of water quality was talked about in rather loose terms, basically assuming that the origin of harmful chemicals and pathogens was primarily in untreated water from various types of sources. When looking at intestinal disease, the multiplicity of moments - and the various means by which - water can be infected, makes monitoring quality a hard task. This, compounded by the deficit laboratory technology that is able to detect all the possible diarrheal pathogens, an accurate estimation of microbial concentrations in water is not always feasible. Despite the difficulties, a good description of the health risks entailed in water consumption and use can be achieved by defining the quality of water at certain crucial points (at source, post-treatment and shortly before consumption).

Water quality of urban piped supply

The water factories in Can Tho City using river water are expected to follow specific water treatment steps, as instructed by the MoC (Fig 2 in Annex). However, as a top official of the water company's branch in Cai Rang volunteered, "Some water factories might change parts of the proposed process according to their capacities [...], but these changes will not affect the basic principles of functioning nor the water quality" (19.12.11, personal interview). In order to control the safety of the delivered water, national regulations foresee the testing of water quality parameters at least once a week by the water factory (MoH, 2009b) and additional independent testing at least once a month by state authorities. The quality of the delivered tap water is also supposed to be checked at the point-of-use (in randomly selected households)[76]. The water quality standards for water companies are stricter than those for CERWASS stations (MoH, 2009b). Moreover, if found non-compliant with water quality standards, water companies are more likely to be sanctioned than rural stations, which are usually just given advice on how to improve their treatment practices (Reis, 2012: 75). Penalties notwithstanding, the problems continue to crop up in

[76] Source: Top official in the Cai Rang branch of the CTCWSC, 19.12.11; personal interview.

many of the water companies around the Delta, as reported by the Institute of Health and Hygiene:

> "The Preventive Health Centre of Tien Giang reports that most water supply stations in the province do not have well-equipped water treatment systems. The number of water supply station facilities that serve more than 500 people is high in the province; therefore the task of water quality monitoring is becoming really difficult. Awareness about how to apply the regulation on water quality monitoring has not been satisfactory from the water factories. Provision of water that meets the standards has not been given enough attention by the facilities. There has not been detailed sanction for the facilities which have not been following the regulations" (IHPH, 2011b).

The detailed results from testing water and inspecting the factories showed that the overall quality of the produced water is good, with up to 80% of the samples complying with national standards (IHPH, 2011a, IHPH, 2011b). Of those failing, a notable 28% was due to microbial pollution (Table 6 in the Annex). The provided water testing results from the water company of Can Tho (CTCWSC) showed microbial concentration of zero at the source following treatment (PHC Can Tho City, 2011d). The same results were obtained by the company's branch in Cai Rang for water that was collected both at source and at point of use from a random selection of households in the district (PHC Can Tho City, 2011e). Independent research from Wilbers (2012) also showed that water provided by water companies was free of microbial pollutants at the point of use in the areas of Ninh Kieu, O Mon and Co Do districts (Ibid. 2012).

Water quality of CERWASS rural supply

Unlike the director of the water company in Cai Rang, who was confident that the produced water is of good quality[77], the representatives from CERWASS-served areas openly admitted that "there is no guarantee for the provided water's safety, unless it is boiled" (top official of district PHC, Binh Thuy district 12.07.11; personal interview). The results provided by the IHPH (2011a, 2011b) from ten provinces in the Delta showed indeed that the quality of tap water provided by CERWASS-stations fails to meet the standards (Table 5.2).

The official results from testing water that is produced in CERWASS-stations in Can Tho City indicated a good quality in terms of microbial indicators at the source of production (water tank), with concentrations lower than 48.0

[77] Source: Top official in the Cai Rang branch of the CTCWSC, 19.12.11; personal interview.

n/100ml for total coliform and below 3.0 for *E.coli* (PHC Can Tho City, 2011c). This is complying with the national standards for domestic use water quality for rural stations. However, the practice of testing water at the point of use (household tap) is not necessary by law, unless there is some outstanding complaint about its quality[78]. Wilbers (2012) found that tap-water from rural households has 5% occurrence of microbial indicators in concentrations that considerably exceed the national standards[79]. Considering the findings of laboratory results from the PHC (2011c) and from Wilbers (2012), it seems that microbial pollution mainly occurs during the distribution of water through the CERWASS-network of pipes.

Table 5.2: Water quality of CERWASS water-stations from ten provinces of the Mekong Delta

Number of water samples found not complying with national standards

(Total)	(From CERWASS rural water supply stations)	
2010:	Physico-chemical pollution	452
931/2497	Microbial pollution	38
(37.28%)		
2011:	Physico-chemical pollution	427
1,105/5447	Microbial pollution	72
(20.29%)		

Data provided by IHPH (2011a, 2011b). Design by the author.

The process of water treatment that takes place in CERWASS water stations was described as similar to that in water companies[80]. Representatives from CERWASS added that "this is the model procedure, but it depends on each station and the capacities to do all this; maybe the methods vary among different water stations" (official in CERWASS Can Tho, 12.12.11; personal interview). Indeed, as the manager of a rural CERWASS-station in Phong Dien

[78] Source: Top official in district Medical Centre, Co Do, 18.07.11; personal interview.

[79] Concentrations of 75 (n/100ml) *E.coli* and 100 - 10^3 (n/100ml) for total coliform.

[80] The manager of a water-supply station described how the process includes: oxygenation, treatment with Fe_2 to get rid of alum residues, filtering through rocks, sand of various sizes and micro-filters, and treatment with chlorine.

describes, the treatment practices follow rough estimations and rely on each station manager's capacities and decisions:

> "The amount of chlorine will be adjusted mainly according to the colour of the water afterwards; just as I was instructed in the training classes: if the water turns out yellow, I will add more chlorine." (Water station manager in rural hamlet of Phong Dien district, 19.12.11; personal interview)

Apart from applying water treatments, the local manager is also responsible for the maintenance of the pipes, for the hygiene of the water tanks and for administrative tasks such as collecting fees and accounting. This person is not exactly a volunteer, but rather an appointed[81] local worker - usually a man - who offers part of his private land and his services in return of a monthly salary not higher than 1.5 million VND[82]. As Reis (2012: 91) describes, people in these posts are usually overburdened with duties related to the station while they engage in other income-earning activities. Similar to water companies, water quality tests are supposed to take place frequently in CERWASS stations (MoH, 2009b). However, in practice, such controls are said to be rather rare[83].

Quality of water privately harvested, extracted or collected

As mentioned before, apart from the piped supply, the water sources commonly used in the region are harvested rainwater, well water and surface river/canal water. The IHPH finds great variations regarding the hygienic status of these water sources but not much between periods (Table 5.3). The number of households that were reported was similar for both years and reaches 2.5 millions. The only noted difference between the samples of the two years was the higher presence of CERWASS water stations in the areas which were examined in 2011 compared to those examined in 2010. It is interesting that this reflects on a significantly lower number of rainwater storage tanks and other[84] utilised sources of water in the 2010-reported areas.

---

[81] The key informant in Phong Dien district, a local cadre in the commune level, claimed that water station managers "are selected by the local government for being trustworthy, for participating in the community activities, and in overall for being renowned as good citizens".

[82] Sources: Official in CERWASS (Can Tho, 12.12.11), Water station manager in rural hamlet (Phong Dien district, 19.12.11); personal interviews. This amount equals to about 52 Euros.

[83] Source: Official in CERWASS (Can Tho, 12.12.11), personal interview

[84] This category is most likely referring to surface water since all the other known sources are already captured by the remaining categories.

Table 5.3: Hygienic status of water sources from the provinces of the Mekong Delta, for 2010 and 2011

	CERWASS taps	Dug-wells	Drilled wells	Rain water tanks	Other	Total
Area examined in 2010 (in thousands):						
Total in the area	115	565	1,298	206	379	2,668
Total tested	114	344	630	65	243	1,396
% (tested) meet standard	99.94%	85.28%	78.29%	97.59%	90.88%	80.87%
Area examined in 2011 (in thousands):						
Total in the area	1.5	97	1,302	515	651	2,571
Total tested	0.7	50	969	431	563	2,106
% (tested) meet standard	82.21%	80.24%	52.71%	9.79%	39.63%	40.65%

Data provided from the IHPH (2011a, 2011b). Design by the author, 2012.

A striking observation from these results is not simply that people "balance" their water strategies and tend to use more rainwater and river water to compensate for the lack of piped-water connections, but that the hygienic status of rainwater and river water drops dramatically in the areas with less access to piped-water (Table 5.3). It is worth underlining that the above results do not refer to water quality, but to the hygienic conditions that characterize water extraction, harvesting and storage. Similar observations come from another study which also found that provinces in the region that had better coverage of piped water connections also had better water quality results in sources that included well water, rainwater and river water[85] (Dang Ngoc Chanh and Nguyen Ngo Thiep, 2010). Although it is not clear if the results concern different water sources from the same households, or if each household was only reporting the main water source, both these studies point to a correlation between community access to tap water and water-related household hygiene.

Among the water sources other than piped supply, rainwater seems to be the one in need of more attention, in terms of perceived versus actual water quality. Interviews and informal conversations revealed that rainwater is considered the tastiest and most preferred water for drinking consumption (look also in section 7.2). The findings by Wilbers (2012) however, show that rainwater stored in clay jugs has the second worst quality after river water. In 35% of the analysed samples, Wilbers (2012) found that the average concentrations in stored rainwater were in the scale of 10^3 - 10^4 (n/100ml) for coliform (Fig 5.4) and 800 (n/100ml) for *E.coli* (Table 5.4).

According to a local NGO worker, rainwater can stay safe in sealed jugs for up to one year[86]. However, research by Wilbers (2012) indicates that when the jug is actually in use, the quality of water deteriorates significantly, as it becomes vulnerable to external sources of pollution. Groundwater and tap water that were sampled at source gave better results than rainwater that was stored in a jug, even though rainwater is generally free of microbial pollution before its collection (i.e. when it drops from the sky). Further findings from Can Tho (Tran Hong Phuoc Tai, 2009) showed total coliform concentrations ranging in rainwater from 17 (n/100ml) when vessels were tightly covered and cleaned at least every week, to even over 300 (n/100ml) for vessels that were left uncovered and were not cleaned more than once a week. Similar findings from Bangladesh (Hoque et al., 2006) support how crucial the intra-house practices and habits can be in changing the quality of water.

---

[85] The prominent pollution factors found to affect the quality of the water were
(i) for well-water: a nearby latrine (65%) and the lack of barriers to protect the well from the reach of animals (78%)
(ii) for surface water: an unprotected/uncovered storage (97%) and the presence of cattle and ducks near it (24%)
(iii) for rainwater: an unprotected/uncovered storage (83%) and the use of water scoops which were located near polluted sources (20%).

[86] Source: NGO representative/WSS expert, 15.12.11; personal interview.

Figure 5.4: Microbial contamination (total coliform) found in four different drinking water sources of households in Can Tho City

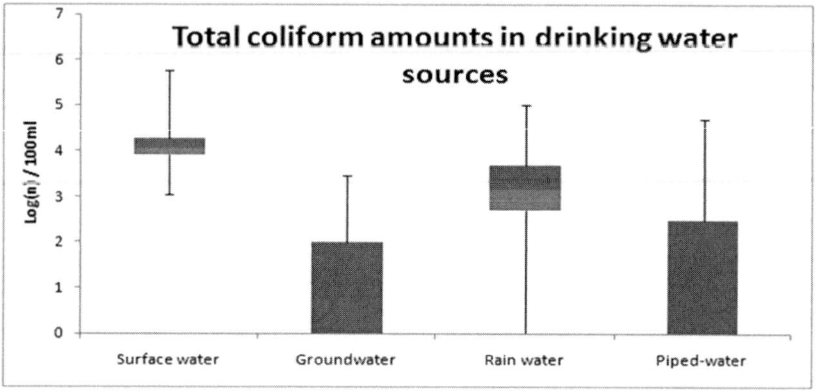

The surface water samples were collected from the canals directly. Groundwater, rain-water and tap water samplings occurred at household level. The box-plots show minimum, 25 percentile, median, 75 percentile and maximum concentrations. Concentrations are log-transformed to reduce the effects of outliers.

Results and figure adopted from Wilbers (2012).

Table 5.4: Average concentrations (rounded values) of *E.coli* in four different household drinking water sources in Can Tho City

Water quality results	Surface water (from the canal)	Groundwater (from the well)	Rainwater (from storage tanks)	Rural piped-water (from the tap)
% occurrence	100	5	35	5
Average *E.Coli* (n/100ml)	6800	175	800	75

* Bottled water did not test positive for *E.coli.*

Results adopted from Wilbers (2012)

Regarding surface water, a source which is still today being consumed by a significant number of people in Can Tho and the wider region of the Delta, Wilbers (2012) finds that microbial pollution can significantly decrease if surface water is treated adequately. Namely, highly contaminated canal water (6800 n/100ml for E.coli and 104 n/100 ml for coliform) was found to be significantly cleaner after it was treated with alum (Table 5.5). In fact, the resulting treated water was found to be of quality comparable to that of stored rainwater. These findings are in accordance with what Wrigley (2007) and Vo Thi Yen Phi (2010) conclude: when surface water is properly treated with alum and followed by boiling or chemical purification, it can achieve microbial quality levels of zero to intermediate risk, which achieves WHO standards (1997).

Table 5.5: Differences in average microbial pollution of canal water in Hau Giang province, before and after treatment with alum

(n/100ml)	Canal water	Jug water (canal water treated with alum)
E.Coli	2500	150
Total coliform	21500	10300

Results adopted from Wilbers (2012)

Finally, the water extracted from private wells (boreholes, deep-drilled or dug-wells) is not suitable for direct consumption according to results provided by CERWASS (2011a), with only 23% of the 309 analysed samples reaching national drinking water standards at the source. Considering the numerous factors that can affect the quality of well-water (depth, years of usage, nearby polluting sources, construction and maintenance, etc), the representativeness of these results is generally questionable. The overall picture of groundwater quality at the source remains very patchy (Vo Thanh Danh, 2008). With more than 50,000 private wells drilled in Can Tho City already by 2002 (DARD cited in Vo Thanh Danh, 2008), it is understood that “checking the water quality of privately drilled wells by governmental authorities is impossible, due to their over-abundance” (top official in YU district branch of Cai Rang, 23.09.11; group interview).

So far, this chapter has discussed water quality prior to undergoing the most commonly used disinfection method, namely boiling. This is not to say that the conclusions thus far have little importance when discussing the risk of diarrheal disease, especially when one considers how water is often consumed raw (i.e. not boiled) when used for purposes other than drinking (see also chapter 7). Furthermore, literature has suggested that the likelihood of contamination is quite high (60.5%) even for water that has been boiled and subsequently stored before consumption (Clasen et al., 2008). It is, therefore, important to know which types of water are more prone to pathogenic pollution under the current habits and practices in the region even before considering disinfection, which may or may not take place effectively.

The collected evidence strongly point to the variability in water quality, which depends on the practices people follow both on an institutional and personal level. While centrally supplied water seems to be of the best quality, access is restricted to the urban residents that can afford it. The quality of CERWASS-water can vary considerably depending on the condition of the network in each locality, as well as on the precision and dedication of the station manager who applies the treatments. Most importantly, literature and secondary results show clearly that water from any source carries the potential of turning unhygienic when it is not handled or stored properly. Rainwater is more prone to external pollution due to its long-term storage, but other sources (like well water and river water) have higher concentrations of pollutants at-source. Intra-household decisions and habits can dramatically alter the quality of water for better or worse. It is, thus, not enough to ensure an "improved" water supply source for each household, as this may become irrelevant in terms of waterborne disease risks. Due to the complex combination of water sourcing and usage that each household chooses to follow for different uses and in different seasons, the public needs to be explicitly informed of the treatment and storage practices that need to be followed for each water source in order to avoid health risks.

5.3 Cultural and structural constraints in sanitation

The national targets of increased water supply coverage are accompanied by the challenge of raising the number of people with access to improved sanitation facilities (GoV, 2006a). The focus on sanitation has been placed side by side with concerns of environmental pollution and health (Rheinländer et al., 2010). As such, the sector has been regulated, defined and promoted in a major way during the last 20 years in Vietnam. The positive impact this has had on the number of improved facilities is evident but various challenges persist. Many people continue to use facilities that pose health risks to themselves and their surrounding community, primarily based on reasoning that is said to be culturally rooted. As this section discusses, the constraints in achieving the expansion of safe sanitation systems do not only owe to people's "bad habits" but also to the malfunctioning of the mechanism that is promoting, supervising and managing the sector of sanitation.

5.3.1 Sanitation types and blaming the "other" latrine

The Mekong Delta presents a mixture of cultural and environmental features that creates a unique landscape for policy formulation and implementation in the sector of sanitation. Having no sewage system developed for the management of faeces and with persistent barriers to accepting the biological treatment and re-use of human excreta in agriculture, environmental sanitation and hygiene face serious constraints. At the same time, great parts of the population are still exercising open defecation, mostly through the use of the so-called 'fishpond toilet' (Picture 5.1).

Picture 5.1: Typical "fishpond toilet" construction, from Dong Thap Province of the Mekong Delta

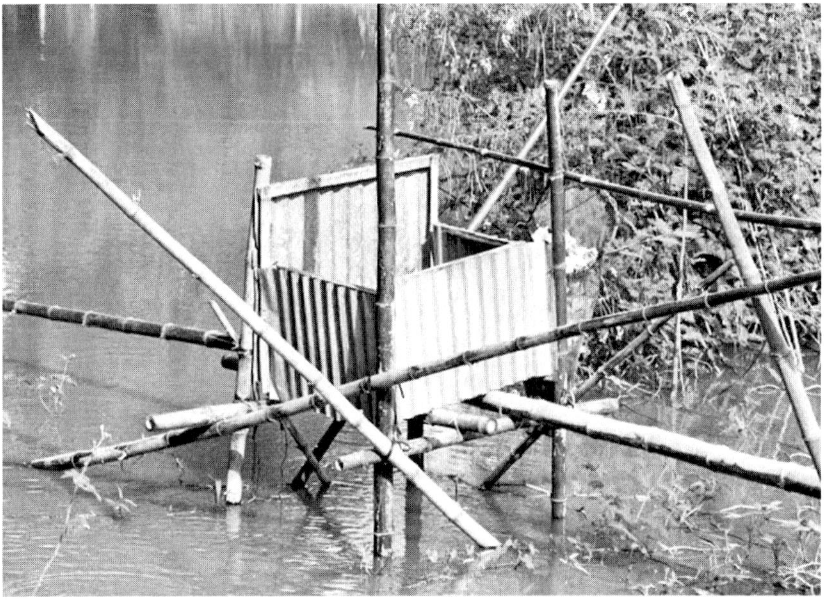

Photo by Dunja Krause, 2011

There are four types of toilets that qualify as hygienic in Vietnam (MoH, 2005): the septic tank latrine, the pour flush latrine, the pit latrine with aeration and the double-vault composting toilet[87]. The first is the type mostly promoted by state authorities in Can Tho City and in the wider region of the Delta[88]. This model consists of a toilet with a flush and of a three-chamber septic tank for

[87] The official instructions on what should characterize these two prominent sanitation facilities (hygienic septic tank and hygienic pour flush latrine) are summarized in Box 3 of the Annex.

[88] Source: NGO expert in Water Supply and Sanitation, 11.12.11; personal interview.

the collection and processing of faeces (CERWASS, 2011d). The construction costs for a septic tank latrine, according to local cadres, slightly exceed the 5 million VND (176 Euros)[89]. However, according to local residents, the costs can be as high as 8 million VND[90]. This cost is often prohibitive for many of the families in the Delta. However, the septic tank toilet is regarded as the best, most hygienic and most "beautiful" latrine (Reis and Mollinga, 2012). The promotion of this type has prevailed as a sanitation solution and has monopolised the allocation of microcredit funds (see also section 5.2.1 above).

The second type of toilet, the pour-flush latrine, comprises a single-chamber collection tank with a perforated wall on the sides and without a built floor. Previous research has indicated that the poorer families in the North of Vietnam prefer this model (Rheinländer et al., 2010) and the same tendency was indicated from informants in the South[91]. This type was not discussed much by health and WSS representatives in Can Tho and was only brought forth as a potential sanitation solution during a public health activity that was held in a rural commune (O Mon district 05.08.11; participants' observation). Only one of the 69 interviewed cadres within the province described this model as suitable and affordable for the poor:

> "It is a kind of an absorbing toilet, where the walls [of the tank] are built of bricks but the middle part is with holes, so that the liquid phase can infiltrate the ground. It costs around 1.2 – 1.5 million VND and thus much cheaper than a 3-chamber septic tank, so the poor follow this model. Only if families have money, would they build a septic tank type." (Top official in PHC of Cai Rang district, 16.12.11; personal interview)

During semi-structured interviews with urban and rural residents, respondents would not refer to either of the models specified above, but to the "hygienic" or the "flush" latrine as their preferred sanitation model (see also section 7.2.2). Only when asked to describe exactly what the term "hygienic" means to them, would people give descriptions that fit that of the septic tank latrine. Nevertheless, the statistics produced by CERWASS for Can Tho (2010, 2011a) clearly indicate that people construct more pour-flush toilets than septic tanks when they decide to make an improvement. Between the years 2010 and 2011 the number of "hygienic" toilets increased by 1% (equal to 1,280 toilets). This includes septic tank latrines, pour-flush, two-vault compost and pit latrines (Table

---

[89] Sources: Top official in IHPH of Ho Chi Minh City (28.07.11), Official in CERWASS (Can Tho, 12.12.11); personal interviews.

[90] Source: Household representative HH2 in Phong Dien district, 21.12.2011; in-depth interview.

[91] Source: Top official in PHC of Cai Rang district, 16.12.11; personal interview.

8 in the Annex). However, it is notable that this increase derives solely from the category of pour-flush latrines and that no septic tanks were constructed in Can Tho during that year. Moreover, it is clear that the users who constructed "hygienic" sanitation were some of those who before used "other"[92] types (CERWASS, 2010, CERWASS, 2011a). In other words, according to CERWASS, no faulty facility was improved to be hygienic and instead, people who invested in sanitation decided to construct pour-flush toilets.

The remaining two alternatives for "hygienic" sanitation are not considered fitting for the region of the Delta. On the one hand, the ventilated pit latrine cannot function hygienically in the wet ground of the Delta. Its construction consists of a simple dug hole in the ground and thus during the flooding season it is not possible to contain the waste. On the other hand, the composting double-vault latrine is incompatible with the mentality of people in the South, who do not accept the use of human excreta as fertiliser in agriculture. However, despite the barrier against the use of human waste compost, the idea of raising fish that feed from human waste - through the use of the fishpond toilet - is very familiar to the people of the Delta.

In the rural commune of Giai Xuan, many interviewees openly described that "everyone has a fishpond toilet" (household interview P13) or that "normally people like to use the fishpond toilet, even if the state guidelines say not to" (household representative P23; personal interview). The local officer in the urbanised ward of Le Binh, however, asserted that "no one uses fishpond toilets here anymore" (household representative P53; personal interview). Even though the use of fishponds has been nationally banned in fear of spreading fish-borne diseases (Rheinländer et al., 2010), both previous literature (Herbst et al., 2009) and empirical results from this study indicate that open defecation in fishponds still comprises a widely exercised practice, and is only recently becoming less frequent in urban areas[93].

Sanitation coverage and the sources of pollution

---

[92] Despite their dominant presence across districts and Provinces, fishpond toilets are not officially recognised as a sanitation reality on paper, being commonly referred to as the "other" type of toilet in the produced reports. Explicit explanations of what the "other" type of latrine refers to, were only found in one document produced by CERWASS (2011b), where it is advised for local enumerators to report as "other", the types of "improved septic fish latrine" and the un-ventilated pit latrine.

[93] Source: UNICEF representative (29.07.11), NGO water expert (11.12.11); personal interviews.

The general picture from 5 million households across the Mekong Delta (IHPH, 2011b, IHPH, 2011a) is that a slight majority of the population has access to a septic tank latrine (51.26%), with the rest being almost equally divided into pour-flush latrine owners and those using sanitation of "other" types (Table 8 in the Annex). As earlier stated, wastewater treatment systems are widely absent from most provinces in the Delta, as well as in Can Tho City. Therefore, it is the technical characteristics of the collection tanks which will determine the environmental sanitation impact of the facilities. This basically depends on whether or not sewage is safely stored and does thus not become a threat for public health.

For the annual surveying of the number and the quality of latrines in the commune and hamlet level, the Ministry of Agriculture and Rural Development has "appointed staff" (MARD, 2008b). Interviewees from the district offices claimed that it is the clinic's health workers who are frequently called upon to check and report on the sanitary situation of every household in their vicinity, including the issues of "toilet maintenance, the existence of bathrooms, the use and treatment of water, etc" (official in PHC of Cai Rang district, 23.09.11; group interview). Representatives from provincial-level offices, however, contradicted this, saying that the maintenance of sanitation facilities is not monitored as it would be very costly[94].

Reports from across the Delta primarily confirm the latter, assigning the lack of post-construction inspections to shortcomings in funding and manpower (IHPH, 2011b, IHPH, 2011a). What arises in the interviews with representatives of health and sanitation authorities is that local health workers and PHC staff only inspect constructions that are built on microcredit financing; the construction and hygienic status of other facilities are not necessarily examined. Despite unclarity about who, when and what to report, sanitation-related reports are continually produced and circulated among health clinics, district PHCs and CERWASS offices (Table 5.6). Given the divergent incentives and resources available for surveying, the contradictions that arise when comparing provincial and district reports are not surprising, even when they reach the extent of local offices reporting double sanitation coverage compared to CERWASS.

Table 5.6: Reported numbers and percentages of households with sanitation facilities in Can Tho City (excluding Ninh Kieu district)

---

94 Sources: Official in PHC of Can Tho (12.12.11), official in CERWASS Can Tho (12.12.11); personal interviews.

District	CERWASS data		Data from other offices
	HH with hygienic toilet	% of total	% of total
Vinh Thanh	11,385	49.33	-
Thot Not	14,211	49.80	-
Co Do	10,144	39.31	45.88 (2011)[95] 70-80 (2011)[96]
Thoi Lai	7,364	27.05	-
O Mon	7,845	35.14	66.09 (2011)[97]
Binh Thuy	4,240	42.92	81.86 (2011)[98]
Phong Dien	7,834	34.06	52.58 (2010)[99] 90.00 (2011)[100]
Cai Rang	12,064	65.28	89.88 (2010)[101] 82.95 (2008)[102]
Total (2011)	75,087	42.11	
Total (2010)	73,807	41.39	

Data provided by CERWASS (2011a, 2010) and local authorities as indicated.

In Le Binh ward of Cai Rang district, it was reported by the PHC that 100% of households had hygienic toilets (2011c). This was proven false not only by ob-

[95] Medical Centre of Co Do 2011. Water Supply, Sanitation and Hygiene Statistics. *In:* Department of Health (ed.). Can Tho.

[96] Source: Head of Medical Centre in Co Do district; personal communication.

[97] PHC O Mon 2011c. Water Supply and Sanitation Reporting for 2011. Can Tho.

[98] Source: Head of Office of Health in Binh Thuy, 08.07.11; personal communication.

[99] PHC Phong Dien 2011. Summary of the Preventive Health Activities for 2009 and 2010. Can Tho.

[100] Source: Head of district office of the Red Cross; personal communication.

[101] PHC Cai Rang 2011c. Water Supply and Sanitation Reporting for 2011. Can Tho.

[102] PHC Cai Rang 2011a. Annual General Reports of Preventive Health Programs for 2008 - 2011. *In:* Department of Health (ed.). Can Tho .

serving "floating houses" in the area, but also from the health clinic director himself, who recognised that at least 63 of the 4,219 households in Le Binh lack any kind of sanitation facility[103]. Official statistics that are generated for Can Tho City clearly show that sanitation remains a problematic issue, with less than 50% of rural inhabitants having access to "hygienic" sanitation. This is much lower than the average rate (70.58%) of the ten provinces in the South (IHPH, 2011b). The vast majority of the people without access to a hygienic facility in Can Tho practice open defecation (Fig 5.5).

Figure 5.5: Reported distribution of household latrine types in Can Tho City by CERWASS

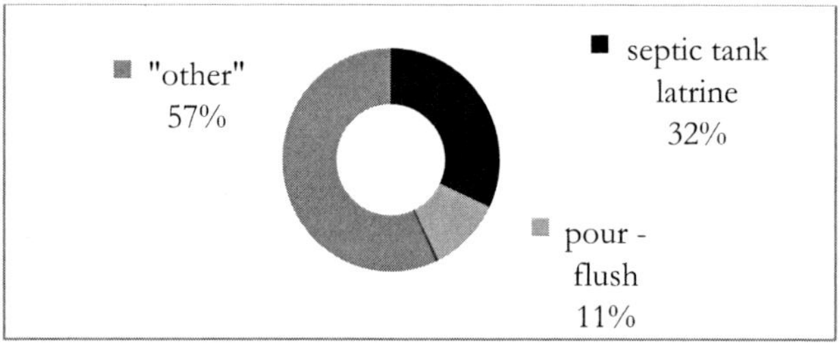

Design by the author; data provided by CERWASS (2011)

Guided by targets outlined in global health and development goals, the central state in Vietnam has identified open defecation as the main enemy to achieving of hygienic sanitation. The abolishment of open defecation habits appears as a central target in public health and environmental sanitation (MoH, 2007b: 118). Nevertheless, the problem in the region is goes beyond the simple practice of open defecation and has roots in the very sanitation facilities that are constructed; these often seem to comply with the standards but are actually "hybrids" of various officially proposed models that may not avoid the problem of contamination:

> "There is a real need for people to have hygienic toilets. The reality is that only 10-15% has one; most people have no other choice but to make a fishpond toilet. Some poor people have other kinds of toilets, but they discharge straight into the canals and the river anyway." (Official in the district branch of the FF, Phong Dien, 13.09.11; personal interview)

However, many cadres base their assessment of sufficient hygienic sanitation in their localities, based strictly on the presence or not of fishpond toilets. When

[103] Source: Top official in central ward clinic, Cai Rang, 13.12.11; personal interview.

asked about the sanitary situation in her ward, the representative of the Women's Union in Cai Rang, for example, supported that:

> "Most of the wards in the district have been characterized as 'cultural wards' which means, among other things, that the sanitary situation is good. There are not many fishpond or river toilets here; only people in some 'deep' rural areas still use them in order to raise fish."(Top official in WU district branch, Cai Rang, 22.09.11; personal interview)

According to data on more than 4 million inspected facilities provided by the IHPH (2011a, 2011b), around 20% of the septic-tank, pour flush, two-vault and pit latrines around the Delta are non-hygienic, proving that the *type* of facility is not a priori a guarantee of its sanitary state (Table 8 in the Annex). Due to the ease of maintaining a fishpond in rural areas, where land is not so expensive and water is abundant, it is an easy and low-cost sanitation option. This has been blamed as the reason why people resist adopting better sanitary solutions[104]. However, some interviewees from within the communes and hamlets believe that the use of the fishpond toilet can be considered a tradition and a cultural practice, which explains why people are unmotivated to change it:

> "People here have fishpond toilets, they like it very much. They feel they are free, airy, and comfortable, whereas in the built toilets the people think the air is suffocating, they don't enjoy it." (Top official of a Health Clinic in rural commune, Phong Dien district, 15.09.11; personal interview)

Local experts on sanitation opine that the use of space and nature in the surrounding environment has also been shaping people's opinions on sanitation. In some areas, local perceptions on hygiene have adapted to the changing environmental conditions of urbanisation and water pollution congestion:

> "In Long An Province, that the fields are empty and people have large spaces; they feel pollution from a fishpond toilet will not reach them so the young and healthy[105] use the outside [fishpond] toilet. Only the old or the sick will use the latrine. In An Giang Province, where the houses are closer to each other, the people appreciate having a [hygienic] toilet and they like using it." (NGO representative/WSS expert, 15.12.11; personal interview)

---

[104] Source: Top official in the district Office of Health, Binh Thuy, 08.07.11; personal interview.

[105] The use of a fishpond toilet requires walking on a bamboo or wooden bridge to reach the cubicle which offers some visual "privacy". One has to balance while squatting and this is not always easy when one is weak, sick or old.

But, according to some, this adaptation is not happening readily or fast enough to overcome traditional habits:

> "People have the custom of not using a [hygienic] toilet. They don't like it and they don't see the reason why it is better. Especially people that live in the countryside and work in the fields all day, they will just defecate out there. Of course when the space is open and the people are few, it is not a major environmental sanitation problem. But the habit remains ingrained in their behaviour and, in the more populated or urbanised environments, it becomes a problem." (Professor at the Institute of Epidemiology in Hanoi, 08.02.2012; personal interview)

A study by Herbst et al (2009) in Can Tho found that most people were satisfied with their sanitation situation (77%) and, at the same time, the majority were fishpond toilet users (74%). Nevertheless, according to the authors (Ibid. 2009), people reacted positively to the idea of having a modern hygienic toilet and many expressed their desire for it. It thus seems that the use of the fishpond toilet does not always take place out of preference, but often as a consequence of financial hardship. As the following section will further discuss, however, the expressed desire for a "hygienic" toilet might simply hide a desire for getting access to a microcredit loan. In that case, financial hardship is still the underlying reason for expressing any interest in sanitation improvements. But if this interest is not guided by an acknowledgment of the benefits of sanitation nor accompanied by a willingness to invest in it, the microcredit funds might or might not be invested in a hygienic facility.

Based on the description above, the question of what would be more effective in helping people improve their sanitation situation could be answered by looking at what constrains them from doing so. Firstly, the singular focus on abolishing fishpond toilets without a concurrent emphasis on upgrading and monitoring the maintenance of existing facilities might overlook significant sources of pollution, especially in urban environments. Secondly, the promotion of the septic tank latrine might not see much success among the region's poorer population, especially when the policies in place to support it tend to exclude the most vulnerable. The next section interrogates why, after the fuelling of so much of central and international capital to support the rural and the poor, the coverage of hygienic sanitary facilities remains low.

5.3.2 Implementing pro-poor programs for sanitation

The Vietnamese government, with the support of international donors[106], has tried to facilitate the expansion of improved WSS through the provision of

---

[106] According to interviewees, the 'East Mets West Foundation' provided funding for the construction of 600 toilets in the Mekong Delta, offering a subsidy of 300,000

subsidies and beneficial loans which, as mentioned before, are largely directed towards the sanitation sector. Subsidies are administered centrally and are distributed to the localities, primarily through a selection of provinces[107]. The provinces more likely to be selected are those which have successfully implemented such programs in the past. As informants further explained, in order for a province to receive NGO support, there has to be proof of demand, and that people that are "ready to implement". In numeric terms, this means that only provinces which present at least 40 households that are willing to build a hygienic toilet will receive subsidy funds. The successful spending of the subsidies, in turn, is also likely to also attract more funds in the future:

> "If the number of people who ask for hygienic toilets is higher than the subsidies offered by the government (40 toilets), then the province will most likely be chosen for the NGO funding. If there is no demand, there will be no funding [...]. It depends on the abilities of the staff to attract the funds, to convince the people. That is, if they can prove that they will realise the goals that they set, that they will pull through the implementation [...]. Every year they have a meeting where the People's Committee comes together with the NGO and the MoH introduces them. Then they talk about the actions for the year to come. For the provinces that successfully implement the tasks, the government will give more money. The government evaluates this through the reports that the provinces produce and through their own observations." (Top official in PHC Can Tho City, 14.07.11; personal interview)

According to the descriptions of informants, once the funds are acquired by a province, the decision-making power about their distribution lies with the localities and is under the guidance and supervision of CERWASS and PHC of the city. However, the responsibilities of these two provincial authorities have been recently undergoing change:

> "We give the subsidies to the communes in need. We know them from the activities that we conduct there, through the hygiene inspection visits, during which we observe and we know." (Top official in PHC Can Tho City, 14.07.11; personal interview)

VND (10 Euros) for each toilet built and a free-of-charge connection to the local water supply network for 400 households. UNICEF and HELVETAS-WATSAN also support the sector, providing funds to the government, which then, through a regulated process of selection, distributes these funds to selected provinces. Usually, the users get relief on about 1/5 of the cost of a septic tank latrine (Top official in PHC Can Tho City (14.07.11), UNICEF representative (Ho Chi Minh City 29.07.11), NGO representative/WSS expert (15.12.11); personal interviews).

[107] Source: Top official in PHC Can Tho City, 14.07.11; personal interview.

"CERWASS receives 2 billion VND[108] each year for the sanitation support, including subsidies and the organisation of information and education activities. We collaborate with the PHC about how we will distribute the funds for toilets to the people. In the following year though, for the NTP III budget, the government will give the funds directly to the PHC and CERWASS will only be responsible for the water supply in the rural areas." (Top official in PHC of Can Tho, 12.12.11, group interview)

Distributing the subsidies for sanitation (up to 500,000 VND[109] per household) was claimed to prioritise beneficiaries according to criteria of poverty, ethnic minority and other socially sensitive characteristics of unprivileged groups. However, there was no regulation provided or found covering the specifics of this distribution. According to informants from within the districts, all the residents are informed of the subsidy and the can apply by putting their names down on a list. Prior to being approved by the commune's PC, this list will be checked by the head of the clinic to make sure that the applicants are indeed in need of a sanitation facility. After the applicants are shortlisted, the names are announced and the beneficiaries are expected to construct the facilities. The local health staff, together with representatives from the PHC, makes sure that the constructed facilities meet the national sanitation standards. Only then can the reimbursements be distributed to the respective families[110].

The criteria for which beneficiaries get shortlisted were not clearly specified apart from the claim that subsidisation is chiefly a pro-poor policy. However, as described above, the support only reaches people after the construction is finished and it only covers part of the expenses in the case of a septic tank latrine (total cost of 5-8 million VND) or a pour-flush latrine (total cost of 1-2 million VND). This is partly the reason why the subsidy is mostly given to people who have already taken up a microcredit loan and are in a position to pay for the rest:

"The subsidy will go to the people who got the loan and built a toilet according to the [hygienic] criteria. The representatives from the Preventive Health Centre will come to check and, if they approve that the construction was according to the regulations, they will give the [subsidy] money to the people as a reward.

[PK: Do people build hygienic toilets with their own money; without a loan?]

---

[108] An amount that is equal to about 70,440 Euros.

[109] Equal to about 18 Euros

[110] Sources: Top official in PHC of Can Tho (12.12.11), top official in CERWASS (Can Tho, 12.12.11), top official in the rural commune health clinic (Phong Dien district, 15.12.11); personal interviews. The process described was cross-checked with representatives from commune, district and provincial authorities.

> Yes, some people do. Some of them will build unhygienic toilets and others that have the money will build proper ones. But the subsidy is for the normal people who get a loan and not for the rich" (Household representative, Phong Dien district 21.12.2011, personal interview).

The head of a commune clinic in Phong Dien district, reported that the number of households receiving the subsidy has grown from ten in 2009 to forty in 2011, but "of course it was always for people who can afford to pay the rest of the cost" (Top official in the rural commune health clinic, Phong Dien district, 15.12.11; personal interview). Evidently, poor households still face steep hurdles in being able to construct a proper toilet: firstly, because the subsidy is not enough and, secondly, because they are not likely to even receive the subsidy if they have not already secured a microcredit loan. The poor are often not trusted to re-paying loans or are not even qualified to apply due to pre-existing unpaid debts[111]. They are therefore in a deadlock situation in which their low financial credibility does not allow them get access to loans and for this reason they are less likely to receive a subsidy:

> "Sanitation facilities are subsidised but the very poor cannot pay the rest of the 3.5 million needed. Also, they cannot get a loan because they are not credible." (Official of the WHO in IHPH, Ho Chi Minh City, 29.07.11; personal interview)

> "Everybody that wants to get a loan can get it, but some people don't want to enter that process. They think a toilet is not necessary [...], of course poverty is also an issue; because they are afraid they won't be able to pay it back." (Household representative HH2, Phong Dien 21.12.11; in-depth interview)

As a result, loans and subsidies are mostly undertaken by middle-income and better-off households and, as Reis (2012: 102) also finds, they do not really benefit the poor.

Sometimes, access to beneficial policies is not only an issue of credibility but also of location. Poor families that live in the urban centres and towns never get the chance to access subsidy programs, as those are not directed to districts with already high coverage of WSS and relative low demand for these types of facilities:

> "Here in this district, 99% of the households have a decent sanitation facility, so there is no policy for subsidies or loans. However, there are people that have no

---

[111] Sources: Household representatives HH1 and HH4 in urban district, 22.12.11; in-depth interviews.

> money to repair or upgrade their toilets which have turned unhygienic, and this is a problem." (Top official of the Area Branch of PC, Cai Rang, 15.10.11; personal interview)

Moreover, it is specifically mentioned in the accounting report of the Vietnam's Social Policy Bank (VSPB) for 2010 that funds are only directed to rural districts (Table 11 in the Annex) and thus, seemingly, urban areas fall completely out of the microcredit policy's scope. A female resident of central Le Binh ward describes how urbanisation and the lack of state support have left her with no options in WSS:

> "We don't have access to a canal or any other surface water, so we get water from the neighbours' hose and we go to the toilet of the factory nearby when it opens up in the morning" (Household representative P40 of classified near-poor household, Cai Rang; personal interview).

Data from the urban Ninh Kieu district showed 95.34% coverage of "hygienic" sanitation facilities, with a striking percentage of 99% of those toilets being septic tank latrines (PHC Ninh Kieu, 2011). Similar to piped water supply (chapter 5.2.2), Ninh Kieu is presented as the 'epitome' of successfully promoted sanitation policy. Nevertheless, there are 238 households in the district with no access to sanitation at all and 246 households with sanitation facilities of an unspecified type which discharge directly into the river (Ibid. 2011). These numbers roughly coincide with the 371 households of Ninh Kieu that are reported to use river water as a primary water source. Upon closer observations of the produced statistics, one can clearly find existing pockets of urban population without access to improved WSS. Despite their significant numbers when comparing to what one finds in rural districts, this part of urban reality is usually lost in narrative of the statistical majority defining successful implementation (Picture 5.4).

Picture 5.4: "Floating houses" constructed at the edge of canals in urban Ninh Kieu district

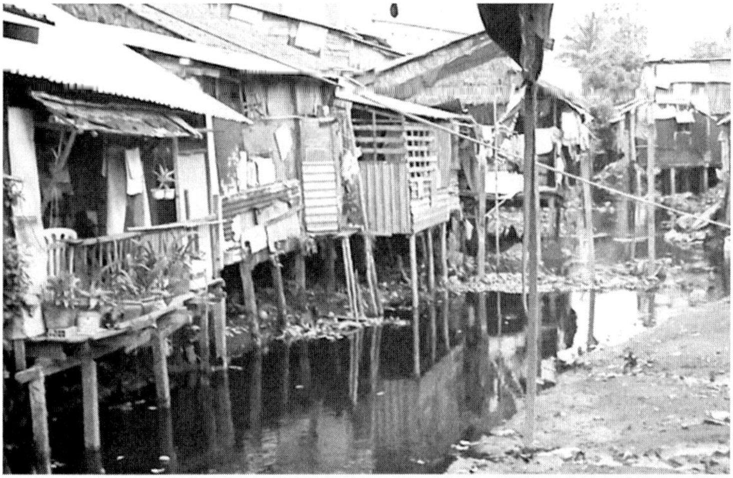

Picture by author, 2011

The "game" of microcredit financing for sanitation

The process of accessing microcredit loans is similar to that of accessing subsidies for sanitation (SNV, 2010), as it firstly includes the compilation of a list with the names of those interested and intending to build a new toilet. The number of people who will eventually receive the loan is fixed by the available budget. The Women's Union is the main organisation facilitating the micro-credit distribution processes (Sakata, 2006). The Union's management will advocate, inform and financially guarantee union members who take up these loans. The Union thus, plays the role of the "middleman" in the lending process, applying and receiving the loans from the Social Policy Bank (VBSP)[112] and then distributing them. According to the head of a WU's group at the commune level, the organisation keeps a percentage of these funds (up to 1 million VND per month) in order to cover administrative expenses from facilitating the whole process. Literature explains that the administration of the loans occurs through the formation of Credit Groups (Cuong 2008 cited in Reis and Mollinga, 2009) but it seems that these groups consist mainly of union members. The head of the Farmers' Union in the commune level specifically de-

[112] Source: NGO representative/WSS expert, 15.12.11; personal interview.

scribed how being a member of a union is the only way for someone to get easy access to microcredit:

> "Everyone belongs to a group [Farmer's Union or Women's Union], or else it means they have their own money to build toilets. As for the poor, some of them build toilets but they are not hygienic ones." (Household representative HH4 and member of the FU; in-depth interview)

Even though the overall activity and the role of the WU in the microcredit lending process was presented by their members as uncomplicated, transparent and inclusive, a female resident from Cai Rang district did not describe this process as so favourable. The interviewee indicated that in order to be a WU's member - and thus eligible to "play the Union's game" for securing a loan - one must make weekly contributions to the Union's common funds which she could not afford[113]. Literature has also suggested that being a member of the WU requires frequent participation in meetings, which is anything but trivial for women who need to work long hours during the day (Schuler et al., 2006). The prerequisite of being a member of a microcredit administering group (Credit Group) for accessing sanitation loans is thus contributing to a further exclusion of the poor as the latter face difficulties in fulfilling the financial, time and participation requirements of being a union member.

Apart from a limited inclusiveness in this sense, there is also little transparency in how funds are distributed and used. It is explicitly stated in the lw that each microcredit loan for WSS amounts to 4 million VND per project and per household, meaning that each household receives 8 million VND to be equally invested in water supply and sanitation improvements (Prime Minister of Vietnam, 2004). Contrasting this ideal, a CERWASS officer (12.12.11, group interview) claimed that the maximum amount for a toilet loan is 4.5 million. District representatives in the office of Labour, War Invalids and Social Affairs (Cai Rang 29.09.11; personal interview) said that the microcredit loan is only up to 3 million VND. A local chief of the FU in the commune level, somehow confirmed the relevant law, saying that "the amount of the loan comes up to 8 million VND, which two years ago was enough to build a toilet that fulfils all the hygienic criteria, but now is no longer enough" (Household representative HH4 and member of the FU; in-depth interview).

According to information that was acquired directly from the VBSP, the loans that were given out during the year 2011 for water supply and sanitation in Can

---

113 Source: Household representative HH4 in urban Le Binh, 20.12.11; in-depth interview

Tho City amounted to 27 billion VND[114] (VBSP, 2011). This was distributed among 4,719 households and thus, each of them received, on average, 5.7 million VND (Table 11 in Annex):

> Total loan money for WSS (27 billion VND) / total number of households benefitted (4719) = amount of loan for each household (5.7 million VND)

As was noted before (section 5.3.1), all new sanitation facilities built between the years 2010 and 2011 in Can Tho were pour-flush latrines (2,745 facilities). The construction-cost of this type of sanitation facilities does not exceed 1.5 million VND. Assuming that all the beneficiaries used at least part of the loan for a latrine construction, there must have been a leftover amount of 4 million VND for each of those 2,745 households who got a loan and built a latrine (not taking into account that they also possibly received a subsidy of 500,000 VND):

> Amount of loan for each household (5.7 million VND) - maximum cost of construction of latrine (1.5 million VND) = leftover funds for each household after constructing the latrine (4.2 million VND)

Moreover, there are 1,974 households who appear to have gotten a loan, but do not appear to have used it for any kind of sanitation facility (Table 8 in Annex). For those households, the whole amount of the 5.7 million VND must have gone for uses other than sanitation improvements:

> Total number of households benefitted (4719) – total number of constructed latrines (2745) = total number of households which received a loan but did not build a latrine (1974)

Since the microcredit loans that were mentioned in the VBSP reports are strictly for WSS improvements(VBSP, 2011), the remaining amounts must have been spent for water supply connections. CERWASS (2010, 2011a) reports only 4,015 newly established water connections during the same period (section 5.2.2) with no other types of improvement regarding water supply. This leaves 704 households who received a microcredit loan, but did not invest the amount in either of it in the two uses it was intended for:

> Total number of households benefitted (**4719**) – total number of water connections (**4015**) = number of households benefitted who did no improvement in WSS (**704**)

A water connection to the piped network does not cost more than 2 million VND[115] and thus, even if all of the 4,015 new water connections were paid

---

[114] Equal to 950,938 Euros

through microcredit loans, there are plenty of leftover funds in each household. Therefore, even with the most generous calculations and under the assumption that every new WSS improvement between 2010 and 2011 was assisted by a loan, the numbers provided by CERWASS and those by the VSPB simply do not match. In numerical terms, the fate of nearly half the WSS microcredit budget for that year in Can Tho (15 billion VND, equal to about 900,000 Euros) remains completely unaccounted for and unjustified (Table 5.7).

Table 5.7: Calculation of the amounts of money spent on WSS improvements compared to microcredit loans given by the VBSP for the sector in Can Tho, during the years 2010 - 2011

	Number of new latrines constructed	Cost of each latrine constructed (VND)	Number of new water connections	Cost of each water connection (VND)
	2745	1.5 million	4015	2 million
Total cost for each (VND)	4117.5 million (sanitation)		8030 million (water supply)	
Total cost for both types (VND)	12147.5 million ~ 12 billion (sanitation & water supply)			
Total amount provided by the VSPB (VND)	27 billion			
Leftover amount (VND)	15 billion			

The calculations are based on the WSS statistics provided by CERWASS (2011a, 2010), the data from the VSPB (2011) in Can Tho for the year 2010 and the prices of WSS constructions as claimed by local informants (see text).

[115] This amount is for a connection fee and a calculation of 1.2 million VND (42 Euros) for pipe extension that is potentially necessary (section 5.2.1).

The above figures and calculations reveal that either the implementing mechanism is allowing for WSS funds to be distributed to people who do not actually invest in WSS improvements - and thus 15 billion VND is spent for other purposes - or these amounts never actually reach any beneficiaries. Decision-making responsibilities on the distribution of these loans are dispersed in authorities along the administrational pyramid of the sector in Vietnam and between different ministries. This makes it hard to trace and clarify the precise loopholes in the implementation of microcredit programs for WSS. Many of the decisions in selecting and monitoring the beneficiaries come down to the health workers and their collaboration with the PHC and CERWASS. The rules around the functions of a health worker are however not clear in the legislation and even differ in each locality (see chapter 4). As a result, their reporting on which facility is "hygienic", which household needs financial support and who is entitled to microcredit loans, can often be unreliable. As a result, while the poor continue to be widely under-privileged in their access to WSS facilities mostly due to financial constraints, much the allocated budget apparently disappears without any clear explanation.

5.4 Conclusions

Following global health-related targets and guidelines, the Vietnamese government emphasizes the development of WSS as the central answer to water-related health problems and especially to the problem of diarrheal disease. This chapter describes how this emphasis is placed particularly on aspects of improving household-based sanitation facilities. Policy and implementation in the sector of WSS is based on the assumption that the statistical coverage of 'improved' facilities is a strong indicator of environmental sanitation and public health. The method of implementation is thus based on a top-down exercise of pressure to local authorities so that the latter might bring about the statistical outcomes that satisfy the centrally-defined targets of the sector. These outcomes are therefore most intimately tied to statistics regarding the presence of household-based WSS developments. The validity of the produced statistics and the health benefits that they are supposed to reflect, however, proved highly questionable in the case study areas.

Significant contradictions came to light regarding the process and the outcomes of producing WSS statistics, which points to a pattern of arbitrary reporting. Personal interviews with staff and experts made it possible to understand that this cannot simply be due to a lack of capacity in the sector, and that the problem of misreporting has deeper roots. The central government sets highly demanding targets, focusing on technical indicators which subsume many characteristics of construction, maintenance and usage (GoV et al., 2006). In their efforts to satisfy these targets, local governments in the communes and districts were often seen to report more "hygienic" constructions than what exists in reality, apparently overlooking details of construction, or simply wanting to present better implementation results. This system of reporting statistics is also connected to the allocation of funds, particularly for microcredit loans and WSS subsidies. Thus, the unreliability of the former engenders fuzzy implementation in the latter. Microcredit and subsidy funds are distributed in a number of selected provinces according to each province's implementation over the previous years. In other words, the reported statistics are supposed to represent the capability of the province's implementing mechanisms to convince people to effectively invest in WSS constructions. Inflated statistics of WSS coverage increase the chance that the province will receive funds in the future. It becomes clearer then that apart from satisfying the high-pressure demands of the higher levels for implementation, the arbitrary reporting in WSS also serves as a means to attract capital. Further findings on the distribution of this type of capital within each province showed that the development of WSS is actually a highly political issue.

Firstly, although the programs of microcredit and subsidisation in WSS are supposed to be targeting impoverished households and assisting the most vulnerable, it seems that the poor remain widely excluded from such programs. This mainly owes to their unreliability for returning credit and their difficulties in joining local groups, which complicates their capacity to play the "Union's game" and gain access to such programs. As a result of this vicious cycle, minorities of poor people without access to WSS remain trapped in an unhealthy situation and are essentially ignored by the current policy and its implementation. Secondly, subsidies and microcredit are connected to each other and are nowadays mainly directed to sanitation because the problem of water supply is considered largely resolved for the majority of people. Even though water hygiene related practices in the household-level appear to significantly affect the quality of consumed water, this issue is downplayed by the implementing authorities, which emphasize the solutions of piped-water connections and the construction of hygienic toilets. Health education activities were rarely taking place in the study areas and the preventive messages communicated to the public were poor in content. The reasons behind this kind of prioritisation of "hardware" versus "software" measures seem to be partly responding to the fixation to statistical indicators that was previously discussed. "Hardware" improvements are easier to quantify than health education outcomes. It is also true, however, that "hardware" WSS constructions necessitate capital investments and thus engender a sector more likely to attract support in the form of external funding.

Research has suggested considerable discrepancies between the amounts of microcredit assigned for WSS and the actual costs of the facilities that were constructed during the same year in Can Tho, with more than half of the province budget for WSS going unaccounted for. Thus, despite the narrative produced collectively from local and national institutions in the sector, which assigns any existing problems to a lack of funds, it appears that it is actually the management of those funds that is problematic. Despite officials claiming that "water supply and sanitation is continuously improving for the benefit of human health", research here has showed that much of the practice in WSS is actually underpinned by the interests of those managing and distributing the sector's funds and is not always serving the purpose of safeguarding people's health or supporting the poor. Satisfied with increasing statistics, the central state turns a blind eye to this inefficiency and mismanagement of implementing mechanisms. Overall, what seems to be lacking from the sector is not money, but a system characterized by meritocracy, inclusion and transparency.

PREVENTING DIARRHOEA: FRAGMENTED POLICY AND THE LACK OF EMPOWERING HEALTH EDUCATION

CHAPTER 6

The previous chapter showed why the preventive sector of water supply and sanitation is still facing many challenges, both in achieving universal coverage and in reaching the health goals related to the prevention of diarrheal disease. The barriers to successfully implementing preventive WSS are related to policy design, institutional deficiencies and an overall distorted concept of managing and reporting within the implementing system. This resulted in perpetuated inequalities of access to clean water and sanitation and, in turn, can be expected to play a role in the distribution of diarrheal disease risks. The preventive success of various promoted programs in WSS was seen to depend on their acceptance by the public, which has often evaluated and implemented WSS solutions differently than what the state has prescribed and expected. The preventive potential has therefore remained ambiguous as infrastructural changes have not always been accompanied by informed practices of hygiene. Advancing this analysis, this chapter will focus on the strategies that the Vietnamese state follows in order to promote diarrheal disease prevention in ways beyond the expansion of WSS infrastructure. The chapter will particularly look at the communication methods that are used to raise public awareness against the spread of the disease, critically examining the empowering potential of health education, as was witnessed in the study area of Can Tho City.

6.1 Merging the gap between local and global approaches to diarrheal disease

As presented in the introduction of this thesis, there are a number of measures capable of preventing the spread of diarrhoea that are known to the international health community (UNICEF and WHO, 2009). These measures highlight, for example, the need for vaccinations, the assurance of food safety and the need to fight children's malnutrition in order to control diarrheal disease. Despite the available knowledge on disease prevention and the legal adoption of many globally suggested measures, diarrhoea persists in many countries of the world, including Vietnam. As this chapter will discuss, the reasons behind the difficulty of incorporating preventive health principles in different societies are to be found in institutional, social and cultural spheres, which are often disregarded by both global advocates and local implementers of such principles and measures.

6.1.1 Vietnamese perceptions about health

In Vietnam, the ideas around health and disease are heterogeneous, as they include both western and traditional medicine approaches. The field of Traditional Medicine[116] has a long history and a strong presence today in Vietnam. It has been shaped by the combination of the northern "Vietnamized" Chinese medicine and southern Vietnamese herbal remedies (Ladinsky et al 1987 and Marr 1987 cited in Gammeltoft, 1999). Traditional Vietnamese medicine considers the healthy body as a dynamic system in balance, which is characterized by strength and stability. Some of the recognised interrelations between symptoms, conditions and cures in traditional medicine do not agree with western principles of biomedicine and vice versa. Gammeltoft (1999: 128) finds that some important determinants of health in traditional Vietnamese medicine, include for example the consumption of certain foods, the amount of rest and sleep, the exposure to wind or other types of weather, as well as personal stressful thoughts or evil spirits.

After decades of interaction between traditional and western medical ideas and principles in the country, the two fields have influenced each other greatly. The study of medicine in Vietnam is mostly based on biomedical principles, but includes entire semesters of traditional medicine theory and practice of methods such as acupuncture, the use of herbal remedies and physiotherapy. The principles of traditional medicine are thus widespread, both in the medical profession and in the extant tacit knowledge about health. The coexistence of the two fields is noteworthy when one considers how, for example, many people consume antibiotics carelessly (see chapter 4) while also maintaining a strong preference for traditional curative means, especially in the case of chronic diseases (Ladinsky et al., 1987). It became evident through everyday discussions with people in Can Tho that the field of traditional medicine is highly appreciated by most Vietnamese, with this appreciation not excluding a strong trust in western biomedical explanations of health and sickness.

Diarrhoea is one of those conditions that are often treated by individuals with traditional medicine at home. Its treatment usually follows the consumption of certain foods, herbs or concoctions, while its causes are also usually assigned to aspects of nutrition. In the herbal garden of the Traditional Medicine Hospital of Can Tho, there are four plants that are considered effective for the treatment of diarrhoea (Picture 6.1).

---

[116] In Vietnamese, traditional medicine is *thuoc Y*, Chinese medicine of Vietnam is *thuoc Bac,* and herbal medicine is *thuoc Nam.*

Picture 6.1: One of the four plants for the cure of diarrhoea, in the herbal garden of the Traditional Medicine Hospital in Can Tho City and the preparation of dried herb mixtures

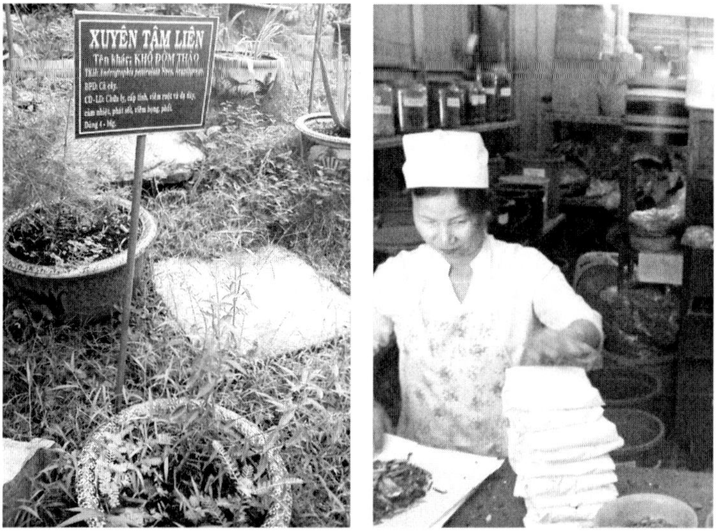

Left: Andrographis paniculata: 4-12 grams of the plant is used in the preparation of a concoction against diarrhoea. Right: preparing herbal mixtures and selling them in the traditional medicine dispensary. Picture by author, 2011

Many people also believe that the disease is a reaction of the body to cold drinks, alcohol, psychological angst or to weather changes that affect the cold/hot balance of the body (see also chapter 7). However useful and accurate this might be, people's traditional knowledge might conflict with the advice provided by the public health institutions which focuses on western explanations and medication. Furthermore, knowledge from the two fields is mixed in an ad-hoc way that does not always lead to the best health decisions. It is often the case, for example, that indigestion or brief gastrointestinal disorders would be placed on the same scale and category with an episode of acute diarrhoea because the symptoms are of the same kind (diarrhoea and intestinal cramps). As a result, a mild episode might be unnecessarily treated with antibiotics while a serious episode of diarrhoea might simply be treated with coconut juice.

Maintaining a strong dividing line between these two fields of medicine, in terms of their value and usefulness for dealing with disease can, understandably, cause confusion in the health behaviours of the public. A holistic approach that considers the history of health understandings, while at the same time integrating global knowledge on disease mitigation, seems to be imperative, especially for issues of public health where people are called to recognise risks and adopt preventive and curative measures. Thompson (2003) observes that during the French colonialisation in Vietnam, the balance between which preventive health messages are embraced by the public, and which are not, was very much shaped by the health communication methods used at the local level, and by the amount of respect paid to the extant cultural values and traditional health conventions:

> "...the Vietnamese quickly lost their initial enthusiasm for western medical techniques due to the forcible imposition of those treatments by the French colonial government. For example, the Vietnamese strongly resisted the French vaccination campaigns (for smallpox) in the 1870s and 1880s. This resistance was due, at least in part, to the exclusion of traditional practitioners from participation in vaccination work. Vietnamese were only allowed to participate in the vaccination campaigns after they had been formally trained in western medicine. Not until after the first class had graduated from the École de Médecine de Hanoi (founded in 1902) were Vietnamese allowed to vaccinate." (Thompson, 2003: 117)

While the two fields appeared to only be accepted by people with considerable conflict and antagonism, the situation now has evolved. A more recent investigation by Jenkins et. al (1996) showed that especially after the wider opening to western influences in the 1990s and the rapid modernisation processes that have been taking place since, people's perceptions have become more balanced. The authors particularly underline that despite the continuing presence of traditional medicine, "the data do not support the hypothesis that these traditional beliefs and practices act as barriers to access to Western medical care or to utilization of preventive services" (Ibid. 1996). In other words, the Vietnamese are open to biomedical approaches to health without losing their faith in traditional explanations of bodily functions. The challenge lying ahead, therefore, is to be able to include and use both these forms of knowledge in the fight against disease to the overall benefit of people's health. As Nichter and Nichter (1996) note, doing otherwise and neglecting aspects that communities believe in, are accustomed to and consider useful, is often the reason of preventive health failures:

> "In the field of health education far more time, energy, and resources have been expended identifying what a population does not know or do, than in assessing what a population does know and the way in which it is known. What is often neglected is a consideration of those concepts of health and images of body processes which underlie the layperson's health practices. Due to this lack of appreciation of tacit knowledge and the cultural common sense (and empirical

observations) upon which it is based, cultural resources are often underutilized by health educators." (Nichter and Nichter, 1996a: 408ff)

6.1.2 The international "toolkit" against diarrhoea

In the face of a relatively static health policy towards the prevention and control of diarrheal disease in Vietnam and the disease's widespread presence, many international NGOs have tried to propose solutions, focusing on vaccinations, sanitation solutions and hand-washing promotion (UNICEF, 2008a, UNICEF, 2012a). One of the most compelling interventions focusing on the legal provisions around the control of diarrheal disease was a project by PATH with the aim to "re-prioritize the disease within the Vietnamese government" (Center for Health Market Innovators, 2012). This resulted in the formulation of new diarrheal disease management guidelines which were then adopted by the Ministry of Health. Nevertheless, establishing new and better-informed high-level documents by no means guarantees their adoption into local practices across the country.

It is not rare that international organisations will produce policy recommendations, taking a rather pragmatic stance that is based on western science and on the belief that their previous application in a number of cases is proof of the adequacy for a number of others. These recommendations often fail to incorporate aspects of local culture (like traditional health understandings) and they rarely ever address the institutional context which will inevitably define their implementation. In the guidelines for the prevention and control of diarrheal disease, for example, some of the emphasized aspects are clearly of a strictly medical nature and refer to western pharmaceuticals, while others more sweepingly mention entire sectors of health prevention (food safety, safe disposal of faeces) without getting into the details of the existing problems within or the institutional structures in these sectors. Both the incorporation of local cultural aspects and the exact manner of implementing what is proposed in the guidelines is left to the judgment and the abilities of the local authorities.

Box 6.1: Summary of the main points in the 'New guidelines for the management of diarrhoea in children' (MoH, 2009c)

Identified risk factors include: food contamination, unclean water, bad kitchen hygiene translated in to dirty appliances, not washing hands in critical times and not disposing children's faeces properly. The recognised pathogens that can cause diarrhoea are listed in categories of parasites (amoeba, Giardia, Cryptosporidium), bacteria (E coli, Shigella) and viruses (Rotavirus, adenovirus, enterovirus, Norovirus).

Novelties of treatment approaches: Emphasis is placed on the usefulness of combining zinc supplements with low osmolarity oral rehydration solution (ORS), on the use of Ciprofloxacin for treatment of Shigella dysentery and on the use of Rotavirus vaccination as a preventive measure. Emphasis is also placed on the measures of proper nutrition, proper hygiene and breastfeeding, not only as part of prevention, but also in complementing treatment and recovery.

Seven key points are listed in order to facilitate a concise communication approach, focusing on the crucial role of the caretakers and the parents. These points are: (i) breast-feeding, (ii) proper nutrition, (iii) the use of clean water, (iv) the frequency of hand-washing, (v) food safety, (vi) the use of hygienic latrines and safe disposal of faeces, and (vii) vaccination.

It is certainly not the position of international NGOs to define the detailed function of a country's institutions. However, it is worth underlining that a policy alone is not sufficient to generate motivation and develop the tools needed for its realisation. The potential of policy guidelines, such as the above (Box 6.1), to bring positive outcomes, is therefore a question of how much political will exists to transform these guidelines into implementable plans. A pilot implementation of the above guidelines started with the guidance of PATH in one province, with the objective of spreading the program around the country (PATH, 2012). Nevertheless, one year later, none of the interviewed health officers or medical practitioners in Can Tho had ever heard of these new guidelines. Despite being aware of some of the measures proposed in the guidelines, most of the medical staff interviewed was using much older material for the case-management of diarrhoea.

To connect with the discussion above, health policy needs to take into account the cultural characteristics of the public whose reciprocal cooperation and feedback it aspires to, but it also needs to address the social and institutional background against which new knowledge is looking to find a way in. Accordingly, failure to incorporate new and useful information in local systems of health might not only be due to the information's disregard of local culture, but also due to the local institutional system's unwillingness to change and transform this new information into practice. Examining both these issues with regard to the prevention of diarrheal disease requires a look into the current public health sector and a questioning of its ability to bridge preventive health knowledge(s) and policy implementation.

6.2 Derelictions of prevention: fragmented measures and weak implementation

This section draws from secondary literature and from empirical evidence collected in Can Tho City to delineate how the proposed measures for the prevention of diarrheal disease are being followed through in Vietnam. By comparing internationally advocated guidelines that are reflected in national policy with what is actually taking place in the local level, this section seeks to elucidate to what extent the above mentioned guidelines (MoH, 2009c) have become embedded in local practice.

6.2.1 The "old story" of diarrhoea: de-prioritising and underestimating a widespread disease

One of the national preventive programs in Vietnam is dedicated to the "Control of Diarrheal Disease" (CDD) and follows the guidelines that had been proposed by the WHO several years prior (WHO, 1987). The main objective of the program had been to educate mothers with children under five years old to readily identify, treat and control diarrheal disease, emphasizing the preparation of Oral Rehydration Solutions (ORS). In order to achieve the objectives of raising such understandings, the program has relied hugely on the health system's communication methods and tools, which, as discussed before (chapter 4), lie mainly in the hands of local health workers[117]. Part of the work that health workers do in relation to the program is to approach mothers individually in the clinics and to provide them with necessary information. Moreover, health workers are said to be frequent attendants of gatherings held under the umbrella of the Women's Union, where they "give some education classes on various issues, including diarrheal disease" (Top official in the rural commune health clinic, Phong Dien district, 15.12.11; personal interview).

Policy documents and reports collected from health organisations as various levels indicate near that the program is nowadays to being shuttered. The foremost indicator is there is no mention of this program in the National Preventive Health Strategy (MoH, 2007b), even though the prevention of diarrheal disease is generally referred to under the program of environmental sanitation. The CDD program was referenced in 2009 by the provincial department of Health in Can Tho (2009) but, two years later, it was already being referred to as "an old story which is now successfully concluded" (Top official in PHC of Can Tho, 12.12.11; group interview). On the district level, however, the pro-

[117] Source: Top official in rural commune health clinic, Phong Dien district, 15.12.11; personal interview.

gram features in annual reports until today (PHC Phong Dien, 2011, PHC Cai Rang, 2011b). These reports include mainly the disease's morbidity and mortality levels for children, but also the type of treatments administered for diarrhoea patients (ORS, intra-venous rehydration or antibiotics) and the number of mothers that were given advice. There was a conspicuous correlation between the reported numbers of child patients and of the number of mothers that received advice in the reports from the wards of Cai Rang district. In other words, the wards most hit by the disease were also the ones where most information-spread activities took place[118] (PHC Cai Rang, 2011b), with the same being observed at the scale of the province[119] (Department of Health, 2009). Though one of the main objectives of the program is the promotion of a correct and timely diagnosis, in order to prevent the disease's worst stages, its current implementation seems to make this type of knowledge available to parents only after a child is already seriously ill and admitted (and thus reported). This demonstrates how the CDD program is actually reactive - rather than proactive - with regard to the disease's occurrence.

It was not made clear whether the one-on-one communication on the premises of the clinic after a diarrhoea episode has occurred to a child is the only way that the health system reaches the public with information specifically about the factors related to diarrhoea under the CDD program. Interviewed young mothers in urban and rural settings of Can Tho said they had never received any related information from health workers or from Women's Union representatives. However, they did mention the communicative efforts of local cadres for the prevention of dengue fever and malaria[120], as well as for the promotion of water supply connections in the rural areas[121]. As one representative of a commune clinic described, another aspect of the CDD program was the free distribution of oral rehydration packs, but this is no longer taking place:

---

[118] These wards were: Truong Thanh, Phu Thu and Tan Phu. They also comprise the poorer and most rural parts of the district, with the lowest rates of access to improved water sources.

[119] In the annual report of Can Tho City, for example, there were 5,382 children patients reported under the CDD program and, similarly, 5172 mothers who were given CDD-related advice.

[120] These activities generally include check-visits to make sure people are complying with mosquito-control practices (no stagnant water in and around the house, the existence of bed-nets, etc.).

[121] Sources: Mothers of young children in Phong Dien (21.12.11) and Cai Rang (22.12.11) districts; in-depth interviews.

> "The Preventive Health Centre will assign communication activities to the commune clinic under the CDD program. We used to give ORESON [a type of oral rehydration solution] for free, but since 2006 we just talk to mothers, instructing on how to treat their kids when they suffer from diarrhoea, to advise them to give ORESON, salt and porridge." (Top official in the rural commune health clinic, Phong Dien district, 15.12.11; personal interview)

The limited extension of communication activities and the withdrawal of free ORS distribution both suggest the limited financial support that is currently provided to the CDD program by the central government. This is also evident in the funding reports from the district levels that do not include CDD in their list of preventive health programs, and is a further indication of its low prioritisation in the county (Table 6.1).

Table 6.1: Budget allocation for preventive health programs in Phong Dien

Content	Allocating budget (in VND)
Food safety and hygiene program	40,000,000
Reproductive health care program	42,000,000
HIV/AIDS program	84,213,000
Dengue fever program	50,000,000
Expanded vaccination program	40,000,000
Vitamin A program	8,000,000
Malaria program	9,000,000

Adopted from the report provided by the PHC of Phong Dien (2011)

It is obvious also in the central guidelines on national preventive health priorities (MoH, 2007b) that the focus lies on lowering the mortality levels of potentially lethal versions of diarrheal diseases, like cholera and typhoid and that diarrhoea (not necessarily classified as cholera or typhoid) is only given attention as a children's disease (see Box 4.1 in section 4.1.3). This is also obvious in the protocol followed in the local clinics, which strictly report on diarrhoea episodes in children with less than five years of age:

> "We only report on children for this program. They don't require us to report anything other than the under-five year olds for diarrhoea. The same is true for the hamlet clinics [...]. For the adults we don't write down diarrhoea. It will ei-

> ther be classified as 'infective diarrhoea' or 'digestive problem'. The levels of dehydration in adults are not easy to differentiate; therefore we will just report the incident as 'diarrhoea – de hydration'. But we only report the kids to the higher levels." (Top official in the rural commune health clinic, Phong Dien district, 15.12.11; personal interview)

Altogether, the implementation and the impact of the CDD program on local communities seems largely weakened. The surveying methods have failed to capture the total burden of the disease in the population, as they ignore the cases of adult patients with milder symptoms and the large number of those who never even turn to public health centres for treatment. Therefore, the final picture regarding the gravity and persistence of the disease is only partly being represented in the reporting of this program. Moreover, the CDD program has become nowadays rather obsolescent, considering that its content has not been updated with more comprehensive and necessary preventive measures proposed globally, such as water access, food safety and vaccinations (UNICEF and WHO, 2009).

6.2.2 Streets to industries: the multilevel challenge of food safety

It was often the case that interviewees would attribute an episode of diarrhoea to the consumption of food that had been contaminated, gone bad or been produced under unhygienic circumstances. In their effort to explain the high incidence of the disease, even in areas of widespread water supply and sanitation coverage (mostly urban areas), health cadres would often discuss the problem of food safety as an urban phenomenon, such as with the following type of explanation: "these [urban] are places where there are more street vendors and more food stores" and "that's why they are more dangerous for someone to get diarrhoea" (Official in the Office of Education, Cai Rang district, 22.09.11; personal interview). Food safety has in this way been used as the scapegoat for existing loopholes in the implementation of WSS policy, so to maintain the narrative of a preventive success-story in WSS:

> "The problem of waterborne diarrheal disease is more intense in rural areas because of the lack of water access and sanitation and because of the poor hygienic behaviour.
>
> [PK: How about the health statistics that show high incidence of diarrhoea also in the urban areas, where water supply and sanitation is mostly improved?]
>
> A lot of people eat out in the cities, street food is not controlled and might be dirty; or the conditions under which it is prepared are non-hygienic. Personal hygienic standards of people that are handling food might be still low; not using soap and not washing their hands. It is very hard to control food manufacture in Vietnam and food safety is now a big problem. Many small factories, and espe-

cially those making ice, use un-treated water and just throw in chemicals to make it look good." (Top official in IHPH of Ho Chi Minh City, 28.07.11; group interview)

Even though the above officials describe indeed many of the leading problems in food safety, they detach those from the rural context. In fact, food-borne risks are not confined to urban areas. While the variety of food products might be less vast in rural and remote areas, there is no proof that rural food products are of better quality. Looking into Can Tho as a province with young urban centres and a traditionally rural character, one can observe how the diversity of food products spreads throughout the territory. Food can be bought fresh or processed, raw or cooked, in rural and urban open markets, small grocery stores and big super-markets and in a number of eateries, restaurants and street corners (Picture 6.2).

Picture 6.2: Example of a street food push-cart in the outskirts of Cai Rang district

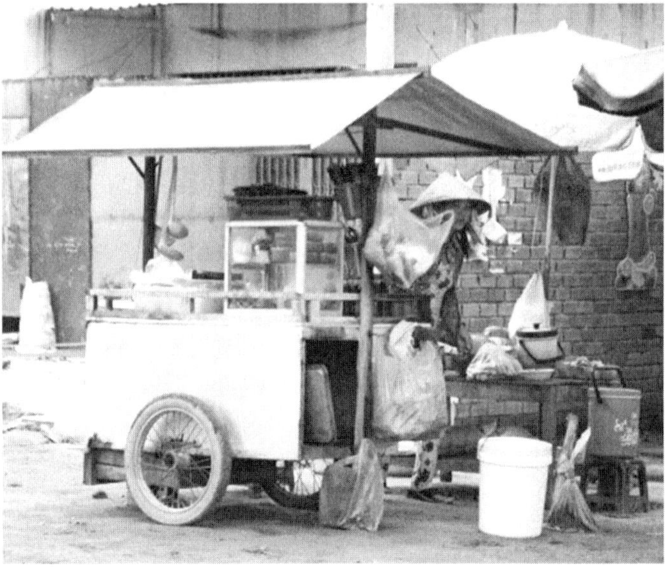

Photo by author, 2011

Rural areas might lack centralised multi-stores with imported products but there are always a variety of open food markets, local cafes or push-cart vendors in immediate access. Moreover, foods, as well as people, travel daily across rural and urban areas, allowing complex food networks to develop and expand beyond administrative borders.

The media have been discussing the issue of food safety as one of increasing concern for the country (Kieu Minh, 2009) and particularly the province of Can Tho, where it was reported that 14% of its food-selling facilities were not complying with hygienic standards and were falsifying expiration dates on their products (Hue Hoa, 2011). The quality of street food is extremely hard to monitor and control, as the vendors are usually poor individuals who the local authorities do not want to fine (Tung and Chau, 2013). At a larger scale, there are very frequent cases of food poisoning and acute diarrhoea across the province in groups of people who attend weddings and other catering events. The lack of regulation and control in the mass production of food and beverages is a burning topic nowadays in the country (Vietnam News, 2007). Food-borne risks are therefore infiltrating multiple scales of production and retail, requiring attention in their multiple forms and expressions.

The Vietnamese government recently took measures to address this problem, establishing the Law on Food Safety (National Assembly of the Socialist Republic of Vietnam, 2010). The provisions in this law call for risk assessment of food products, as well as for the forecast and communication of these risks to the public (Ibid. 2010:31). However, the legal framework outlining the responsibilities for checking and sanctioning food industries has scattered jurisdictions to five different ministries[122], as well as local governments and local health units, which complicates coordination and efficient implementation (Vietnam News, 2007, Kieu Minh, 2009). The only governmental body that was found to be actively enforcing food safety regulations was the Food Safety Unit in the province level (MoH, 2008). However, the activities of this body are limited to high-level businesses and companies that are registered under the province; thus, its jurisdiction does not include the numerous smaller food-selling units, which continue to escape the control of any authority[123].

One of the business sectors that often falls under the control of the provincial Food Safety Unit is the production of bottled-water and ice. This sector has been looked at with much concern and suspicion in Vietnam regarding its pro-

---

[122] These are MARD, MoH, MIT, MoNRE and MoST.

[123] The representative from the Food Safety Unit in Can Tho (16.12.11, personal interview) claimed that it is the health clinic's responsibility to inspect these small food vendors, but this was not verified by any clinic worker within Phong Dien or Cai Rang districts.

duction quality standards[124] and safety, with many companies having been accused of evading regulation (Duong et al., 2009, Thanh, 2009). Nevertheless, the current legal framework around the sector's control and the imposition of sanctions in case of non-compliance appears rather weak (Box 4 in Annex). Escaping sanctions has also been witnessed in smaller scale food businesses, as local authorities are intentionally sympathetic to their owners for reasons of interpersonal familiarity and acquaintance (Hue Hoa, 2011). There are similar practices of turning a blind eye to food safety violations of local businesses "because it would seriously endanger their livelihoods" and, regarding higher-level businesses, sanctions are avoided in order "to maintain good relationships"; this phenomenon is not limited to food vendors, and has also noted in the water polluting activities of the fish-sector in the Delta (Waibel et al., 2012). Therefore, even though the ineffectiveness of the sector is usually assigned to shortages of personnel, with "only 127 specialised people being employed in the sector for the year 2011" (Nguyen Qui Don, deputy director of education and training in Can Tho City, cited in Hue Hoa, 2011), it is also a matter of elastic implementation from the side of the existing authorities.

In an attempt to address food safety risks in a preventive manner during the peaks in their appearance, the government recently established three periods of the year to deal with extremes in food safety control[125] (Central Interdisciplinary Committee for Food Safety and Hygiene, 2011). One of these is the period of four weeks between mid-April to mid-May, which are considered "hot" for food poisonings because of the high temperatures and humidity levels of that time of year. The consumption of beverages - with ice of low quality - is expected to increase during hot days and the food-spoiling rate is accelerated, especially in areas lacking proper refrigeration (Thanh Nien online, 2010). Both of these factors are considered to contribute to the high number of children with diarrheal disease observed in the paediatric Hospital of Ho Chi Minh City during such hot periods of the year (Ibid. 2010).This period is the hottest and most humid also in Can Tho (Fig 6.1) and is accompanied by the highest reported incidence of disease (PHC Can Tho City, 2011b). The average

---

[124] Sources: Top official in the district PHC (Binh Thuy, 12.07.11) and top official in IHPH of Ho Chi Minh City (28.07.11); group interviews.

[125] These are (i) the 'Month of Action' (Tet celebrations in February), (ii) the four weeks period of mid-April to mid-May, and (iii) the autumn period of lunar celebrations, usually in October. During these times, appointed teams from the districts are assigned to run snap-checks in food establishments and to intensify the dissemination of food safety information to producers and consumers.

monthly cases of diarrheal disease in all of the southern provinces of the Delta tell the same story (Fig 6.2), with their maximum numbers being noted for May.

Figure 6.1: Average temperature and humidity per month in Can Tho City for 2011

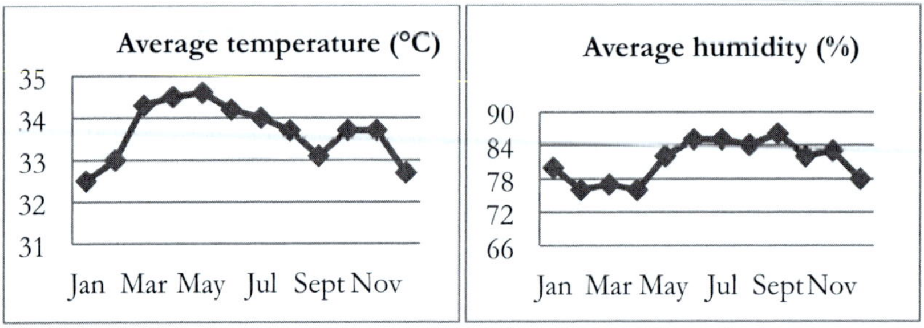

Data from the Statistical Office of Can Tho (2011)

Figure 6.2: Monthly cases of diarrheal diseases in the southern provinces, averages for the period 2005 to 2010

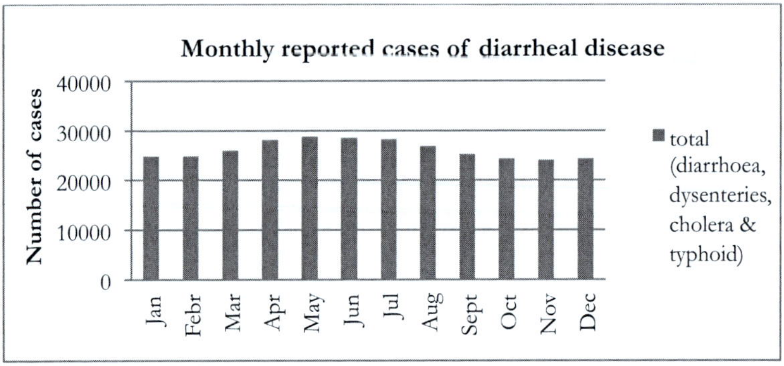

Source: Institute of Hygiene and Public Health (HCMC), 2011

The other two periods targeted for food safety are the days of the moon celebration (October) and the period around Tet holiday (February). This is because the consumption of food that has not been prepared in the household increases during these times[126]. However logical this periodical preventive action might be, it remains restricted in scope and duration as it leaves much of

[126] During these periods of celebration, people attend social events and are likely to drink and dine outside. Cultural habits also include disproportionate consumption of traditional confections and pastries which are sold in stores and stalls along the streets.

the food sector relatively uncontrolled during the remainder of the year. As briefly discussed above, the effectiveness of the checking and sanctioning mechanism is also highly questionable, with legal gaps leaving a large fraction of the food retailing business as "everybody's and nobody's" responsibility. Apart from controlling and sanctioning, the focus of food safety campaigns is also claimed to be informative for the consumers.

As this chapter will later discuss in detail (see section 6.3), the content of the communicative material consists largely of a list of prohibitions. In terms of food behaviours, instructions about what *not* to do leave people with few options, and they tend to leave out what people *can* do in order to ensure food safety in the household. Frewer et al. (1994) found that especially in the field of food safety, people tend to overestimate their knowledge on the potential hazards and thus fail to accurately assess the risks they are exposed to. As a result of this "bias of optimism" people take for granted that information from preventive health campaigns is not directed to them, but to those who do not already know (Ibid. 1994).

6.2.3 Anti-diarrheal vaccination: an inaccessible and unknown solution

One type of diarrheal disease that can be prevented through vaccinations is Rotavirus (Glass et al., 2006). Rotavirus diarrhoea lists among the eight most lethal vaccine-preventable diseases in the world (Dittmann, 2001). The Rotavirus type is also the most prevalent cause of diarrhoea in Vietnam (Van Man et al., 2005). Experts confirm that the incidence of Rotavirus-induced diarrhoea has outgrown diarrhoea caused by *E.coli*, *Salmonella*, *Campylobacter* and other pathogens[127], particularly in the South of the country where up to 40% of children under the age of two have suffered from it at least once.

According to the vice-director of the PHC in Can Tho, the vaccine protecting against the Rotavirus became available for purchase in the province during the year 2010. Since then, attention has been called to its usefulness via the local media. However, anti-diarrheal vaccination was not mentioned as a preventive measure by any of the health cadres in the district and was even confronted with complete ignorance by representatives in the PHC of Ninh Kieu district (23.06.11, personal interview). Moreover, as a reflection of the poor awareness about this vaccination, none of the 140 interviewees from rural and urban households recognised Rotavirus vaccination as a preventive measure against diarrhoea.

---

[127] Source: Top official in the Pasteur Institute, Ho Chi Minh City, 06.02.11; personal interview.

Rotavirus vaccines are currently produced in Vietnam[128] but they are not included in the national vaccination program offered free to children. The commercial price of the vaccine also makes it inaccessible for the masses, with the required double dose costing 700,000 VND (25 Euros)[129], an amount close to the average monthly income of a rural inhabitant (GSO, 2011b: 249). It is actually said that, in Vietnam, the vaccine costs five to seven times more than its average international price (Kuanpoth 2007 cited in Anh Tuan Nguyen et al., 2009). Even though it has been distributed for free in some pilot project areas (PATH, 2012), these areas have never included the Mekong Delta. Literature on the issue indicates that a free Rotavirus vaccination policy would bring benefits to the overall economy of the country, significantly reducing the number of inpatient and outpatient cases of diarrhoea and would thus financially relieve the healthcare system (Fischer et al., 2005, Kim et al., 2009). However, the Vietnamese government is still reluctant in taking a step towards making the Rotavirus vaccination free for all:

> "Whoever wants to get them [Rotavirus vaccines] has to pay for them and they are not cheap; only middle class people can get them. The government at the moment doesn't have enough money to provide for nation-wide vaccination. Maybe in 5-10 years we will be able to do that." (Top official in the Medical and Pharmaceutical University in Ho Chi Minh City, 28.07.11; personal interview)

The case is similar for the 'killed oral cholera vaccine'[130], which is also locally produced and was successfully used during the cholera epidemic of 2007 – 2008 in Hanoi (Trach et al., 1997, Anh et al., 2011). However, it is not a widely known to the local residents of Can Tho and was brought up as a preventive measure by only one interviewed medical professional:

> "The Preventive Health Centre manages the vaccination program. Here in the hospital we only provide treatment. Vaccination is not for free, but vaccines exist for cholera and for typhoid but not for diarrhoea. I don't know how much these vaccines cost, but one has to pay for everything in Vietnam; no medicine is for free." (Top official in the Central General Hospital of Can Tho, 20.06.11; group interview)

---

[128] The vaccines are found under the commercial names Rotatex and Rotarex.

[129] Source: Top official of PHC of Can Tho City 12.12.11, group interview.

[130] Killed oral vaccines are called this way because they contain killed whole cells of the *V.cholerae* organism in order to induce the process of immunization. The commercial name of the vaccine produced and locally available in Vietnam is mORCVAX but it is yet to be pre-qualified by the WHO (Ryan, E. T. 2011. The Cholera Pandemic, Still with Us after Half a Century: Time to Rethink. *PLoS Negl Trop Dis,* 5, e1003.).

The promotion of Rotavirus or cholera vaccinations appears not to be considered a realistic preventive measure for the masses and consequently it is not widely promoted by the public health system. As a result, there is overall very little awareness about this measure among local level health professionals and citizens, making them only an option for those who are well-informed and financially better-off.

6.2.4 Diarrhoea and malnutrition: the disregarded links

The links between insufficient breast-feeding, children's malnutrition, and an increased vulnerability towards diseases such as diarrhoea have long been studied and established (see chapter 1). A person's nutritional status strongly shapes the perpetuation of diarrhoea or leads to premature death, which is especially evident in children. It has been acknowledged that well-nourished kids are less likely to fall sick, and if they do, they are physically more apt to recover (WHO, 2001b). Likewise, diarrheal disease can lead to a rapid loss of nonreplaced nutrients and eventually to a malnourished stage, especially when a wholesome eating regime is not followed during the illness. Either way, malnutrition and diarrhoea can form part of the same vicious circle if not prevented in an integrated manner.

In Vietnam, food supplementation and breast-feeding are measures that figure prominently in the national health strategy plans for strengthening children's health and preventing malnutrition (Department of Health, 2009). However, those aspects have not been explicitly linked to diarrhoea. This lack of an explicit connection is also evident in the state's approach to communication, where messages focus on the importance of nutritional food and water provision when children are suffering from diarrhoea but not on how a good nutritional status contributes to prevention[131]. The concept of proper nutrition seems to generally be confused with food abundance, as malnutrition was often mistakenly understood as under-nutrition and famine. Some interviewed young mothers in Can Tho often reacted with expressions of horror when asked if

[131] Some representatives of the Women's Union referred to the 'Nutritious Porridge' program that teaches mothers what ingredients to use and how to properly cook rice for their kids (Top official in WU's commune branch, Phong Dien district, 19.12.11; personal interview) and other interviewees mentioned the efforts of commune clinic workers on advising them to breast-feed their newborns for at least six months after birth (Representatives of households HH3 (Phong Dien, 21.12.11), HH1 (Cai Rang, 22.12.11); in-depth interviews). However, the benefits of these practices in the prevention of diarrhoea were never mentioned.

their kids suffered from malnutrition and attached the disease to countries where children suffer from extreme poverty, but not to Vietnam.

Contradicting these public perceptions are the statistical realities in Vietnam: the rates of malnourished five-year-olds remained significant in samplings from both 1998 and 2011. In 1998, 39% of children being underweight, 34% stunted and 11% wasted[132] (Dearden et al., 2002); in 2011, the WHO (2012c) found that stunting decreased, with UNICEF reporting 31,9% stunting and 18,9% under-weight (HEMA and UNICEF, 2011). Notwithstanding year-on-year differences, the disease not only still exists, but it also reflects significant inequalities in the population. The poorest are the hardest hit and the gap in malnutrition rates between rich and poor has been widening from double in 1993 to over 3.5 times in 2006 (GSO 2008 cited in WHO, 2012c). Similar disparities are noticed in child malnutrition rates in rural areas, among ethnic minorities and in kids whose mother's education level is low (GSO, 2011a). The current malnutrition rates reported for Can Tho City are much lower than those of the whole country and the rate of underweight children has been continuously decreasing over the last ten reported years (Fig. 6.3).

Figure 6.3: Reported rates (%) of malnourished children in Can Tho City for 2000 - 2010

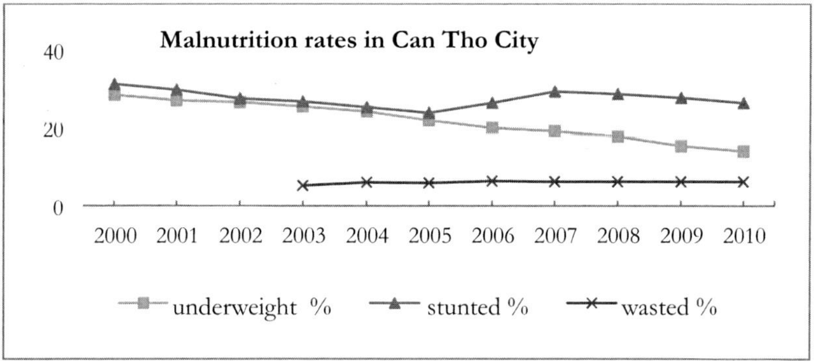

Data source: PHC of Can Tho City (2011a). Design by the author.

However, the rate of stunted children has remained high in the last five years, indicating that a higher calorie intake (increase of weight) is not necessarily equal to a better nutrition and body development (increase of height). While more studies are needed to substantiate the connection between weight, height,

132 underweight=low weight-to-age ratio, stunted=low height-to-age ratio , wasted=low weight-to-height ratio

nutrition and poverty, the data above already indicate that although food is generally not hard to access in Vietnam, nutritional food is not equally available to all, with consequences for the poorest and minorities.

The observed disparities between urban and rural areas, but also between the rich and the poor, that were noticed in malnutrition are strikingly similar to those noticed in the sector of water supply and sanitation (section 5.1.2). Literature on the Vietnamese case has already highlighted linkages between malnutrition and low rates of breast-feeding, lack of proper feeding practices and poor hygiene (Dearden et al., 2002); implicit in these results is the connection between malnutrition and diarrhoea. A recent study examined exactly how malnutrition relates to hygiene in Vietnam (HEMA and UNICEF, 2011). The study found correlations between malnutrition and factors such as having latrines and maintaining them properly, using a clean water source, exercising hand-washing and maintaining good hygiene practices in the house (i.e. cleaning objects used for feeding, cleaning breasts before feeding, feeding freshly cooked food), concluding (with 95% confidence) that:

> "(i) the rates of underweight and stunting among children under five years old could be reduced by 0-23% and 0-33% respectively if all households used hygienic water sources; (ii) [...] by 1-10% and 4-16% respectively if all households used hygienic latrines; and (iii) the rate of underweight among children under five years old could be reduced by 1-10% if all mothers/caregivers practiced hand-washing with soap before and after preparing food for children" (HEMA and UNICEF, 2011).

Addressing the problem of malnutrition by recognising its connectedness with issues such as hygiene and diarrhoea seems not to be yet part of the national policy or of the local discourse in Vietnam. The same lack of integration is also noted in the case of breast-feeding; a key practice in the battle of the vicious malnutrition-diarrhoea circle (Dearden et al., 2002). Namely, only two out of five children in Vietnam are breastfed within one hour after birth and less than 17% are breastfed until the recommended age of six months (GSO, 2011a). The number of infants younger than four months old that are exclusively breastfed has actually decreased in recent years, from 31.1% in 2000 to 28.8% in 2010, which is still below the national targets (National Institute of Nutrition and UNICEF, 2011). The choice of mothers not to continue breastfeeding for the recommended period of months was examined by Dat Duong et al. (2004). The authors found that mothers were influenced by family members and healthcare providers in hospitals and clinics, with the latter generally emphasizing the benefits of breastfeeding (Ibid. 2004). However, the benefits of maintaining breast-feeding have not yet managed to be taken up into a common discourse that will also address malnutrition, hygiene and their connections with diarrhoea.

6.2.5 Polluted hydro-environments and weaknesses in advocating personal hygiene

Sanitation is one of the main factors recognised as important in bringing down the prevalence of diarrheal disease (UNICEF and WHO, 2009). Sanitation refers to household-level facilities but also to the sanitary management of surrounding environments. In Vietnam, however, the term has come to mistakenly be equated with the construction of "hygienic" toilets (see section 5.3) that are able to store sewage and does not address issues of environmental pollution through the unregulated disposal of untreated sewage into river water networks. As was explained in more detail above, even if toilets are constructed, the issue of integrated water management often remains unsolved. Apart from households, water pollution occurs from the activities of farming and agriculture, as well as from urban industrial waste. The section 'environmental health' in Vietnam's Preventive Health Strategy (MoH, 2007b: 118) is rather silent on aspects of sanitation that depend on services and decisions that need to be state-led.

The only aspects of environmental sanitation that are reported by local PHCs concern the hygienic condition of barns (reported by CERWASS) and the methods of garbage disposal (reported by district PHCs). According to reports, both sectors have rather poor performance, with most small-scale farming establishments being unsanitary and with a an absence of proper garbage collection and treatment systems remaining in most areas (PHC Binh Thuy, 2011, PHC Cai Rang, 2011c, PHC Ninh Kieu, 2011, PHC O Mon, 2011c). The lack of waste collection services in many rural communes has been assigned to some areas' remoteness and difficulty in access. The only alternative for the management of household garbage, apart from disposing it in the rivers and canals, is to bury or burn it. These practices are officially recognised as "hygienic" and are found to be exercised by 85% of households in Cai Rang and Phong Dien districts (2011, 2011a). According to a health official in Co Do district the practice of throwing waste into the environment "has become people's everyday habit" (18.07.11, personal interview). A representative from the WU in Phong Dien described, with similar nonchalance, that without better solutions, people are naturally expected to pollute the waters:

> "[Laughs] what can they do? When they are working in the floating market, where are they going to throw the waste? There is no system of collecting rubbish in the river, only inland and only in some areas where the trucks can reach.

In the rural areas people might burn or bury." (Top official in the district branch of Women's Union, Phong Dien, 08.09.11; personal interview)

Waste from households, food residues from the markets, garbage from stores, sewage from toilets and multiple other kinds of waste are all recognised sources of water pollution by authorities, experts and the public[133]. Numerous media reports have underlined the gravity of this problem, especially in urban areas (Ha Van, 2010a), underlining the negative consequences for the environmental sanitation of households that are agglomerated along the edges of polluted canals (Ha Van, 2010b). Resulting from this scenario, many people are exposed to water environments that are highly polluted. This has been also well documented and discussed in section 5.2, which deals more explicitly with the water quality of different sources in the region of the Delta. Since the exposure to contaminated environments is high, the prevention of disease necessitates informed behaviours from the side of the exposed public. Apart from practices of water treatment, which were previously discussed, the adoption of precautionary hygienic habits appears to be imperative in limiting disease risk.

One of the main aspects of personal hygiene that relates to the spread of diarrheal disease is the practice of hand-washing with soap. Despite its widely recognised preventive health potential, Vietnam lacked any state-generated initiatives to promote hand-washing with soap until the year 2006, when a pilot project was initiated with the help of international donors (Nga Nguyen et al., 2011). The project included promotion campaigns in 40 selected communes around the country using the established network of the WUs as the platform for communication. The WU used to receive funding to specifically spread this information to mothers and caretakers (Ibid. 2011), mostly with the aim of reducing the mortality and morbidity of diarrhoea in children. Research in Can Tho City indicated that the hand-washing initiative is now rather moribund, considering that there is no active hand-washing campaign and there is no reporting taking place by the PHCs on this issue. Many interviewed representatives of WUs from the district and commune levels claimed that they receive no funding or material for the promotion of hand-washing anymore. Interviewees claimed that they occasionally discuss the importance of keeping good hygiene

[133] Source: Representatives from PHC of Can Tho, in IEC activity O Mon, 05.08.2011.

when talking to their members without, however, particularly referring to hand-washing[134].

After what was considered to be a successful first phase of the project, the hand-washing initiative expanded to be included in the content of primary-level education, integrating principles of hand-washing into school curriculum (Dutton et al., 2011a). However, the approach remains solely focused on children, aiming then for a domino-effect of awareness and practice from children to their parents. Literature has suggested that these effects are strongly inhibited by the contrasting habits and decisions defined by adults, such as the persist lack of designated hand-washing facilities in the household (MARD, 2003, Dutton et al., 2011b). This absence was highly noticeable in most of the visited homes in Can Tho, but also in many schools, public offices and hospitals. Secondary results from An Giang province of the Mekong Delta (UNICEF, 2008b) showed how low the adoption of the practice is in the region: only 48% of respondents claimed to wash their hands with soap, most of them only doing so when hands were "visibly dirty".

6.2.6 The lost chance for an integrated approach: the policy of "healthy and cultural villages"

As the discussion of the findings has shown so far, despite some targeted efforts to promote preventive measures, the spread and adoption of preventive behavior by the general public appears constrained. The different aspects of preventing diarrheal disease present distinct challenges requiring more support from the central state and more transparent engagement from local authorities. More importantly, however, these aspects need to be addressed discursively in a more holistic manner in order to enable the public to understand their interdependence and to develop a skill for detecting, avoiding and acting against the risk of disease. Interestingly, the policy of the 'healthy and cultural village" includes many of the aspects that relate to the prevention of diarrheal disease (MoH, 2004).

Despite the apparent potential of framing these issues under one policy umbrella to foster a holistic understanding, there are three major obstacles standing in the way of such progress. Firstly, the interdependence of the various aspects (i.e. sanitation, malnutrition, clean water, food safety), is neither explained in the policy nor in the public campaigns that are meant to support the policy's implementation. The nature of the targets in this local policy is derived from

---

[134]Sources: Top official in the district branch of Women's Union in Phong Dien (08.09.11), top official in WU's commune branch, Phong Dien (19.12.11); group interviews.

the centrally produced quantifiable indicators of progress in WSS and the control of epidemics (The Prime Minister of Vietnam, 1994, GoV, 2006a). Thus, instead of discursively bridging issues together, the 'healthy village' policy remains simply a haphazard accumulation of some centrally produced but nevertheless fragmented pieces of legislation. Secondly, although the 'healthy and cultural village" policy consists mainly of targets, it does not include any consistent plan of action. While the implementation of these targets is transferred to the local levels of the hamlet and the commune, there is no funding assigned exactly to those levels and no material or methodology tailored to their needs and capacities. The "cultural and healthy village" basically scales down national targets to local ones by handing over responsibilities without mobilising any central resources for their implementation.

Box 6.2: Selected criteria for being a 'cultural and healthy village' that relate to diarrheal disease (MoH, 2004)

(i) there is no disease epidemic in the area; (ii) the rates of morbidity and mortality of some common infectious diseases are reduced at least 10% in the urban areas, and 5% in delta, midland and mountain areas, compared to the previous year; (iii) at least 95% of children under one year of age get the provisioned vaccinations, according to the regulation; (iv) food poisoning cases do not surpass 30 people per case; (v) the rate of malnutrition in children under 5 years of age is being reduced by 1.5% each year; (vi) the percentage of households that use clean water and have a bathroom is at least 90% in urban areas, 80% in the Delta and middle regions of the country and 60% in the mountainous areas; (vii) the percentage of households that have a hygienic latrine is at least 80% in the urban areas, 60% in the Delta and middle regions of the country and 50% in the mountainous areas.

Thirdly, while many of the objectives in the above policy (Box 6.2) depend to a significant extent on people's personal choices (sanitation habits, hygienic practices, nutrition of children), there is no target for general health and hygiene education. Although national plans nominally address the importance of awareness-raising for better informed health decisions (MoH, 2007b), this objective is not explicitly mentioned in this policy. Despite its mention, hygiene education is rarely ever given quantifiable targets in national policy documents. This might be part of the reason why this otherwise very crucial aspect of preventing disease is hard translated into local targets. Even in the one instance where health education was given a specific target rate (MoH, 2007b: 118), there was no description of how to measure "health education". The weakness in defining and assessing communicative activities is also reflected in the reports of local health offices, which cannot provide any substantial information on their awareness-raising impact (see also section 6.3). As a result of all issues presented above, the dispersed and unsupported targets that the 'healthy and cultural village' proposes can hardly be turned into commonly understood health objectives for the wider public.

6.3 Health education and the public communication of disease

It was previously highlighted that health education can give individuals the power to make healthy choices and to sustain those choices in the long-term (see section 2.3.2). This section examines the manner in which knowledge about diarrheal disease is passed around by experts, the state and the public. Given the problems in the disease's control and the weaknesses in achieving a widespread adoption of preventive measures, the mechanism that provides the related information to the public is questioned. By closely looking at the content and the dissemination of the messages produced by that mechanism, some possible reasons explaining their poor reception by the public and the impacts thereof are examined.

6.3.1 The Vietnamese approach to health education

Following the specific objective in the National Health Strategy of the country "...to change the awareness and raise the sense of responsibility for disease prevention and health protection in all of Party Committees and administrations at all levels, in mass organisations, in the community and every citizen" (MoH, 2007b: 81), most preventive health programs in Vietnam claim to have communication components. Awareness-changing is also portrayed as a central goal in the strategy against the spread of infectious diseases (MoH, 2007b, GoV, 2007). As mentioned above, the necessary methods for achieving this awareness-change are left undefined. Instead, legislators and policy-makers seem to leverage notions of ethical obligation in order to motivate implementers to invent their own means and methods, for example by pointing to values such as state solidarity, unity, the community and the people's sense of common good (see Box 5 in the Annex). Blending hygiene with social responsibilities is a pattern that seems to have trickled down to the local levels, often framed in a widely proclaimed vision of modernity:

> "The 'National sanitation and clean water week' policy is organised as a response, to provide extensive propaganda to the masses and gradually raise the awareness of people, in order to improve their living conditions, to create healthy communities in rural areas and to contribute to a more modern and civilised society. This can be achieved if each of us in the social communities is aware of their hygiene practices" (PHC Binh Thuy, 2011).

The frequent use of ideologically charged words such as 'propaganda', 'socialisation' and 'community organisation', is a motif that Laverack and Dap (2003) also detected in the communication material used across Vietnam. Without wanting to demonise the term as such, the use of 'propaganda' when referring to communication activities is suggestive of an understanding of communication as a unidirectional means to persuade, instead of an interactive process to enable discernment and to empower. Whereas the community is presented as having a distinguished role in safeguarding healthy and cultural ideals, the actual participation of local people, both in health education activities and in the formulation of preventive strategies, is not mentioned anywhere.

This prominence of the notion of social and moral obligation when framing the preventive health approach is not new in the country. Bloom (1998: 235) notes that public health was literally an obligation and that, ever since the 1980s, local leaders would punish anyone who did not attend the organised health education activities, demonstrated individualistic behaviour against public health priorities. Many respondents claimed that due to health workers' feelings of social responsibility and moral obligation during the war, the Vietnamese managed to survive many plagues. Marr (1992) also observes that "hygienic education and preventive medicine were woven into the larger revolutionary ethos from 1945, becoming an integral part of both the anti-feudal and anti-imperialist struggles" (Hoang Dinh Cau and Le Anh cited in Marr, 1992). However, the attitude of the Vietnamese, to safeguard their health and help in the survival of others, emerged from the grassroots peasantry and had its roots in feelings of brotherhood and unity. Contrarily, the responsibility or obligation that is prescribed by central authorities and is positioned coercively in the law has little to do with such feelings. As Marr (Marr, 1992) (1992) further notes, "this momentum was lost from the mid-1970s onwards" when the war was over and people did not feel threatened anymore. Even though messages against disease have been echoing in the country ever since Ho Chi Minh's encouragements to "maintain very good hygiene" (Ho Chi Minh 1961 cited in Rheinländer et al., 2010), the impact that these messages have today on the population is questionable.

As Glasgow et al. (2004 cited in Panter-Brick et al., 2006) recognise, an effective and sustainable behavioural change can be hard to achieve, especially when ideological and moral flags are waved above messages of health prevention. The actual essence of those messages can be diluted if they are not received by the public as useful instruments, but merely as obligations towards the state. As Curtis et al. (2000) pinpoint: " 'good' hygiene, in the moral sense, is not the same with 'safe' hygiene in the epidemiological sense". Building on better understandings of health risks such as disease has the potential to enhance one's sense of self-efficacy and allow for conscious and informed choices in health (Strecher et al., 1986). However, replacing these choices with simple compliance to rules undermines this potential. It has been commented how, in Vietnam today, "Information, Education and Communication (IEC) is a more controlled process of coordinated action toward a national approach within guiding ideological principles" (Laverack and Dap, 2003: 364). As it will be described below, the legal texts produced under this ideology maintain a top-down character, pre-empting the possibility of issues to be discussed and adapted to the capacities and the desires of local communities (GoV, 2007: 60).

6.3.2 Directing funds, expertise and information

In the legal framework, the terms information, education and communication are interchangeably or concurrently used, and are understood as a necessary instrument to achieve behavioural change (Box 5 in the Annex). However, the instrumentalisation of these terms, as well as the methods for implementing them and allocating funds is left open to the localities. The PHCs of the provincial level decide to allocate a certain percentage of their funds for the communication part of each program, while some of that budget derives from central support. In the sector of rural water supply and sanitation, for example, it was decided to direct 9% of the national funds to communication activities (GoV et al., 2006). This was with the purpose of raising the demands and the willingness of the people to invest in sanitation facilities:

> "[...] the main future role for the government is to focus on implementing IEC and management activities rather than be directly involved in the construction of RWSS facilities [...] to create a much higher awareness around hygiene and around the link between sanitation, hygienic practice, water supply and health." (MARD and MoC, 2000: 17)

In Can Tho City, the promotion of water supply and sanitation expansion received central funds of 200 million VND[135] for the year 2011; double the amount that was directed to the prevention of malaria[136] and four times the amount that was directed to the communication of food safety and hygiene in the same year (Food Safety and Hygiene Unit, 2011). A top official from the PHC of Can Tho City (14.07.11, personal interview), said that these funds are mostly used for executing public communication activities (conducting training classes, producing radio and television spots and printing brochures). Moreover, he claimed that despite the complete lack of funding for the CDD program, the topic of diarrhoea is being addressed during the promotion of water supply and sanitation.

---

[135] An amount equal to about 7,043 Euros

[136] Source: Head Top official in PHC Can Tho City, 14.07.11; personal interview.

Despite the funds that the PHC receives for public communication activities, there is no reporting on exactly how this budget is spent. It was made clear, however, that no part of this budget is being transferred down to the district or grassroots authorities[137]. The organisation of health education activities in the districts is therefore dependent on their local capacities. As the head of the PHC in Cai Rang district explains, this leaves them with limited options:

> "We don't spend any money on information and education activities, we only gather people and talk to them. When the City's Preventive Health Centre organises activities, they have funds, they offer people water, pay for the rent of a place and also sometimes they give money to the people who do the training, because some programs provide funding for that." (Top official in PHC of Cai Rang district, 16.12.11; personal interview)

The "training-of-trainers" in health education

Although central funding support for preventive health is restricted to the provincial level, there are education and communication activities taking place within the province that serve the purpose of transferring knowledge and material to the lower administrative levels. These activities follow a successive process of 'training-of-trainers', according to which information and guidance flows vertically. Targets of this process are the staff of district PHCs and commune health clinics, the members of unions and the wider public (Picture 6.4). Findings indicated that the staff of central health organisations do not actively take part in this 'training-of-trainers'[138]. However, material is centrally produced to guide the content of public health messages in the provinces and districts. This material is reproduced and circulated mostly through the provincial Centres for Health Education and Communication (CHEC); this centre is also

---

[137] Ibid.

[138] Examples of central health entities that do not actively contribute to "training-of-trainers" are the Institute for Hygiene and Public Health (IHPH) and the Pasteur Institute in Ho Chi Minh City. The latter has an established department of Health Education that is in charge of designing and planning training activities for the provincial staff under its jurisdiction, but currently this department remains under-staffed and is not functioning (top official in the Pasteur Institute, Ho Chi Minh City, 06.02.11; personal interview). Some interaction between the expert staff of these two institutes and the authorities within the provinces might take place, but only in times of serious epidemic threats. During these times, the experts will investigate whether disease-management protocols have been correctly followed by local authorities and thus the process is one of inspection rather than of knowledge transfer (Top official in the Pasteur Institute (Ho Chi Minh City, 06.02.11) and top official in PHC Can Tho City (14.07.11); personal interviews.

responsible for guiding public communication activities and to help in capacity-building at the grassroots.

Picture 6.4: Directions of training and material on health prevention, within the province

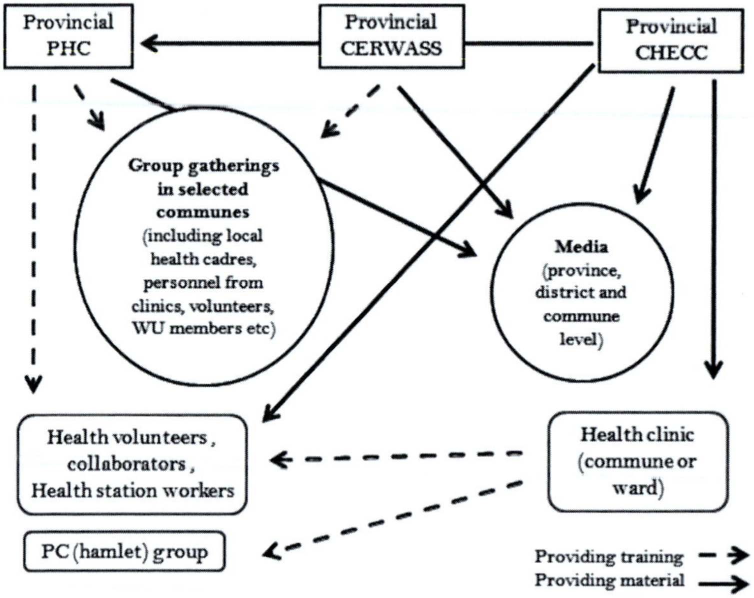

The above framework is not meant to be part of the legal framework in its entirety, but is a depiction of the research findings (qualitative interviews conducted with preventive health staff, civil society representatives and health workers from the Ministry of Health to the commune level). Design by the author, 2011.

According to the representative from the regional Institute of Hygiene and Public Health, however, the CHECs have not effectively taken up their responsibilities:

> "At the moment the task of guidance in information and education activities has been assigned to the CHECC, but because of limited funding and their lack of capacity, they do not execute anything else other than some administrative tasks. They give out brochures to the communes and the districts, which remain on their shelves and do not get distributed. The process is not educational; it is rather a box to be ticked, a process of handing out pieces of paper." (Top official in the Pasteur Institute, Ho Chi Minh City, 06.02.11; personal interview)

The topics addressed in the material that the centre distributes follow the priorities set by the Ministry of Health. Information regarding the prevention of diarrheal disease was found sporadically in some of the material produced during the last five years. However, the exact content and the quality of the information were found to significantly differ (see section 6.3.3). One of the most effective examples of informational material on health issues was claimed to be a monthly published magazine of the MoH entitled 'Health for a Cultural Village'. Some of the articles in this magazine were found to cover topics of diarrheal disease, including the use of chloramine-b for water treatment (Tran Giuu DS, 2007), the correct steps for treating and curing diarrhoea (National Center of Preventive Health, 2007), the control of flies as a transmitting agent (Hanh Nguyen, 2007), advice regarding food-borne diarrhoea (Pham Kim, 2007) and other preventive measures against the disease's spread (Tran Vu, 2007). However, all of these articles were in issues published during 2007, a year when a cholera epidemic broke out in the country (MoH, 2011). It is therefore possible that this thematic orientation about the prevention of diarrheal disease was affected by the general alarm about cholera. Unfortunately however, these were the only issues made available to the researcher and thus, comparisons with other years were not possible.

According to the director of the CHEC in Can Tho, 100 copies of this magazine are distributed every month around the province (CHECC, 2011), reaching every health unit, commune clinic, district hospital and PHC[139]. Observations from the province revealed, however, quite a different picture. Only two district PHCs (of the five visited) were found to have a copy of this magazine and both of them were in urban districts. Moreover, the utility of this material was diminished to decorative, as they were placed in a showcase behind glass doors and were thus not available to the visiting public. Contrary to the director's claims, none of the representatives in the visited clinics or health stations had ever received any kind of public health communication material at all. These magazines are, in fact, well-written and thematically rich, printed on high-quality paper quality and with a careful layout. However, their limited distribution diminishes their impact. Other types of material[140] was also claimed to be distributed by the CHECC (2011), but was similarly found to be absent from all the (five) visited clinics and (six) district hospitals. Exceptionally, the staff of

[139] Source: Top official in the IHPH, Ho Chi Minh City, 06.02.11; personal interview.

[140] This included 3000 posters promoting hand-washing and 130 CDs with information on food-safety and hygiene, distributed monthly within Can Tho (according to the reports provided by the CHECC in 2011).

the provincial PHC in Can Tho appeared to have a variety of materials at their disposal, although not in large quantities. This made clear that public health communication faces problems to achieving widespread distribution, particularly at the levels of the district-and-below.

Beyond issues of quantity, the usage and the impact of visual-oriented communication material (posters, leaflets and brochures) is also dependant on its appearance. While illustrated posters were available at the provincial level, the local health units provided mostly photocopied reproductions of the original material. This was usually of smaller size, lower printing quality and harder to read, thereby reducing the strength of the preventive messages (see Pictures 3-5 in the Annex). MARD is aware of this, noting that, for one thing, the sector of WSS needs more attractive IEC material and larger availability of this material for the intended audience in the local levels (MARD, 2003).

Gaps exist and seem to be growing, not only concerning the amount and the quality of the available material, but also in reference to the capacity of the local health staff who are meant to use it. Seeing how the educational requirements for grassroots health posts are not demanding[141], the low expertise in specific issues of disease and health prevention is understandable:

> "Preventive health sector staff are trained in the university (college level) to serve for the district and the provincial level. These people need to have a university degree. For the commune level and below, a vocational training is enough - for the pharmacists as well - and there is one such school in each province. In the South however, there is only one in Ho Chi Minh and one in Can Tho City." (Top official in the Medical and Pharmaceutical University in Ho Chi Minh City, 28.07.11; personal interview)

> "Many of the people at the local levels are not capable of answering or explaining things on the topic. They just pass on some printed information to the public." (Top official in the IHPH, Ho Chi Minh City, 06.02.11; personal interview)

The changeable requirements and the lack of medical professionals especially in the rural areas (see section 4.1.2) exacerbate the phenomenon of limited health capacity at the grassroots. This reflect the capacity to perform effective preventive health communication, as it has been emphasized in the past in Vietnam (Laverack and Dap, 2003, MARD, 2003). Nevertheless, the main actors in the spread of public health messages are claimed to be exactly the health workers of the grassroots (volunteers, collaborators, health station workers). As interview-

---

[141] In the legislation, the minimal educational requirements for health workers in the hamlet demand no more than three months of vocational training (MoH 2010b. On Prescribed Standards, Functions and Duties of Village Workers. *39/2010/TT-BYT*).

ees in these posts described, they learn how to perform such tasks through their involvement in preventive health programs and through their occasional attendance at monthly meetings in the commune health clinic. This involvement only takes place at particular times of the year and mostly during periods of elevated risk of disease spread[142]. As mentioned before, despite their duty to approaching the population and raise awareness on public health issues (GoV, 2010b), health communicators do not receive any of the funds that are available for preventive activities in the provincial level. The lack of expertise and guidance from higher levels, on the one hand, and the imbalance between their available resources and their responsibilities, on the other hand, can easily result in a reduction in the quality of service that the health workers can offer (see also section 4.1.3).

Another strong player in disseminating information to the local level is the network of the Women's Unions (WU), which was repeatedly mentioned as being central in communicating health-related information to their members. The government used to provide funds in order to encourage this kind of training within the organisation, but this policy has now concluded[143]. Representatives from the local branches of the WU said that diarrheal disease is now being addressed through the focus on household hygiene:

> "We assign women working in each ward as volunteers for fulfilling prevention tasks and promoting health via the 3-clean model: clean house, clean kitchen, and clean surrounding environment." (Top official in WU district branch, Cai Rang, 22.09.11; personal interview)

> "Indeed, we promote the 3-clean model to our members, who are obliged to follow it in their homes and are being checked on it... we also advice people to follow this model through our IEC activities." (Top official in WU's commune branch, Phong Dien district, 19.12.11; personal interview)

Apparently, there is not much printed material or other supporting information meant to frame this focus on household hygiene and thus the WUs basically act as "loudspeakers" for some of the core messages for the female community that is under their umbrella. However, the members of the unions are also not expert in medical issues and their ability to provide substantial health education on a complex topic like diarrheal disease is rather questionable.

---

[142] Source: Top official in health station of a rural hamlet (Phong Dien district, 15.12.11), top official in rural commune health clinic (Phong Dien district, 15.12.11) and top official in PHC of Cai Rang district (16.12.11); personal interviews.

[143] Source: Top official in PHC Can Tho City, 14.07.11; personal interview.

If capacity at the local level is low and the material are in short supply, how are people to exercise their right of "access to information, education and communication for disease prevention and control" (GoV, 2007)? Representatives from the PHC of Can Tho often referred to education classes that take place at the commune level (Picture 6.4), through which information is provided to the participating public. The participants of these classes then have the responsibility to spread around this information within their communities. As it was made clear from informants, these classes only invite a certain number of people, who are usually members of unions, health workers and local government officials. After many interviews and observations, it became clearer that apart from the confined audience, the frequency of these classes is also very limited. There are 30 to 40 such classes organised by the PHC of the province each year, but the location is different every time. There are about 50 attendants in each class[144] and as the vice-director of the PHC claimed:

> "We cannot afford for more. The refreshments offered cost money. The number of the people is set, or else we wouldn't be able to afford it. The people that come are people from offices or somehow that hold a position in their localities" (Top official in PHC of Can Tho, 12.12.11, group interview).

These classes include a long lecture, which is given by designated experts of the provincial PHC, followed by a short session of discussion with the public. The whole process is accompanied by the handing of some material (media articles, audio-texts, brochures and booklets), which are produced and provided by the CHECC. Many different topics are covered during each of these classes, ranging from the proper construction of water supply and sanitation facilities to various types of waterborne diseases, household hygiene, food safety and healthcare-seeking advice. In this way, a number of boxes are ticked for many different preventive health programs, saving time and expenses for the executing body (primarily the PHC of the provincial level). However, the whole event is dominated by expert talk, which last for over 1.5 hours in a lecture format. Observations from one of these classes (in O Mon district 05.08.11) indicated that the audience is rarely ever given the opportunity to participate[145]. When the floor opened for the audience to ask questions, people were very hesitant. The only comment arising after some moments of silence was from a lady that made her concern waveringly known:

---

[144] Ibid.

[145] The presenter asked if there were fishpond toilets in the community. Upon the audience's confirmation, the point made by the presenter would be on the need for more "hygienic" sanitation facilities and the stronger implementation of the subsidization and microcredit policy.

> "My family has two disabled people and we got the subsidy five years ago. Now the toilet is full and we need to build another one, can I get the subsidy again?" (Woman participant in group gathering, O Mon district 05.08.11, personal observation).

After the end of the training, local informants assigned this lack of participation to people's shyness, in other words in order to avoid appearing ignorant by posing questions or demonstrating that they were not paying attention. But why would the presence of a health educator cause feelings of hesitance or fear, instead of familiarity and interest? The answer can be found in the notions of superiority that the provincial PHC has, solely by being an institution ranked in a higher administrative level. Hierarchy plays an important role in the Vietnamese state and in social interactions. This is also reflected in the didactic way in which the above activity was carried through. Namely, the speaker stands at a pedestal, distant from the audience which is seated in rows of school desks. The speaker is not interrupted, as interaction is not encouraged. The opinions of the audience on the topic are not given the opportunity to be heard, as there is not enough space for feedback within the established structure of the training. The lack of people's active inclusion in the design and the planning of preventive activities and practices has also been observed by MONRE and the UNDP (2008: 41). In the example of hand-washing promotion, Dutton et al (2011a) have also noted that the so-called "consumer-research stage"[146] is being left out when designing campaigns, despite this stage proving to be the most important for the success of the project, particularly in the Vietnamese context.

After the process of 'training-of-trainers' described above and through the activities of union members and health workers, the flow of preventive health information is supposed to be eventually channelled to the wider public. As was briefly mentioned on the topic of diarrhoea, the dissemination of preventive health messages to the public is based on face-to-face communication through household visits. The frequency of these visits is vaguely described by health officers and local cadres to take place "with every given opportunity". However, interviewees from rural and urban communities in Phong Dien and Cai Rang districts described this interaction with "health communicators" as small interventions performed by local cadres, who drop by their households to in-

[146] The consumer-research stage in a hand-washing promotion project, for example, refers to the research work done before designing the material and executing the campaigns. Such research is trying to identify and assess the existing motivations, restrictions and preferences of the targeted audience.

spect how well they comply with certain practical public health instructions[147], but rarely ever discussing more on the risk and the prevention of disease. As a result, in best case, the public will receive unconnected information on practices that they should follow, without having much explanation on why they should do so. Therefore, it is questionable whether the understanding and behaviour that people end up shaping about a disease like diarrhoea have much in common with the central guidelines that frame its prevention.

6.3.3 Content and quality of the produced messages

There are different levels of accuracy and explanation in the content of communication material used in disease prevention. A number of published samples of this material on diarrheal disease were collected during fieldwork in Can Tho. As an exercise, samples from three types of organisations were rated for content. These included district PHCs, the PHC of the City and the CHECC. After the selection and listing 15 preventive messages around diarrheal disease that are commonly circulated by public health communication mechanisms (drawn from exemplary CHECC-produced material), each sample was analysed and rated based on these messages (Table 6.2).

Table 6.2: Selected messages related to the prevention of diarrheal disease, in documents circulated by preventive health organisations in Can Tho

- Consume cooked food and boiled water
- Wash hands before having meals and when preparing food
- Wash hands after going to the toilet
- Do not eat fish and seafood, especially not raw
- Use a hygienic toilet
- Do not defecate in open areas
- Use clean water for cooking
- Use chloramine B or alum to disinfect water
- When someone in the family gets acute diarrhoea, inform the nearest healthcare centre
- Do not eat raw vegetables
- Avoid eating out in mass servings like weddings, funerals etc.

[147] The points most often mentioned concerned the existence of bed-nets for the prevention of malaria, the avoidance of stagnant water spots and open water containers, the connection to the piped-water network and the presence of a toilet.

- Keep your latrines clean, have enough water and soap
- When getting diarrhoea, use the toilet and apply powdered lime or chloramine-b and flush with water
- Don't throw garbage or dead animals into the rivers, lakes and ponds
- Control the spread of flies

Based on material collected during fieldwork in Can Tho City, 2011

The rating was done with regard to whether samples included each of the messages and to how much explanation was provided about these messages[148]. The purpose of the exercise was to show what kind of preventive advice about diarrhoea is in circulation and how this information varies according to the organisation where it is produced encountered. One of the difficulties in this attempt was that different organisations in different administrative levels often recycle and use the same material. Thus, what was found in a district PHC had usually originated at a higher-level organisation. Nevertheless, duplications could be traced by revisiting offices and collecting material in three research phases and most of the material could be traced back to its institutional origin within the province. Although not all of the examined sample documents were of the same kind, they are seen as synergistically contributing to the formulation of messages of each type of organisation (Table 6.3).

[148] Details of the rating scores can be found in the Annex (Table 3).

Table 6.3: Information on the examined material from the different organisation types

Source	#	Type of material (# of each)
Distr. PHC	5	Training material - WSS - staff in the district (2) Radio reading text - public health (1) Recommendations - prevention of diarrhoea (1) Food safety instructions - staff and public (1)
PHC Can Tho City	3	Booklets for training on water and hygiene related issues (2) Plan and instructions - 'food safety action month' (1)
CHECC	8	Leaflet - diarrheal disease (1) Articles - 'Health for a cultural village' magazine (5) Food safety leaflets (2)

Material collected and analysed by the author, 2011.

Overall, the results showed that the message of '*eat cooked food and drink boiled water*' prevails among the preventive messages (Fig 6.4). Regarding the topic of hygiene, the practice of hand-washing is generally emphasized but the need to use soap when washing hands is not stressed, and, if so, only implicitly (point 12). Regarding sanitation, the preventive messages seem to focus on the need to discourage open defecation (point 6) and to have hygienic toilets in the households (point 5). The promoted use of chloramine-b for disinfecting water and the advice of seeking medical care in case of diarrheal disease were also quite prominently present in the overall content of the material. In contrast, much of the food-related measures and other detailed habits of hygiene were less prioritised (points 10 – 15).

In addition to the overall trends, differences came into view regarding the prominence of messages in the three distinct types of organisations. Material coming from the CHECC was seen to guide the overall distribution, which is an expected result, as the list of messages was formulated based on this centre's material. This was particularly evident regarding information about what to do when the disease occurs (points 13) and on the importance of hand-washing after defecation (point 3). The messages coming from the provincial PHC, in contrast, focus primarily on sanitation and the use of clean water (points 5-8 and 14).

Figure 6.4: Frequencies of messages mentioned in the material from the three organisation types

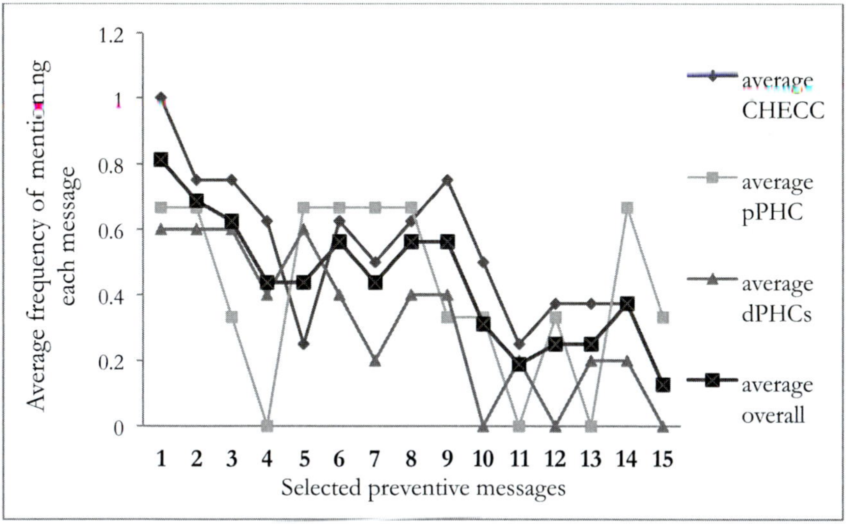

y = number of documents with a mention/total number of documents collected in each level. x= reference to the selected preventive messages, as listed in table 6.2. (pPHC= provincial PHC, dPHC= district PHC)

Considering the emphasis on sanitation (see chapter 5) and the particularly high budget that the WSS sector receives in comparison to other preventive health priorities (see section 6.3.1), this finding is not surprising. It is expected that the topic of WSS development would be even more represented if material coming from CERWASS was also taken into account. However, since CERWASS is mostly responsible for the technical side of solutions, rather than for the 'software' of hygienic behaviour measures (Rheinländer et al., 2010), material from CERWASS was not included in this analysis. The promotion of hygienic toilets (point 5) was also seen to be overly emphasized at the district level, the trend of which was noticeable similar to the average overall, in how topics were prioritised, but in a much lower frequency. In other words, the district level material was found to be inclusive but more fragmented in relation to the messages it produces about diarrheal disease.

The institutional origin of the material was distinctive not only in the diversity of topics (which decreases in number successively from the CHECC to dPHC), but also in the extent of explanation that it involves. The majority of the messages were poorly framed as bullet-point instructions of 'does and don'ts'. The exceptions to this were the well-written and informed articles of the 'Health for a Cultural Village' magazine and some training booklets provided by UNICEF[149]. The latter, however, were only found at the provincial-level PHCs, as the cost of their reproduction and wider distribution was claimed to be too high for the preventive health budget to be able to cover. Curtis et al. (2000) suggest that it is wise to be frugal with preventive health resources, for example by saving funds for transmitting the most essential messages about health. However, what can be seen in Can Tho is an oversimplification of diarrhoea-related messages during their journey from experts to trainers and to the public, resulting in a mere set of instructions with minimal educational quality, which can hardly be said to be well received and essential.

Apart from the limited explanation and the commanding tone that prevails in many of the communicated health messages, many of them also contradict aspects of the Vietnamese culture. For example, it would be a challenge to follow the advice not to eat fish and raw vegetables (point 4 and 10), which are a staple component of the Vietnamese diet, and not to dine outside in social events and celebrations (point 11), which is very common in Vietnamese social life. Facing difficulties in addressing the multiple challenges of food safety (see section 6.2.1), the state seems to resort to a prohibitive approach, which apparently goes against its the state's commitment to encourage preventive activities that are "suitable for the target groups and their cultural and national traditions" (GoV, 2007: 59). Prohibiting anything that the state cannot directly control is destined to face implementation obstacles if it goes against people's rooted habits and cultural practices. Another way in which the state ignores salient aspects of the Vietnamese culture is in the complete exclusion of Traditional Medicine from the approach against diarrheal disease. Despite the strong respect and the trust of many Vietnamese in eastern and herbal medicine, the principles, methods and remedies are not included in the official policy of preventing and curing diarrhoea and is also, needless to say, absent also from the content of the communication material.

---

149 Two such booklets were collected, entitled: 'Clean water: Personal hygiene, Family hygiene and Community hygiene' and 'Safe Water Supply and Sanitation for the Community'. They focus on guiding community-level education about water, health, hygiene, environmental sanitation and about linked behaviours through the interactive use of illustrations and provocative questions. However, such interactive usage was not reported and the representative of the PHC unit in Can Tho said that the booklets are used simply as a manual in training-of-trainers activities (14.07.11, group interview).

Awareness on diarrheal disease within health organisations

Semi-structured interviews with staff from different health organisations indicated that there are significant differences in the level of institutional knowledge that those organisations have concerning the risk and prevention of diarrheal disease. A systematic analysis was undertaken to reveal how this knowledge "travels" about the different types of organisations by comparing the responses from five administrative levels (Table 6.4).

Table 6.4: Distribution of interviewees from health organisations and offices in Can Tho

Administrative level	#	% of total interviewed	Types of institutions
the hamlet	2	4%	Health stations
the commune	4	8%	Health clinics, group gathering activity
the district	20	43%	PHCs, Offices of Health, Hospitals, Red Cross offices
the province	5	11%	PHCs, Hospitals, CHECC
the MoH	10	34%	IHPHs, DoPM, Pasteur Institutes, VIHEMA, HSPI, Medical Universities

The assessment of the responses was based on whether or not certain key aspects (Table 6.5) were mentioned, discussed and further elaborated by the respondents during the course of each interview. The selection of the nine key aspects was based on a review of the literature, with the pre-condition set that each aspect should be mentioned at least once. During the analysis of the transcripts, one point would be assigned to each interview if an aspect was mentioned at least once by the informant, either after small prompts by the researcher or spontaneously. After this was done for all the interviews, the rate of mention was calculated for each administrative level in relation to the total number of interviews that took place within this level[150]. A certain bias exists when comparing the different levels due to their very different numerical repre

[150] See Table 2 in the Annex for the detailed results of this analysis.

sentation (Table 6.4), but complementary qualitative analysis provides additional evidence and explanation about how meaningful and representative the resulting scores really are.

Table 6.5: Selected key-aspects describing a good level of awareness about the risk and the prevention of diarrheal disease

- There is a high rate of diarrhoea cases in the region
- There are different epidemiological causes and – accordingly - different symptoms
- The dehydration stages and the recommended treatments steps
- The possible means of spread (faeces-fingers–water-food-digestive system)
- There exist connections between water safety, sanitation and diarrhoea
- Intra-household hygiene is an important preventive measure
- Promoting hand-washing is an important preventive measure
- There exist connections between diarrhoea and malnutrition
- Communication and education activities are crucial for building understandings and fostering behavioural change (not only promoting WSS constructions)

The results provide an idea of the presence of these key aspects in discussions with expert authorities in Can Tho (Fig 6.5).

Figure 6.5: Scores for mentioning the key aspects of diarrheal disease risk, by administrative level

Design by the author, based on 41 semi-structured interviews with health authorities, 2011-2012

Despite its limitations, the analysis indicates indeed that higher-level institutions are relatively better informed on the topic than lower-level ones, but that this difference is not of great magnitude. The difference between the scores of interviewees from ministerial posts and those from provincial, district or commune offices was barely over 10%. Overall, staff from organisations directly under the jurisdiction of the MoH did not achieve even a 50% score in mentioning the selected key aspects. That being said, the relatively small gap between of the results from the different organisations might have been smaller if interviewees had been given the opportunity to elaborate on these key aspects more fully.

Qualitative analysis of the interview transcripts suggests that almost all interviewees in district-and-below offices and organisations (80%) avoided discussing further the significance and the interconnectedness of the key aspects. Even though awareness-raising activities were constantly mentioned as evidence of well-implemented health policy, particularly from representatives of district-level offices, when they were asked to elaborate on the content of these activities, their answers were often reduced to catch-phrases such as "boil the water and cook the food". When interviewees were encouraged to provide more explanations on the necessary preventive measures against diarrheal disease, their answers were usually incomplete and limited:

> "Diarrhoea comes mostly from water, but also from food. Clean water is a key issue to prevent it [...] Household behaviours are also important because the water is severely polluted nowadays. It is a serious matter." (Top official in the district Hospital, Cai Rang, 06.07.11; personal interview)

> "Yes, there is a relationship between the water supply situation and the water-borne diseases. Water supply alone though cannot solve the problem. The authorities have to control and guarantee the food safety of the products and goods that people consume. [After being prompted]... sanitation is also related. There aren't many people now using the fishpond toilets; the number is very small." (Top official in district PHC, Phong Dien, 21.07.11; personal interview)

At the grassroots level of the commune and the hamlet, respondents seemed more talkative and more aware of the problems that encompass the spread of diarrhoea, speaking more from experience than expertise, and using descriptions from everyday life to explain the disease's spread. Nevertheless, knowledge of the complexity of personal measures for the prevention of diarrhoea was largely absent:

> "Mostly kids get diarrhoea. I think is because of the behaviour of kids: not washing their hands, eating everything with their hands, touching the ground

and everything they have around. Also because they eat everything, they don't follow any rules. Their parents have to work to make a living so they leave them at home alone and uncontrolled. [After being prompted]... water is polluted nowadays, especially due to the untreated waste going into the river from the animal barns of the households. A large number of people don't have access to water supply and have to use river water which is polluted. They live in the rural parts which are not near the main road. They use alum to treat the water but they do not always do it properly. Some families don't have the time to boil the water and they just drink it like that. In the past, we used to have cases of cholera and typhoid but now not anymore." (Top official of a Health Clinic in rural commune, Phong Dien district, 15.09.11; personal interview)

At the provincial level, the amount of elaboration by the respondents varied significantly between respondents, ranging from extended explanatory descriptions to more restricted answers following the narrative of official regulations and guidelines, such as the following:

> "Diarrhoea is always happening, the frequency is always high and especially during the flooding and the dry season. We write and inform about it frequently." (Top official in the CHECC of Can Tho, 14.12.11; personal interview)

> "We report on malnutrition following the national regulation on malnutrition indicators issued by the Institute of Malnutrition in Hanoi. For the relationship between malnutrition and diarrhoea, we are not sure; we don't have any data or proof about that." (Top official in PHC of Can Tho, 12.12.11; group interview)

In contrast, most of the interviewees from institutes directly under the jurisdiction of the MoH willingly discussed many of the aspects that frame diarrheal disease in its complexity, being also able to trace the drawbacks and the imperatives in the policies for prevention:

> "The clinical signs between the different types of diarrhoea are very different. Diarrhoea is characterized by watery stools at least 3 times a day. Dysentery can lead to defecation up to 20-30 times per day, but with a different morphology of the stool: small, with blood and mucus [...] Food poisoning is not a disease; it describes where one got the pathogenic agent from. Usually it appears with severe abdominal pain, vomiting and maybe some diarrhoea. Usually patients come in groups within a day. When we ask them when they ate and what they had, they say they ate in the factory cantina, at a wedding party, a birthday party etc.
>
> [PK: What do you think are the main causes of diarrheal disease?]
>
> It is caused by the consumption of unclean water or food. When people are not treating food properly, not following necessary hygienic processes like handwashing, not boiling the water, using untreated water to wash the dishes etc... Also when they are not being careful with what they consume, how it was pre-

pared, or the hygienic conditions in the places they live, eat, cook, or choose to buy food from. Especially in the rural areas, where sanitation is limited, water-borne diseases really are a serious problem; people are very prone to getting them." (Top official in IHPH of Ho Chi Minh City, 28.07.11; group interview)

The noticeably increased levels of awareness that is demonstrated by the elaboration in responses such as the above, suggests that central institutions are more knowledgeable and have greater expertise. However, again, the issue of hierarchy in the country's administration and the power relations that it entails need to be considered. Being a health worker in the district or commune level, one is under the supervision of superiors at the next level of administration and is, therefore, "vulnerable" to their judgment. To contrast, ministry-level staff that are at the level of the central government wield more socio-political capital and are thus more comfortable tracing the weaknesses of central policy and the problems in implementation. During every single interview with state representatives, there was an air of discursive caution and hesitation in expressing one's opinion. This was, however, particularly conspicuous during interviews with representatives at the district and the provincial levels. The amount of explanation that informants were willing to provide was possibly not only a consequence of their awareness levels, but also of how much criticism towards the government they feel free to volunteer. Overall, it would require further investigation to discern whether the laconic nature of some answers was due to a lack of knowledge, lack of time, or was a sign of personal disinclination to further elaborate. It became clear, however, that awareness concerning the prevention of diarrheal disease is more likely to be found at the high-level organisations (where it is considered expert knowledge) than in the provincial and district authorities (where it is compartmentalised) or in the levels of the commune and hamlet (where it is rather experiential).

6.3.4 The hollow construction of a success story

The term 'awareness-raising' has been used as a banner for preventive health campaigns and the touted as the means to bring about behavioural change. However, the level of people's awareness is hard to measure without with qualitative research and extensive surveys. According to the representative of the Health Strategy and Policy Institute of the MoH, behavioural evaluation studies are mostly carried out by donor agencies, but their results are hard to translate into advice useful to local governments. This informant attributed the problems in evaluation to the lack of means for channelling such knowledge from experts to policy-makers[151]. Government officials and health representatives from provinces and districts, however, often use statistics on diarrhoea mortality, and on water supply and sanitation coverage, to discursively "measure" and evaluate awareness-raising campaigns. As it was discussed in previous chapters, this use of statistical indicators hides a lot of assumptions about the trustworthiness and representativeness of the data which often prove problematic. In other attempts to present evaluation outcomes, respondents from central offices would equate the impact and success of communicative activities with the execution of simplified activities, presenting, for example, the amount of flyers distributed or the number of training classes held as a proof of public awareness-raising.

In the few cases where interviewees did not try to paint a picture of awareness-raising success and went so far as to recognise the high incidence of diarrheal disease, they would assign the problem to people's unhygienic habits and not to the state's false approach in public health education. Interestingly, however, the respondents recognised that even though some messages reach the intended audience, they admit that they have little impact on their actual behaviours.

> "In general most of the people nowadays seam to have a better perception and a change in their level of awareness. When they are asked what they should do, they can give the right answer. When it comes to actual actions though, people still seem to stick to their habits and the results in reality are not satisfactory." (Top official in district PHC, Binh Thuy, 12.07.11; personal interview)

> "I will give you the example of the doctor that smokes... He knows that it is bad for his health, but he does it anyway; it is the power of the habit [referring to people not practicing hand-washing with soap]." (Top official in PHC Can Tho City, 14.07.11; personal interview)

The usual way to escape elaborating on such issues was to assign all related failures to the poor. The poor would be depicted as the only group that is unable to escape bad health, independently of the content or the quality of health communication efforts. Most interviewed officials would recognise that the residents of remote, rural and poor households are more vulnerable to suffer from disease, but this problem tends to be attached to the poor (as a group of people) and not to poverty (as a social phenomenon). Poor people would be described as having low hygienic standards and not willing to prioritise or pay for access to clean water and improved sanitation:

> "Those who don't follow our advice are mostly in the rural areas and it is because sometimes the conditions are unfavourable for them. For example when they don't have clean water access because the piped water system doesn't reach

---

[151] Source: Official in the National HSPI, Hanoi, 09.02.12; personal interview.

them, how are they going to protect themselves from unclean water? When people are really facing poverty problems, they don't seem to care about their health that much." (Top official in the district Office of Health, Binh Thuy, 08.07.11; personal interview)

"The poor are in a more disadvantaged position and more likely to suffer from diseases. This is so with diarrheal disease is because they cannot afford to preoccupy themselves with hygienic standards and behaviour. They face financial problems and so they don't care about their health. They know what would be better to do, but they cannot afford it, or don't bother thinking about it; they don't have good living conditions or eating and drinking habits." (Top official in district PHC, Cai Rang, 06.07.11; personal interview)

"The people know that they should use soap for washing hands but in real life they don't do that because they don't care about their health that much." (Official in PHC Can Tho City, 14.07.11; personal interview)

Firstly, these arguments contain a complete disregard of all the other preventive measures (breast-feeding, vaccinations, better hygienic behaviours in treating and storing water, etc) that the poor, just as everyone else, could adopt if they had better health education and if these measures were better supported by the state. Thus, the problem of awareness-raising about diarrhoea is falsely presented as a problem of water supply and sanitation, and in doing so portrays the poor as a vulnerable group only because they cannot invest in such constructions. Despite the amount of truth that this claim contains, it implies that the risk of diarrheal disease is avoided by those who have invested in such improvements. As it has been already demonstrated, data on WSS[152] and on the disease's spread[153] do not confirm this argument. Secondly, poor people are not presented as a group that needs more support, but as being insensitive to their own health and well-being. This way, the problem of governmental policy turns into a problem of the poor, who are maligned as dirty and indifferent and thereby become the scapegoats for state negligence.

Moreover, the blaming of the poor articulated above is based on the assumption that the public health communication mechanism is effective. The results of in-depth interviews with residents of rural and urban areas widely contradicted both the availability and the impact of this mechanism, at least concerning the issue of diarrheal disease. The role of the clinic and the health works praised by the state as reference points in health education were categorically refuted by interviewees from the rural Phong Dien district:

---

[152] See Table 5.1 in section 5.2.2 and Table 5.6 in section 5.3.1

[153] See Figures 4.9 and 4.10 in section 4.3.1

> "PK: Have you ever taken any advice as a young mother from the local clinic on any issue regarding the health of your child and in relation to diarrheal disease?
>
> "Respondent: Yes, but seldom does this happen. The commune clinic staff came to my house to ask about the baby when it was born. Each month they will come to weigh and measure the height of the kid and they will also talk to me. They ask me about the birthday of the kid, how much the kid weighs, and if there is something wrong with his health. They have never talked about how to treat diarrhoea." (Household representative HH1/mother of three, rural commune, Phong Dien district; in-depth interview)
>
> "No, there hasn't been anything like that ... Some people come here for counting the population, making a survey, and some other people will come to check about baby-mosquitoes in the house and they will show us how to kill them. They do not talk about good or bad drinking or eating habits. There is also a man that goes around the households to ask whether people are connected to the water supply network, and if not he tries to convince them. He is the man who works in the hamlet and collects money from the tap water bills. He will try to convince people to use clean water and keep their environment clean to protect themselves from disease. The commune clinic staff doesn't come here, only the hamlet leader, who is also the one managing the water supply station." (Household representative HH2/grandmother of one, rural commune in Phong Dien district; in-depth interview)

Based on the words of the interviewees, the main interaction taking place between the local communicators and the public boils down to an activity of inspection and persuasion. The fact that health workers are not actually active in discussing preventive measures with the public was not only noticed in the rural context, but also in urban areas. Respondents from Le Binh ward gave answers similar to the above, while only one of the interviewed mothers reported seeing material in circulation that included information on measures against the spread of diarrheal disease:

> "The brochures talk about the killing of mosquitoes, teaching kids to wash their hands and carefully boiling water and cooking food. The television or the radio is also a source of information, but I will not remember everything they say. If they came to the house it would be better, because I would remember and I would follow their advice. This has never happened, we only receive some brochures. I do follow the advice of boiling water, and cooking food and I also use salt-water to wash the vegetables." (Household representative HH1/mother of one, urban ward in Cai Rang district; in-depth interview)

From the words of a WU representative (quoted earlier in section 6.3.1), a change of behaviour with regard to hygiene is considered an obligation for members of the union, particularly the 3-clean model which they "are being checked on" (Top official in WU's commune branch, Phong Dien district,

19.12.11; personal interview). It was generally the case that people holding public office positions in the district or commune level would project a paradigmatic profile of their household and their family's habits, trying to reflect the requirements set in the "healthy and cultural village" policy[154]. Possibly due to the notions of social morality, unity and citizenship that the state often attaches to hygienic priorities, local cadres embody these expectations by using "healthy behaviours" as proof of their loyalty to their community and the Party. Despite their efforts to realise a successful policy implementation and to portray a functional mechanism of health education, local cadres and government representatives cannot hide the reality of a weak public health sector which leaves many people vulnerable to disease.

As it became clearer though the systematic analysis and the qualitative synthesis of results, what is being transferred from high-level departments down to the people that are facing health problems is not knowledge but feelings of superiority and supervision. The localities struggle to fulfil the prescribed targets of preventive health, charged with duties but given very little support. At the same time, local communities are very hesitant to voice concerns about the challenges that they are facing. Similar to the sector of water supply and sanitation, local cadres struggle to meet the targets on paper and often resort to disregarding key aspects in the policy's objectives, such as making health education accessible to all, reporting truthfully and benefitting the most vulnerable.

6.4 Conclusions

The Vietnamese government has aligned parts of its national legislation to world-class guidelines for the integrated prevention of diarrhoea (MoH, 2009c). Drawing evidence from Can Tho City, this chapter describes why, despite this positive step, there are still core impediments in the way of achieving success in disease prevention. The implementing mechanism was found to treat diarrheal disease in a fragmented manner, attributing its risks to separate and non-interacting spheres (of water, food, children, poverty or rurality). Failing to recognise the holistic dynamic of the problem, the state fails to appreciate the scale of the problem. The official discourse around the control of diarrhoea is serving the construction of a success story in public health to parallel that of the water supply and sanitation sector, which is, in reality, proving to be rather hollow.

---

[154] This is referring to the 'cultural and healthy village' policy, part of which is described in Box 6.2.

The main weaknesses of the approach followed can be traced to the methods and the content that are being used in health education campaigns. The principal implementers of public health communication are supposed to be the health workers and the volunteers in the communes and hamlets. Regardless of their willingness to perform those tasks, the people in these posts usually command very limited resources and have weak educational backgrounds in medicine. In most cases, the communication approach relies entirely on the training material and publications from higher-level health organisations. Regarding the availability of materials, cadres from higher-level administration would claim that they are in shortage of funds and thus cannot provide enough support to the public health mechanism at the local levels. As this chapter discussed, central funds do exist but they are received exclusively by the Preventive Health Centres (PHCs) in the provincial level. The results indicate that, in fact, hundreds of millions Vietnamese dong are assigned annually to the sectors of WSS, malaria control and food safety in Can Tho City. Based on the claims of PHC's representatives, these funds are exhausted in the annual organisation of 40 training gatherings around the province, each of which manages to invite a maximum of 50 attendants. It is therefore highly questionable whether and how the provinces actually spend the budget assigned to them for preventive health activities.

Regarding the quality of the communicated messages, research indicated that the ability to scale down scientific knowledge without reducing the essence of its content is not developed sufficiently in the case study regions. The expertise that is needed to address the issue holistically seems to fizzle out with the current system of training local trainers. With limited expertise, trainers depend on the printed material that reaches them. Examining the content of this material revealed a pattern of guiding action in a top-down manner through a bullet-point set of instructions that does not promote understanding, let alone health empowerment. Health communication becomes, in practice, a process of convincing, rather than promoting, participatory action. In fact, the channels of health-related communication are used to further promote priorities of water and sanitation constructions, paying little attention to the extent to which the public understand certain health risks and how much people actually adopt adequate preventive behaviour.

Findings further demonstrate how discourse around the risk of diarrheal disease can often be alienating and disempowering to the public. Firstly, in a process of blueprinting western biomedical science, the government's "modern" public health policy has excluded Traditional Vietnamese Medicine approaches, which many Vietnamese consider valuable and meaningful. Disassociating new approaches from the ingrained systems of understanding might have played a role in the poor engagement in preventive education that health educators have encountered. Secondly, research indicated how diarrhoea-related information can actually be felt as an obligation, and thus a burden, rather than a helping hand for the public. Given the commanding tone of preventive guidelines and through the use of politically charged language, aspects of health and hygiene are connected to values of socialism and to a sense of responsibility towards the government, the Party and the country. These notions of social morality, which are embedded in a top-down paradigm, do not leave room for health-related information to be questioned or adapted on its way to local implementation. Through the moralistic and patriarchal manner of delivering public health communication and promoting healthy practices, the state reinforces the idea that problems are solved solely through its central knowledge and expertise, without needing input and feedback from the population at the grassroots.

Despite the stability in the state's hierarchy, which is perhaps reinforced by implementing health education in this manner, the Vietnamese government risks perpetuating a situation in which a nation of people remain vulnerable to preventable disease, confused about what makes them sick and how can they best protect themselves from disease. By de-prioritising diseases of low mortality, the country compromises the everyday well-being of its people. Moreover, by not paying much attention to what the public knows, but to what the public does, Vietnam also jeopardizes the future of health literacy and is vulnerable to future emerging epidemics.

PRACTICES, PERCEPTIONS AND BEHAVIOURS AROUND DIARRHEAL DISEASE IN URBAN AND RURAL HOUSEHOLDS

CHAPTER 7

One of the main claims that have emerged from the statements of interviewed state representatives in the sector of water and health can be summarised in the assertion that the high coverage of piped water supply and hygienic sanitation facilities in urban areas demonstrates that the residents of those areas have higher levels of awareness around the risk of diarrheal disease. Interviewees further confirm that urban areas do not face problems of diarrhoea disease anymore, using official health statistics. In previous sections of this work, it was explained why the above claim is false and how accepting the assumptions behind such claims impacts health policy. Firstly, health statistics that are produced in the region do not show the actual number of diarrhoea cases and are therefore a weak basis for drawing conclusions about its distribution. Even if health statistics were seen as a valid indicator for comparing how the risk of disease is distributed in different areas, they do not show a clear differentiation between rural and urban areas (section 4.3.1). Secondly, a higher rate of access to "improved" water sources does not exactly speak of the quality of water people consume, as the latter depends on the water supplier and the intra-household practices, as well as on the complementary sources of water used by the people in the household (section 5.2). Accordingly, the presence of a toilet that rated as "hygienic" does not guarantee proper use or improved environmental sanitation in the wider community.

In the light of the institutional set-up and implementation of policy described previously, this chapter looks at how the institutional weaknesses reflect on the perceptions and the practices of the population, bringing together empirical material from in-depth and quantitative interviews at the household level. Focusing on people's behaviours, the findings illuminate the problems and the constraints that urban and rural inhabitants face in protecting themselves from disease. The following sections will show, firstly, how aspects of water access, use and treatment at the household level were encountered (7.1). The way people access, perceive and exercise "hygienic" sanitation will then also be introduced and discussed (7.2). Finally, the chapter examines the ideas that people have about the source of diarrheal disease and the strategies that they follow in order to prevent and treat it (7.4).

7.1 The complex diversity of water use and treatment

Having previously discussed the spectrum of options that people have in terms of water supply, this section reviews the real-life situation of 131 households in Can Tho[155]. The collection of data not only documented their primary water sources, but also drew attention to the various simultaneous water strategies and treatment methods that were followed in each household. Compared to officially generated data and discourse, the results clearly portray how complex and diverse water usage is in the region, underlining the need for more support, not only in the form of infrastructure but also in the form of information on water treatment and safety.

7.1.1 Household water sources and water preferences

The results of the household survey point to the diversity and flexibility concerning people's water use strategies that prevail among households in both rural and urban areas. Most people claim to use more than one source, including rainwater, tap water, groundwater, surface water and bottled water. These water strategies shift slightly between the dry and rainy seasons, but not to an extreme extent. Questions regarding the source of water, as well as regarding its treatment methods and its storage, were asked separately for drinking water and for daily-use water. As illustrated below (Fig 7.1 and 7.2), some water sources are used widely for both purposes (noticeably piped supply and well water), while others are mostly designated for drinking (see bottled water and rainwater).

The statistics produced by CERWASS on the rate of piped supply connections in Can Tho (50-60%) and the total percentage of households using river water, whether "hygienic" or not (30%), do not seriously contradict the results of this household survey (CERWASS, 2011a, CERWASS, 2010). However, there is a significant difference between the official data and the survey on the issue of rainwater use. Specifically, according to CERWASS, the rate of rainwater use is in the scale of 3% (Ibid. 2010 & 2011), which diverges from the results of the survey showing rainwater use as high as 30.5% (with some seasonal variability, and mostly for drinking purposes).

---

[155] For more details on the household survey, see the section "Trajectory of Fieldwork Methodology" in the Annex.

Figure 7.1: Distribution of responses on the water sources used for drinking, by season

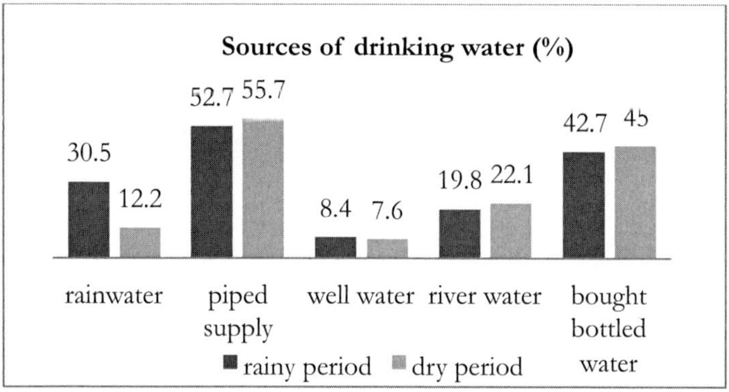

Multiple-answer question (N=131). Data from household survey, 2011

Figure 7.2: Distribution of responses on the water sources used for daily-use, by season

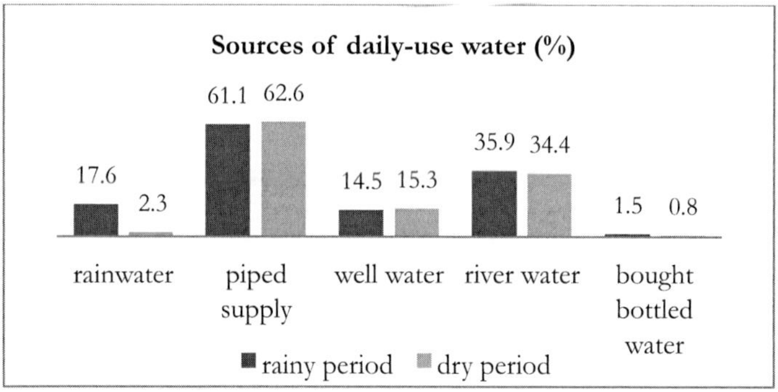

Multiple-answer question (N=131). Data from household survey, 2011

CERWASS reports a very low percentage of rainwater use probably because rainwater collection is a complimentary strategy and thus rarely captured by CERWASS's surveys, which report only the main water sources (see also section 5.2.2). The rate of households using well water in the survey was also found to be quite different from what is captured in the CERWASS reports (15% versus 27.4%, respectively). What can explain this difference is the illegal state of many wells, which might make people hesitant to reveal their presence to the researcher. CERWASS enumerators, unlike the researcher, are expected to have the authority to inspect each household's premises and reveal the presence of such wells.

Given the insistence of state representatives to discuss water access and the prevalence of disease on the basis of urban and rural administrative divisions, the above answers were also analysed by region. Since there were no significant changes observed in the use of water sources between the rainy and dry periods, except a decrease in the use of rainwater in the dry season, the analysis was based on the answers given concerning the rainy season. The results showed that although most households appeared to have good access to piped water connections (63%), either through a water company (urban) or one of the CERWASS mini-supply stations (rural), this rate was not equally distributed in the two case studies. While most of the urban households were connected to the central water network, less than half of the rural ones had access to CERWASS-provided piped water (Fig 7.3).

Figure 7.3: Distribution of households with piped water supply in the rural and urban study regions

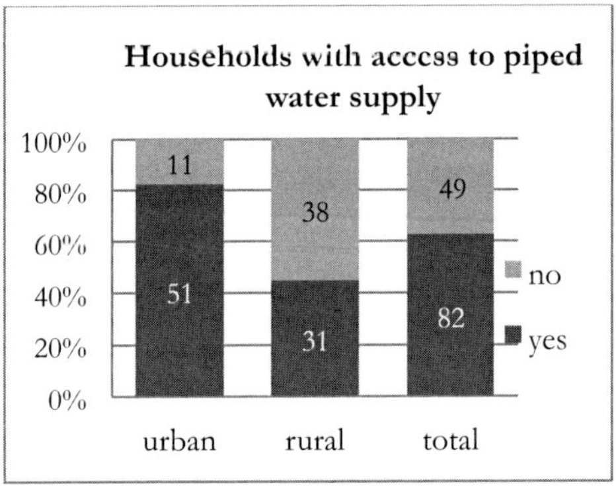

Numbers in the bars are absolute numbers of responses (N=131). Data from household survey, 2011

Comparing the two sets of answers concerning the access to piped water and its use particularly for drinking, it appears that while piped water is accessed by 63% of respondents, it is used as a primary drinking source only by 55.7% of them. Of the 82 households that claimed to have access to piped water, some stated that they also drink bottled water (34), rainwater (17), well water (5) or even river water (6); this indicates that some actually do not prefer to drink piped water. These results can be better explained when looking at each household's location and thus, the type of piped water that they have access to. Most of the households supplied by the Cai Rang Water Company (98%) indeed choose to drink the piped water. On the other hand, the percentage of people drinking the water provided by CERWASS is only 68%, making it clear that the quality of piped water provided in the rural areas is not preferred (or trusted) for drinking. Considering the water quality results that were obtained from secondary literature (section 5.2.3), this behaviour can be seen as wise.

The interviewed residents from rural areas seem to compensate for their lower use of piped water with drinking more rainwater, well water and river water (Fig 7.4). Urban residents, on the contrary, seem to use these sources significantly less. The exception to this were the poor people living in the "floating houses" in Yen Binh urban area, who do not have access to piped water. While the survey did not capture the exact financial situation of the families interviewed, observations and qualitative documentation made it clear that the majority of households without access to piped or well water were families belonging to the poorer part of the population (even if they were not always officially classified as poor)[156]. As it was discussed before, people that face financial problems are particularly hesitant to invest in piped water connections, especially when a cheaper solution is available. Such choices often depends more on the costs than on the actual quality of each source's water (section 5.2.1). As the collection of rainwater or river water requires only a storage jug for year-long supply, it is of no surprise that people in "floating houses" and in the poorer parts of rural areas tend to exercise more these practices than their better-off urban counterparts.

---

[156] It is described in the Annex (Trajectory of Fieldwork – Household Survey - sample selection) that the selection of poor, nearly-poor and 'average' households was not only made on the basis of official classifications of poverty, but also on the advice provided by local cadres and on personal observations from the case study areas. This manner of selection owed partly to findings indicating how fuzzy the process of official poverty classification really is (Box 4.2 in section 4.2.2) and how challenging collecting data on people's incomes proved to be (especially when considering the complex ways of distributing income among the members of a household and extended family and various informal and unstable income sources that are hard to define). Overall, the official classification of poor households was often found to contradict with the observed reality. For these reasons, unless otherwise specified, the mention of "poor" in this chapter is not only based on official classifications but also on research observations and on interviewees' own attestations.

Figure 7.4: Distribution of water sources for drinking in rural and urban households

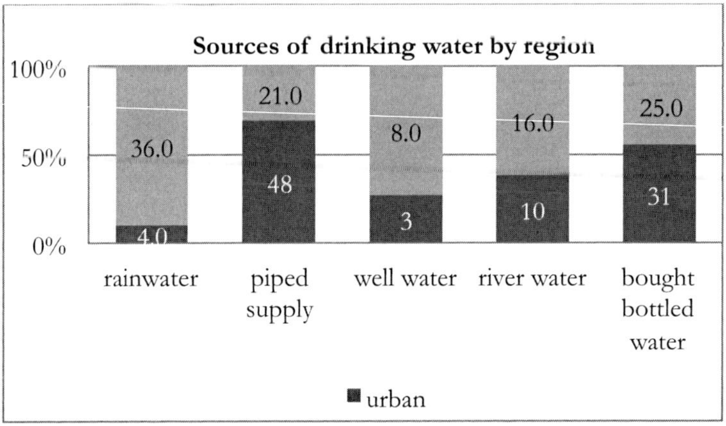

Numbers in the bars are absolute numbers of responses to a multiple-answer question (N=131). Data from household survey, 2011

The purchase of bottled water was found to be a very common practice (Fig 7.1), despite its high price and the unsafe production standards often discussed in the media. Bottled water for drinking was almost equally popular in rural and urban areas (Fig 7.4), but also between households that had access to piped water and those that did not (crosstabs analysis). A detailed look in the results of the household survey showed that, actually, many of the rural and urban poor tend to buy bottled water for drinking. According to these respondents, however, bottled water is mostly a complementary source for times when river water is too dirty or when rainwater is no longer available. With regard to drinking water preferences, bottled water was the third preference (12.2%), while piped water was the first (Fig 7.5). The question above was intended to capture people's preference and desires without taking into account constraints of practical nature. It aimed to understand which water sources people value the most. In general, however, respondents were rather despairing when justifying their answers, claiming for example that "we have no other choice [other than river water]" or that "this [piped water] is the type of water that we get here, and it is good". There was, therefore, an observed difficulty of people conceptually separating their desired preferences from their realistic constraints.

Figure 7.5: Distribution of given answers regarding the most preferred drinking water source

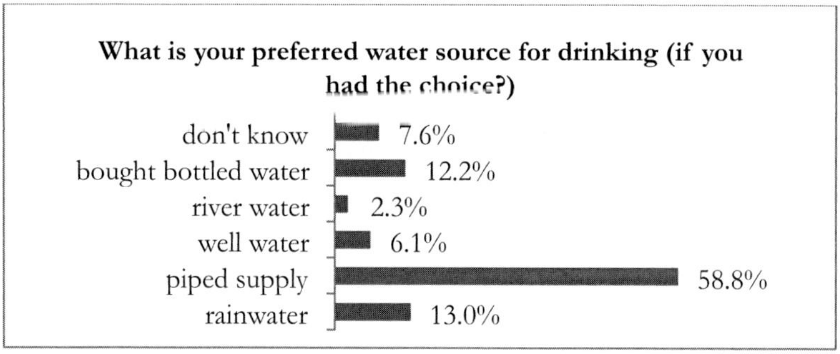

Data from household survey, 2011

Some might have had the impression that the researcher was somehow able to realise their expressed desires for water supply and thus there was a tendency, especially from those without access to tap water, to eagerly claim their preference for it and to explain how useful this would be for their daily activities. These attitudes are particularly indicative of the constraints that many people face in accessing a year-long piped supply and of their dependence on external support. Many would also describe their water choices as a matter of habit, convenience, or socially-induced influence ("other people do it"). Altogether, 31% of the respondents did not refer in any way to a source's quality or safety when justifying their water options (see also section 7.3.1).

Apart from its source, drinking water quality is considerably shaped by the way it is collected and stored in the households before consumption. Literature has suggested that one of the practices defining the quality of stored water is the covering of the storage jugs (section 5.2.3). Therefore, the habits defining how storage vessels are kept and how they are covered were also surveyed. In most of the households, vessels were being kept outside of the main house (67.9%). However, the limits of 'inside' and 'outside' were sometimes hard to position, as the back parts of many households (usually the kitchen) were open to the yard and did not have a built floor. This means that, in some cases, the water vessels were claimed to be "inside" while they were actually in an external environment, exposed to dust, insects, domestic animals and weather conditions such as flooding. Regardless of where they were placed, the majority of the vessels were said to be kept well-covered (84%). However, in the households where direct observations of the vessels were possible, findings would often contradict the given answers and vessels would be be visibly half-covered or completely open. Of all the different types of vessels that were used for storing drinking water, clay jugs were the most likely to be well-covered (with special sealing lids), while other types of vessels would, more often than not, be only loosely covered with pieces of plastic, or not covered at all (Picture 7.1)

Picture 7.1: Jugs and containers used to store water for drinking purposes in the rural case study

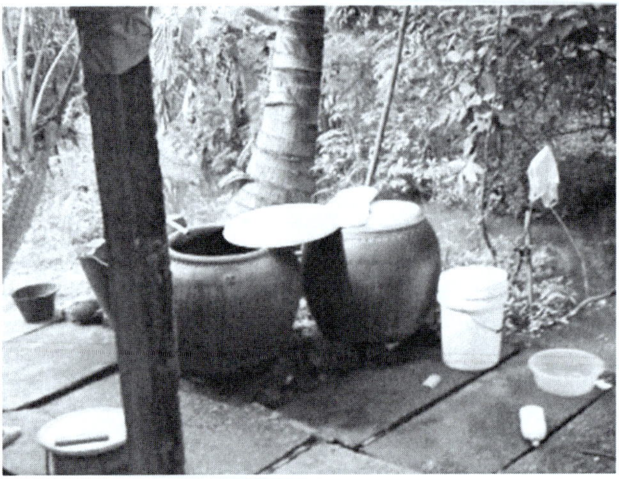

Pictures by author, 2011

Clay jugs are used for various types of water, but mostly for the long-term storage of rainwater. This explains why clay jugs were also mostly present in rural areas. The study of Özdemir et al. (2011) in the Mekong Delta showed that the number of clay jugs each family owned was linearly connected to their monthly income levels, showing how jugs also become a commodity that is not easily accessed by everyone. Despite their relatively high price, however, they are - by far - preferred to other vessels due to the pleasant taste they give to the water (Ibid. 2011). As discussed before (section 5.2.3), water that is being stored in clay jugs is prone to external contamination which can abruptly changes its hygienic state (Tran Hong Phuoc Tai, 2009, Wilbers, 2012). With rainwater being a very popular water source among rural residents (Fig 7.1) and clay jugs being one of the most preferred storage means, the use and maintenance of the latter, proves of great importance regarding water safety in the rural areas.

7.1.2 Drinking-water treatments

Even though there are not many options regarding home-based water treatments, the manner in which they are applied can differ between households and for each water source. Moreover, not every member of every household seems to apply these methods in the same manner. Considering that most households are also using more than one water sources for drinking, evaluations of water quality at the point of consumption are difficult to make. The analysis, therefore, focused on the water treatments applied to the primary source of drinking water, excluding bottled water (to which treatments are never applied), at the household level (Table 7.1).

Table 7.1: Types of water treatment methods applied to the primary drinking source in each household

	Rainwater	Piped supply	Well water	River water
Alum	2.5%	*not used*	54.5%	92.3%
Cloth filter	57.5%	*not used*	*not used*	*not used*
Purifying machine	10.0%	15.9%	9.1%	*not used*
Boiling	55.0%	92.8%	54.5%	84.6%
Chemical disinfection	*not used*	1.4%	*not used*	3.8%

*The rates (%) are: people using (x) method/people using (y) primary drinking water source * 100. Data from household survey, 2011

The results show that the people carefully treats drinking water, with almost all of the respondents claimed to apply some method of treatment before consumption. Most people said that they boil water for drinking (113/131), which significantly reduces the chance of microbial contamination. Nevertheless, a more careful analysis of the results showed that while people are consistently careful to boil river water (84.6%) and tap water (92.8%), this is not the case with well-water (54.5%) or rainwater (55%), which the many do not filter, flocculate or boil before consumption.

Worryingly, wells are easily exposed to surface pollution, which can enter the reservoir due bad construction or improper maintenance. This often renders well-water unhygienic at the source (Thang, 2002, Nuber and Stolpe 2008 cited in Fortier, 2012), a dynamic that has been observed also in the Delta (section 5.3.2). Consuming untreated well-water is, therefore, highly risky for this small - but significant - percentage of people who use it for drinking (Fig 7.1). Apart from not applying the recommended treatments, respondents also claimed to intentionally leave well-water in uncovered containers or buckets, in order for it to "air"[157], a practice that possibly has further negative effects on its quality. A similar set of risks arises in the consumption of rainwater, as only 57.5% of the respondents mentioned the use of a cloth filter during collection and only 55% considered boiling rainwater to be a necessary treatment before its consumption (Table 7.2). Previous research in Can Tho by Köster (2008: 52), has found an even lower percentage of people boiling rainwater before drinking it (46%), confirming the health risks that surround its consumption.

When comparing the results from rainwater and well-water, it appears that people who apply a primary treatment, like filtering rainwater with a cloth or flocculating well-water with alum, would not necessarily boil water before drinking it. Categorically, well-water that has been treated with alum is also boiled if it is destined for drinking. This, however, was not true for rainwater (crosstabs analysis). Moreover, the number of households applying both treatments before drinking was rather small (6-7 for each source) and thus, insufficient for concluding whether there is a behavioural correlation between initial filtering and boiling water for drinking. Regarding other treatment methods, the survey showed that chemical disinfectants such as chloramine-b or purifying (Aquatab) tablets are not commonly used. Similarly, purifying appliances with incorporated sand micro-filters were regarded as expensive and thus rather scarce among the interviewed households (Table 7.1).

Surprisingly, although the tap water that is provided through a piped water network has already undergone some disinfection (chlorination), the vast majority of respondents claimed to boil tap water before drinking it (92.8%). One of the interviewees commented on this practice:

---

[157] By "airing" water, respondents mean that water would be left in an open container so that most of its surface would be exposed to open air and the "bad smell" would disappear. The "bad smell" was referring to the odour of sulphur or aluminium that groundwater often carries. "Airing" would also be applied to tap water, either from CERWASS or from central supply, in order to remove the unpleasant "chemical" smell of chlorine.

"When my household was first connected to the water mini-station, the running water was impure and I could see the dirt settling at the bottom of the storage vessel. Then, together with other people, we decided we had to boil the water before drinking it and now most people do. The messages from the television and the radio have enhanced this practice a lot by repeating the motto of 'boil your water before drinking'." (Household representative HH3, Phong Dien district 21.12.11; in-depth interview)

It is important to note how the above respondent evaluates water quality based on visual indicators. After the water's quality is identified as low (due to turbidity), an imperative to apply the state-promoted advice of treating the water arises. Similar to tap water, the rates of treatment with alum (92.3%) and boiling (84.6%) were high also for river-water. Microbiological analyses from the region have shown that these methods can significantly reduce the loads of pathogens in river water, if applied correctly (Vo Thi Yen Phi, 2010: 85). Although most state officials maintain that these practices are universal applied[158], many experts and local health workers share different opinions:

"A lot of people, especially in the Delta, have the traditional habit of using surface water to cover their needs of water consumption and daily activities. Now they still do it, but the water is polluted. Most people just treat the water with alum and do not even boil it before using it." (UNICEF representative, Ho Chi Minh City, 29.07.11; personal interview)

"A lot of people do not have access to water supply stations and have to use river water, which is polluted. They live in the rural areas and not near a main road where the station can easily deliver water. So, they use alum to treat the water, but they do not always do it properly. Some families do not have the time to boil the water and they just drink it like that." (Top official of a Health Clinic in rural commune, Phong Dien district, 15.09.11; personal interview)

If common assessments of water purity (or impurity) rely on visual indications (like turbidity), then persistent habits such as not boiling rainwater or well-water can be better understood. Rainwater and well-water are usually not as muddy and turbid as is the water in the canals or the water provided by the CERWASS station (which has flowed through badly maintained, dirty pipes). The same principles of evaluating water purity might explain why river water is often treated with alum to get rid of visual impurities (particles settle) but is then not usually boiled before consumption. Questions of water quality perception and the kind of health risks that are associated with water consumption are dis-

---

158 Source: Top official in the Red Cross branch of Phong Dien district, 07.09.2011; personal interview.

cussed in following parts of this chapter (6.3). The analysis generally indicates that people's senses (sight, odour and taste) are more determinative of their water treatment practices than is the circulated information on water quality and safety.

The results indicate that there is a somewhat confused public awareness regarding the health risks that certain water choices and practices entail. Some respondents were very strict with the habit of filtering and boiling water before drinking. Some others would make tea with unfiltered water or would drink water that has not been boiled. Some of the claimed constrains in applying water treatments were the costs and the time required for treatment:

> "When we have the time we will boil the water [tap or rain] but if we are coming back tired from the field, we won't bother." (Household representative P35, Phong Dien district; personal interview)

> "If I don't have wood, I don't boil tap water, I just drink it like that." (Household representative N9, Phong Dien district; personal interview)

In other cases, people expressed different sorts of beliefs about making water safe to drink, indicating that there are still many misunderstandings on how and why water treatments improve the quality of water:

> "I will sometimes add some boiled water to the vessel where I keep rainwater to kill the worms." (Household representative A11, Phong Dien district; survey interview)

> "I add some special type of mushrooms in the jug in order to clean the water." (Household representative, T20, Phong Dien district; survey interview)

The survey results are based on what the respondents *said* they do. It is probable that this might not have always been truthful or fully accurate[159]. A number of observations showed, for example, that tea is brewed and not boiled; thus, the disinfecting impact of it might not be thorough. Moreover, the amounts of alum that are being used to treat water differ widely from one household to the other and are often not enough.

Generally, it can be concluded that urban residents with piped water face the lowest risk of waterborne diarrhoea, since they mainly use tap water which they tend to boil before consumption. On the contrary, rural inhabitants often rely

---

159 Respondents were often under pressure, when local cadres also attended the interview. The observed tendency was that respondents would try to give the perceived "best" answers and claim to perform "optimal" behaviours.

on sources other than piped water and do not consider the careful application of disinfecting treatments that are equally necessary for all the different water sources. The poor - in either rural or urban areas - are usually not in a position to freely make choices about water access and are usually dependent on surface water, with a complementary seasonal consumption of bottled water

7.1.3 Water for daily use

As it was demonstrated before, the sources of water used for daily activities follow roughly the same patterns as drinking water, with a comparatively higher use of river-water and well-water compared to rainwater and bottled water (Fig 7.2). The majority of households that had piped-water supply use this for all of their main types of daily activities. Households without this access use mostly water from a well or from the river (Fig 7.6). There was not a great difference between water source used for each of the daily activities and it seems, therefore, that once a source of water is assigned for daily usage, it covers all of the household's needs. There was only a small tendency to use rainwater for cooking and cleaning the food/kitchen from a few households, while using another source for showering or washing hands. Moreover, it was made clear that when access to surface water is easy, independent of what types of water people used for other daily activities (Fig 7.6), river water would be the used for cleaning the floor.

Figure 7.6: Usage of different water sources for the various daily-use purposes

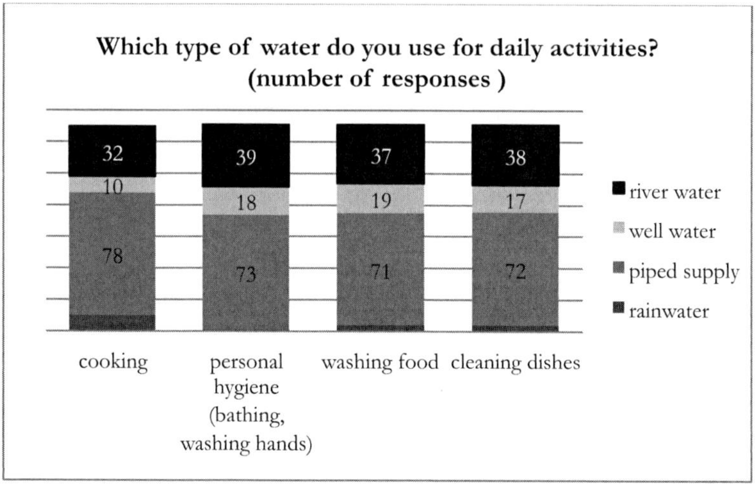

Data from household survey, 2011

Regarding the water treatments applied, survey results indicate that tap water is generally considered to be safe enough for daily usage and is not treated any further (Fig 7.7). River water, on the contrary, was seen as polluted and thus, always treated with alum by the majority of the respondents. However, there were some people who said they never treat their river water. Similar to what was found for drinking purposes, almost half of those using well-water or rain-water for daily use purposes will not apply any primary treatment to it (alum or cloth filter, respectively).

Figure 7.7: Frequency of followed treatment practices for daily-use water, by source

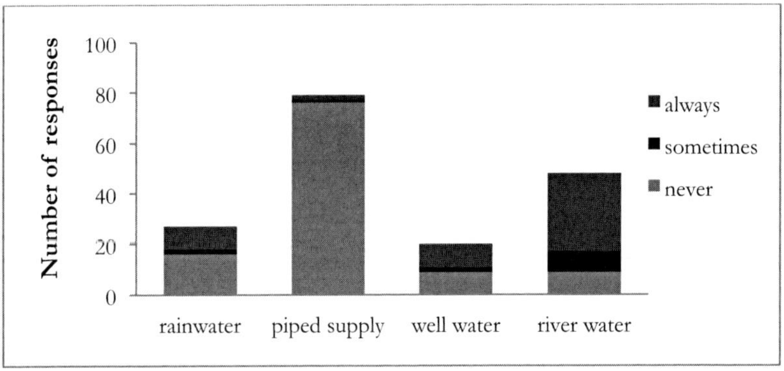

Data from household survey, 2011

When analysing data comparatively (i.e. by crosstabs analysis), it became apparent that the people who applied treatments to well-water or rainwater for daily usage also applied these treatments before using the water for drinking. As observations from the households confirmed, this is due to the fact that all the collected (rain or well) water is treated and kept in one container, from where it is used for either daily activities or drinking. As it was discussed earlier, the boiling of water before drinking is more likely to take place in the case of well-water and was less likely for rainwater. Overall, it seems that concerning these two water sources, public awareness is rather mixed and confused regarding their water quality at-source, as well as the risks involved consuming them untreated.

7.1.4 A web of waterborne risks of disease

The region of the Delta presents a great diversity of water source choices and behaviours, which became only partly visible through data presented so far.

Apart from the different strategies of water access that are followed by each household, there is also quite a variety of water behaviours within each household. Many sources of water can be in use concurrently in a household and can change according to season and the habits of each family member. Taking the case of a rural household that depends on river or well water, for example, it is likely that water will be stored in one vessel, whether for daily use or for drinking. According to the previously discussed findings, alum will then be most probably used to flocculate the impurities in that vessel. Some of the family members might choose to drink this water without applying any further treatment because they think it is safe enough, or because they have no time to boil it. Apart from the health risks of directly consuming untreated water, significant health concerns arise when untreated river - or well - water is used for showering, cleaning fruits and vegetables that are eaten raw, and washing kitchen utensils or making tea; all of these practices that were common among the respondents

However, these types of water behaviours seem to change with the season, following perceptions of water safety. A number of respondents[160] described how, during the period of the year when the tide is high, and there is a lot of new water in the river canals, they will shower or wash their vegetables with surface water because they believe that this water is then fresh and clean. During the dry and low-tide months of May and June, on the other hand, people say that river water is of very low quality and would thus treat it with alum before using it for these kinds of activities. Likewise, many people choose to drink rainwater during the wet season, but switch to bottled water after the stored rainwater stored supply has been exhausted in the dry season. This was especially true for those rural households without access to piped supply and which did not have enough storage capacity to save more rainwater for the dry period. However, some respondents said they drink bottled water even if they have CERWASS-supplied water access, which makes clear the distinction between availability and preference. Households located in the urban areas that had access to central water supply, however, tend to be more consistent in their exclusive use of tap water for drinking and for other activities, both because it is convenient but also because they trust the quality more.

Water behaviours can vary between members of the same household due to their diverse daily habits. Children spend much of their time at school while grown-ups might work in offices or at the rice-field, with each accessing differ-

[160] Sources: Household representatives P15, P16 and P23; personal interviews.

ent types of water. Trying to understand the risk of waterborne disease by only evaluating the primary source for each household is thus oversimplifying their complex lifestyles. The trend that emerges through research observations and the responses of local people, however, showed that most of the water used for daily-use, and much of what is used for drinking, is not being properly treated. Thus, the purity of the water is not guaranteed and the risk of diarrheal disease is increased. According to the results, well water and rainwater prove to be of particular concern for public health, as their treatment and storage are much dependent on each household's capacities and behaviours. While the preventive message of "boil the water" seems to have become ingrained in the minds of rural and urban inhabitants, it appears to be conceptually connected only to piped and river water, but not to rain or well water. Despite the diversity that exists in the way water is collected, treated, used and consumed, it is worth underlining how the latter two water sources deserve more attention in terms of health education, in order to better prevent the risk of waterborne diseases such as diarrhoea.

7.2 Sanitation realities

Previous chapters discussed the difficulties faced by most people in the region of the Delta and in Can Tho with regard to the construction and maintenance of sanitary facilities. This section presents empirical findings that not only illuminate their geographical coverage, but also the concept of safe sanitation that local residents have based their claims and practices upon. The analysis unfolds by looking at the differences between the type of sanitation that people prefer, those that they can access and those which they are actually using.

7.2.1 Household sanitation and community hygiene

The household survey results revealed a distribution of sanitation types similar to what was documented by CERWASS for the whole of Can Tho City (see sector 5.3.1). Septic tank latrines were found to be the most prevalent toilet type (31%), but the number of people practicing open defecation (including in river toilets, fishpond toilets and no toilet at all) was much higher than expected: 46%. Indeed, the number of people using a fishpond toilet was almost the same as those owning a pour-flush toilet or a pit latrine (Fig 7.8), suggesting at the gravity of the problem in the region.

The analysis of the results by region demonstrates that only 14 of the 62 urban households did not have a hygienic latrine. Most of these 14 households were floating houses of Yen Binh area (see section 3.2). One might argue that the urban "floating" households are not representative of urban inhabitants. However, their inclusion in this study was intentional and meant to emphasize the existing problem of urban poverty, a problem that is not exclusive to Yen Binh, but exists throughout the Mekong Delta.

Figure 7.8: Total rates of different sanitation types in households of the two case-studies

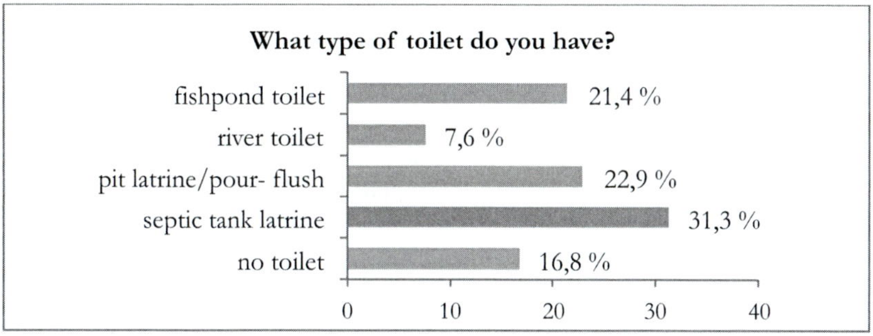

Data from household survey, 2011

Since open defecation in the region is mostly connected to surface water, it demands the presence of a fishpond or direct access to a river or canal. Considering the high price of land in the urban areas and the tendency to construct houses more and more inland, open defecation is becoming increasingly impractical for urban residents. Of the interviewed households with direct access to a canal or the river, 64% were rural (in Phong Dien district) and only 35% were urban (in Cai Rang) (Table 7.2). This matches the percentage of people that practiced open defecation, including those who declared having "no toilet". Overall, there was a tendency for fishpond toilets to be mostly located in rural areas. This by no means implies that all the urban residents maintain hygienic sanitation facilities (Table 7.3).

Table 7.2: Cross-tabulation of the variables "proximity to canal" and "type of toilet"

Proximity to canal	Type of toilet							
	No toilet	Septic tank	Pit/ pour flush	River toilet	Fish-pond toilet	total	rural	urban
no data	9	5	3	1	4	22	22	0
Yes	12	18	15	5	23	73	47	26
No	1	18	12	4	1	36	0	36

Number of responses. Data from household survey, 2011

Table 7.3: Distribution of toilet types in the urban and the rural case study

	Type of toilet				
	No toilet	Septic tank	Pit/ pour flush latrine	River toilet	Fishpond toilet
Rural	19	12	10	1	27
Urban	3	29	20	9	1
Total	22	41	30	10	28

Number of responses. Data from household survey, 2011

Merely abolishing open defecation is not enough to ensure proper sanitation in the community or to mitigate public health risks, even in urban areas. Many constructions that can be nominally called "hygienic" by their owners, because they carry some characteristics of a septic tank or a pour-flush latrine, are actually unsafe because they do not store or dispose of faeces properly. When asked which type of toilets they own, respondents would often reply with abstract terms, saying that they have "hygienic" or "flush" latrines. These descriptions, however, did not speak to any technical details or hygienic standards. In order to cross-check the accuracy of the answers, a question regarding the disposal of sewage was also posed to each respondent. The questions probing the issue of open defecation verify each other across the two sets of answers (Fig 7.8 and Fig 7.9). Results show that only 45% from the expected 54% (pit latrine, pour flush latrine and septic tank latrine users) actually have a sewage collection tank.

The rest (9%) of the "hygienic" toilet owners are likely to be disposing of their sewage directly into the river stream (see also section 5.3.1).

Figure 7.9: Rates of different disposal methods of sewage by households in the two case-studies

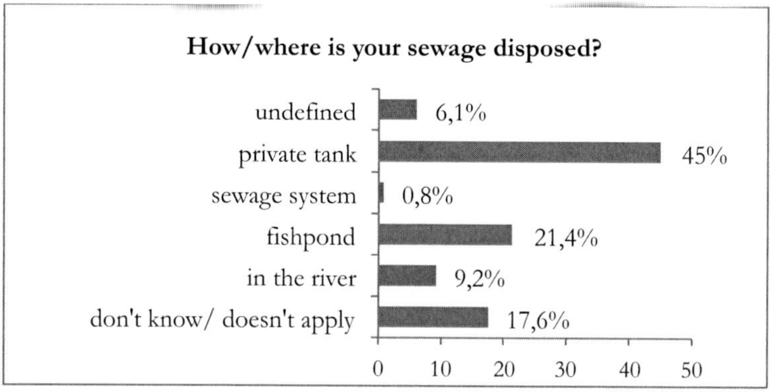

Data from household survey, 2011

Only one respondent openly admitted that their "hygienic" facility had serious technical shortages:

> "We have a tank that keeps the solid faeces and the rest goes into the river. This is not a septic tank, because that would cost five million [VND] to construct. This type of construction costs one million only." (Household representative P62, Cai Rang district; survey interview)

Looked at collectively, more than half of the respondents in the study areas seem to contribute to the contamination of surface water sources, posing a significant risk to the environmental hygiene of their communities. A study from the coastal provinces of Vietnam by Sijbesma et al. (2010) found that such polluting practices are very common. This was confirmed for various provinces of the Mekong Delta, by experts who discussed how untreated sewage disposal is contributing to the deterioration of the river's water quality, especially in its small canals and in areas with a slower water flow and limited water circulation[161].

[161] Source: Water quality expert, University of Can Tho 30.06.11; personal communication

Even in cases when a proper septic tank is in place to collect the sewage, the issue of emptying this tank and managing its content eventually arises. Having the tank emptied would demand a contract with the Urban Works Company of Can Tho and a payment of three million VND (105 Euros) by each household. Firstly, this can constitute a considerable expense that people will try to avoid. Secondly, the big collection trucks cannot reach the households in remote rural areas, since there are no suitable roads for them to follow. Local authorities have in the past avoided addressing this foreseeable problem (Reis and Mollinga, 2012). Recently interviewed CERWASS officials suggested that sealing of the tanks that are full and the constructing new ones would be "an easy solution" (30.06.11, group interview). However, seeing how many households struggle financially to meet the expenses of constructing one tank, any additional costs do not appear to be as "easy" as the cadres present it to be. It was claimed by a water expert in the region that, under normal use, a single household owned septic tank would need more than eight years to fill up[162]. None of the interviewed families have needed to empty their tanks so far and therefore it appears that this problem is deferred to the future.

7.2.2 Sanitation ideas and preferences

The problems of bad sanitation do not go unnoticed by the local residents. The majority of respondents (53%) expressed a desire to improve their sanitation situation, including almost all of those who practice open defecation. Of those owning a latrine already, 63% of the pour-flush or pit latrine owners asserted satisfaction with their situation and did not express any desire to upgrade or change their facilities. This satisfaction was even more widespread among septic tank latrine owners (85%). The reasons why people did not initiate improvements or construction of a new and better and hygienic sanitary facility, even though they wanted one, were predominantly financial (Table 7.4).

[162] Source: NGO expert in Water Supply and Sanitation, 11.12.11; personal interview.

Table 7.4: Cross tabulation of present sanitation situation and declared constraints in changing

Type of toilet (present situation)	Constraints in changing				Total
	don't know	financial	not necessary	other	
no toilet	1	19	0	2	22
septic tank latrine	1	5	33	2	41
pour flush/pit latrine	0	6	16	8	30
in the river	0	7	0	3	10
fishpond toilet	0	22	2	4	28
Total	2	59	51	19	131

Number of given responses from the household survey, 2011

Data from household survey, 2011

When respondents were asked directly which type of toilet which they consider the most pleasant and preferable to use, most said listed the "hygienic latrine" (Fig 7.10).

Figure 7.10: Rates of preference for different toilet types among households in the two case-studies

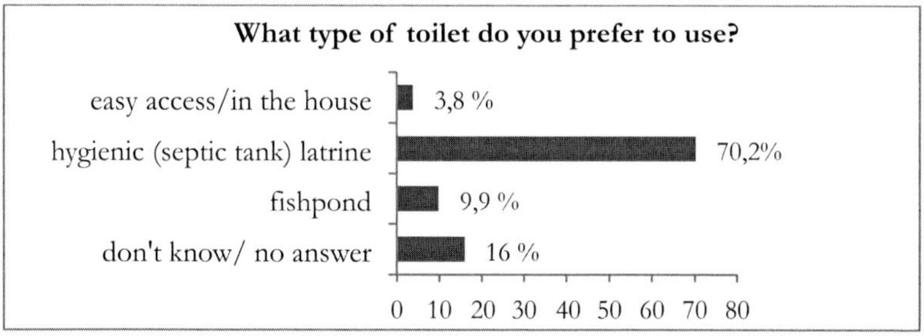

As it was previously explained (see section 5.3.1), this description often refers to the septic tank latrine. However, this reference does not guarantee that when constructing a septic tank latrine that the sanitation requirements will actually be met. In short, results show that the desire for the most modern and proper latrine does exist but people seem to lack the funds and/or the knowledge on the construction details that will render their facilities hygienic and safe. The findings, therefore, contradict what local cadres have repeatedly claimed about people preferring open defecation and about the latter being the reason why the coverage of sanitary facilities remains low in the area.

Nevertheless, the survey's possible limitations in revealing the true thoughts and feelings of people when local cadres where present need to be registered here. It would be against state recommendations to give an answer that would be different than the promoted preference for the septic tank latrine and it would even be illegal to admit the use of a fishpond toilet. However, local cadres where not always present throughout each interviews. In any case, the fervour with which people supported their preference for hygienic toilets was noticeable and suggests that most of the interviewees indeed wanted access to improved sanitation facilities.

The question remains, however, what 'hygienic' and 'improved' really means for people who are not sanitation experts. Some respondents specified that by 'hygienic' they were referring to the septic tank latrine, but many simply described 'hygienic' facilities as those having a "strong water-flush" or a "closed room with a toilet seat and not just a hole in the ground". In most of descriptions, criteria of community and environmental sanitation are not included in the judgments people make or in the shaping of their desires regarding sanitation. It is more the concept of individual comfort and household hygiene that governs people's preferences. Considering the mismatch previously noted between the facilities people claim to have and the disposal systems that they actually have (Fig 6.7 and Fig 6.8), there seems to be some confusion about three interrelated issues: what is a hygienic toilet, why are hygienic toilets beneficial for the individual users and for the community, and what is the difference between the individual (personal hygiene) and the community (environmental hygiene) benefits of sanitation.

For communities which widely use surface water and groundwater, these questions prove particularly important in relation to the spread of waterborne diseases, such as diarrhoea. In the study region, despite the continuous pollution of surface and groundwater resources from human activities, the residents appeared confused about the connection between improper sanitation, consuming groundwater and surface water and the spread of diarrhoea. This confusion was particularly clear in the answers regarding the issue of fishpond toilets. In the few cases (10%) when a fishpond toilet was preferred over other modern toilet models, this was not due to a lack of interest towards hygiene, but a result of different, personalised perceptions on sanitation-related health risks. Namely, those practicing open defecation revealed that defecating in open air carries a sense of cleanliness and freshness. On the contrary, the idea of defecating in a small room was described by them as "suffocating", "hot" and "uncomfortable". The preference to open defecation is, therefore, not clearly a case of ignorance or indifference towards hygienic sanitation, but a matter of personal criteria about what 'clean' and 'sanitary' feels like. Considering that most toilet rooms in public offices or common spaces (cafes, restaurants, and other households) often do not dispose of faeces properly and are also not aerated nor kept clean, the preference of a fishpond toilet appears - on the surface - not completely irrational from a hygienic sense. Nevertheless, these answers continued to view personal health risks separately from environmental sanitation. Public health risks associated with the untreated disposal of faeces therefore contradict such feelings.

From the description above, it is better understood that the choices people make regarding sanitation are shaped by the interplay between their personal hygienic perceptions, their community sanitation concerns and their capacity to improve. Apart from awareness-raising campaigns that can encourage sanitation improvements, there are also the financial constraints that people need to overcome. As the interviewee below describes, sanitation can be a particularly tricky dilemma for those who cannot afford it:

> "Three years ago I could drink water from the river but now it is too dirty. In general, floating houses do not have a toilet. People realise they are causing the water to be dirty… but there is no other choice for us. I recognise the risks of getting diarrheal disease from this water." (Household representative T17, Cai Rang district; personal interview)

To summarise, while the desire for sanitation improvements seems to exist, people's financial constraints and their unclear understandings of the nature and the usefulness of hygienic toilets are hindering their spread. The lack of a sewage treatment system is further posing major constraints for the area to achieve safe and sustainable environmental sanitation.

7.3 Identification of risks and local awareness about diarrheal disease

The difficulties in tracing patterns of water-related behaviour and in understanding the reasons behind everyday decisions about water and sanitation have been covered so far. This section explores the beliefs and the perceptions that underpin the strategies people employ. It focuses on people's understandings of hygiene, water safety, disease and health. These issues are examined in connection to diarrheal disease, looking particularly at how this disease is being discussed and what kinds of measures are followed for its prevention and treatment.

7.3.1 Where does diarrhoea come from?

Previous chapters have discussed the connections that the preventive health mechanism draws between the spread of diarrheal disease and issues of water use, water treatment and drinking water safety (section 6.3). This section questions the impact that such an approach has had on public understandings of the disease. When respondents were asked directly about the relationship between water and disease (Fig 7.11a), the vast majority did not recognise water as a potential carrier of disease (76.3 %) and some of them declared complete ignorance on the issue (9%). The question about diseases that are associated with water highlighted even less awareness, with 21.4% of respondents not able to provide any answer (Fig 7.11b). Notwithstanding the above, when people were specifically asked about the causes of diarrhoea, they recognised water as the possible source of risk (64.1%).

The timing and context for posing the above questions can explain part of the contradiction in the answers. The preceding discussion was focused on *household* drinking water sources and the water treatment methods followed by the members within the household. It is therefore possible that the respondents automatically assumed the discussion was continuing in the same basis, assuming that 'water' was referring to the water used and consumed in the household, even if the actual question (Fig 7.11a) was not meant in that way. It is possible, therefore, that the given answers were reflecting the respondents' protective stance towards their household, leading them to deny any connection between household water and disease. This stance shifted, however, when the researcher provided specific examples of general conceptualisations of water, such as "water that has not been boiled" or "water from the river". This was also the case for food, which was recognised as a disease-causing factor when placed under the frame of "food that is being sold on the streets" or "that has gone bad" (Fig 7.11c).

Figure 7.11: Distribution of answers regarding the relationships between water and disease

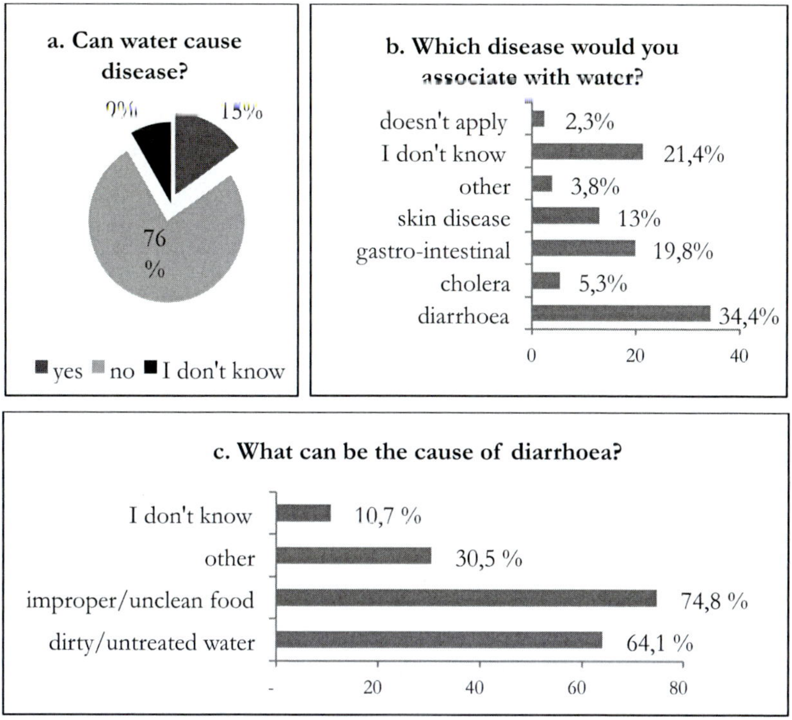

Note: When answers (a) and (c) contradicted each other (denial of water-disease relationship but recognition of water as the cause of diarrhoea), enumerators would return to question (b) and ask which disease one associates with water. When answers did not contradict, question (b) would not be asked and would be marked as "doesn't apply".
Data from household survey, 2011

When discussions were clearly about water outside of one's households, many respondents would be very descriptive and critical about the quality of surface water. People often said that "water in the river is very dirty, polluted and fish die in it" and that "people throw everything in the river, even dead animals and waste from livestock"[163]. Some respondents were also of the opinion that even CERWASS-supplied water is of low quality and carries pollutants dangerous for

[163] Sources: Household representatives (P1, P2, P3, N1, A1, P5, P6, P9, P12, T2, P17), Phong Dien district; survey interviews.

human health. For this they would mostly blame the work of the mini-supply station managers:

> "The water is contaminated. I told the officer at the mini-supply station but they do nothing about it. When we were getting water from the city centre, it was much better." (Household representative T12, Cai Rang district; personal interview)

> "Water is unclean, with impurities, because the people responsible [for the mini/supply station] are being lazy and they do not clean the tank." (Household representative P26, Phong Dien district; personal interview)

Food that was "dirty" or "improper" was the most prevalent perceived cause of disease (Fig 7.11c). Respondents often blamed canteens, street-vendors and restaurants for the unhygienic food that they serve[164]. Unlike what was claimed by health officials, the risk of food-borne diarrhoea was equally recognised by urban and rural inhabitants, both of which spoke of food poisoning experiences and food safety problems. Defining what "improper" food is, in terms of diarrheal disease risk, turned out to be a quite varied and personal issue. Many blamed alcoholic drinks for causing diarrheal episodes. When they were asked to be more specific, they mostly mentioned "beer that is served with ice", pointing back to the issue of bad water quality in ice production. The consumption of seafood was also commonly mentioned as causing food poisoning. This was attributed this to its long transport distances and the inevitable spoiling along the way. Beyond these epidemiologically explained perceptions about food-borne risks, there were also a number of responses which reveal another type of understanding about the relationship between food, the body and disease; namely those that related closer to principles of traditional medicine. Such were, for example, the claims that certain types of food are causing diarrhoea because they are "too oily", "indigestible" or simply because some people are sensitive to them. Certain other types of food, on the other hand, were considered to be helpful for the body to recover from diarrhoea, as will be described in one of the following sections (7.4.3).

The levels of awareness about the sources of diarrheal disease (Fig 7.11) did not differ significantly between rural or urban households, nor between those with access to piped water and those without, or between households dependent on surface water and those with access to other water sources. It is therefore evident that public health campaigns have been equally unsuccessful in establish a

[164] Sources: Household representatives (T9, N13, P42) from Cai Rang district and (N3) from Phong Dien district; survey interviews.

clear understanding about the basic connections between unclean water and the incidence of diarrhoea in all the above groups. After years of water-focused communication efforts and hygiene-promoting activities, it is rather disappointing that no more than 59.1% of respondents associated diarrheal disease (including cholera and gastrointestinal problems[165]) with water. Another observation with regard to the prevailing perceptions of people about diarrheal disease is that they are often based on experiential knowledge and traditional beliefs. As was discussed before, this is something rather disregarded in public health campaigns (chapter 6) and not used as a basis upon which to build new or complementary understandings.

7.3.2 Senses of water safety and hygiene

The most preferred source of drinking water among the respondents was tap water (Fig. 7.5). This preference was almost equally distributed amongst urban (40/62) and rural (37/69) inhabitants. The next preferred water source for drinking was claimed to be rainwater, followed by bottled water, well water and river water. Finally, some respondents chose not to answer that question. Prior its distribution, tap water has typically undergone some kind of treatment. However, as discussed before, this does not always guarantee its hygiene. Piped-water supply, especially water that is provided centrally from a water company, was found to be of much better quality than river, well or rainwater that is collected and stored in the households. Looking at the responses regarding preference, it seems that most people have a good grasp of which water is of better quality.

Despite the fact that more than 40% of the respondents were using bottled water for drinking, only 12.2% prefer it to other sources. Compared to a piped-supply, buying bottled water also does not make financial sense. The reason that many households do not yet have a water connection - and thus buy bottled water for drinking - is, most probably, because the water-delivery network cannot reach them and not because they do not want to be connected. When

---

[165] The variety of answers provided when asking what kind of disease one associates with water (Fig 7.11b) indicated a distinction between what people call "diarrhoea" and what they call "gastro-intestinal problems". The differences between the two are blurry, but could possibly be on the basis of people's own experiences (strong or mild symptoms, accordingly for diarrhoea or gastro-intestinal problems). They could also refer to the distinction between "serious" and "everyday" diarrhoea that was commonly made by health staff and officials. However, research did not find clear connections between what people call "gastro-intestinal problems" and the category of "everyday" diarrhoea, which goes unreported in the local (and national) health system.

people were asked about the specific reasons for preferring one water source over another, the most common answer concerned the quality of the water and specifically the treatment the water has undergone (Fig. 7.12). However, the answers were spread between various other reasons, including the water's taste or smell (13%)[166], the convenience of accessing some type of water (10.7%) and the habit of using it (7.6%).

Figure 7.12: Distribution of reasoning the choice of preferred drinking water source

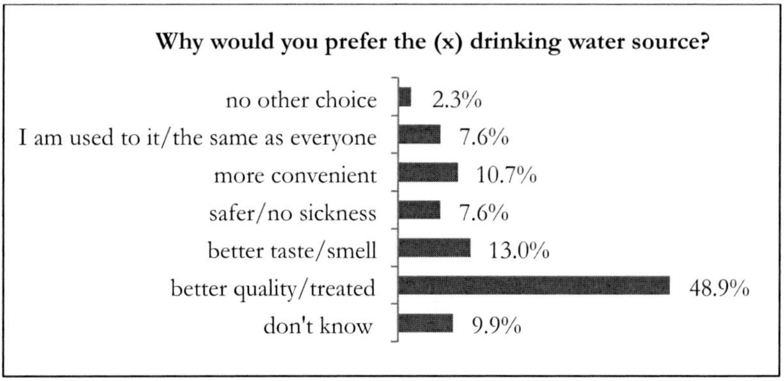

Data from household survey, 2011

Closer analysis (crosstabs) showed that most people who claimed to prefer a certain water source due to its better quality, treatment, or safety, were referring to tap water. For those who base their preferences on the water's taste or smell tend to like rainwater (Table 7.5). Despite the distinction between the concepts of quality and that of taste (or smell), which the researcher introduced by creating these categories, these concepts are not necessarily separated in the categories used by respondents to justify and describe their water preferences (Fig 7.13).

166 Taste and smell are very close terms in Vietnamese language and are eve used interchangeably in everyday speech (taste (n.) = mùi vị / thị hiếu ; smell (n.) = mùi /mùi hôi thúi / khứu giác). For this reason, the above indicator included them both.

Table 7.5: Cross-tabulation of "justification of drinking water choice" and "preferred drinking water source"

Preferred source	Reasoning of drinking water							
	don't know	quality/ treated	taste/ smell	safer/no sickness	conve-nient	used to it/ same as everyone	no choice	Total
rainwater	1	3	11	0	2	0	0	17
tap water	7	49	3	7	5	5	1	77
drilled well	0	5	0	0	1	1	1	8
river/ canal	0	0	1	0	1	1	0	3
bottled water	1	6	2	2	4	1	0	16
don't know	4	1	0	1	1	2	1	10
Total	13	64	17	10	14	10	3	131

Data from household survey, 2011

The distribution of answers on quality (Fig 7.13a) and taste (Fig 7.13b) of drinking water are evidently similar. In fact, more than half of the respondents (59%) gave the exact same answer when evaluating the quality and the taste/smell of their drinking water, including people who drink tap water. This shows how these two categories are somehow interwoven into the manner of evaluating drinking water sources. In other words, *taste* and *smell* are important indicators of water quality for people in the study region. Tap water is evaluated as of good quality, because of its prior treatment, even though people often said "it smells bad because of the chemicals [chlorine] they use to clean it". Rainwater, on the contrary, was often described as having a "sweet" and "cooling" taste and is preferred by precisely those people who base their evaluations on taste and smell (Table 7.5).

Figure 7.13: Distribution of responses concerning the evaluation of drinking water quality (a) and water taste (b)

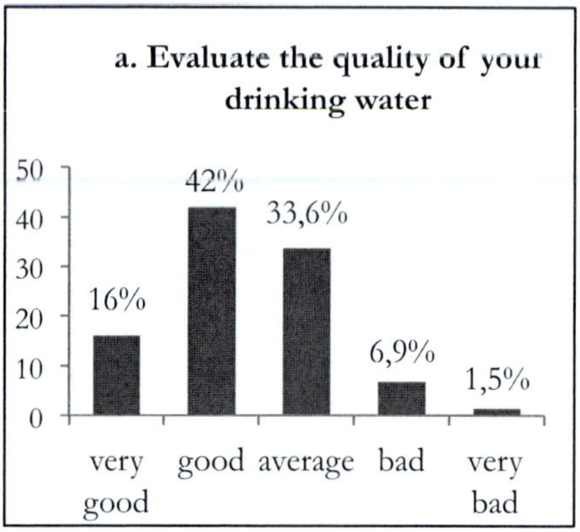

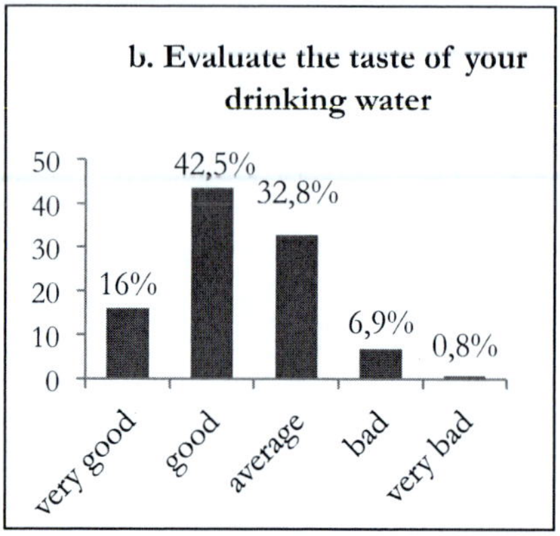

Data from household survey, 2011

The question that arises is whether water of good quality and water that is tasty is also understood as water that is safe for consumption. The related question revealed that most people judge safety based on their direct senses (including smell, taste and visually apparent clarity or turbidity) compared to those who consider previous treatment to provide safety (Fig 7.14).

Figure 7.14: Distribution of answers characterizing criteria distinguishing between safe and unsafe water

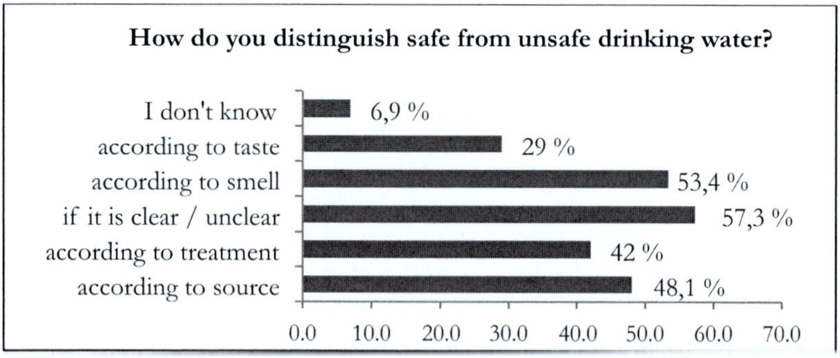

Note: Multiple-answer question. Data from household survey, 2011

This strong association between odour and safety was also evident in the study of Knudsen et. al (2008), which showed that farmers strongly believed that if harmful 'smelly air' enters their bodies, it will make them sick. Herbst et al. (2009) also found that it is difficult for locals to make judgments about water-related health risks and impurity if pollutants are not traceable by vision or smell. The importance experiencing impurity in a tangible way as a method for determining health risk can also explain why the habit of hand-washing with soap is mostly practiced "when hands are dirty" (Fig 7.15).

Figure 7.15: Distribution of given answers regarding the practice of hand-washing

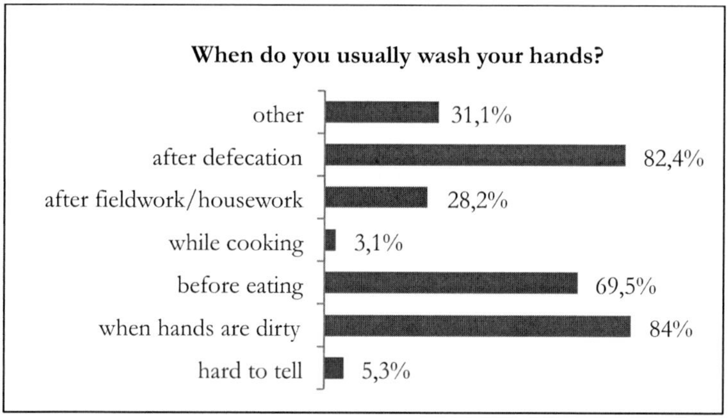

Multiple-answer question (N=131). Data from household survey, 2011

Despite the open-ended nature of the hand-washing question (Fig 7.15), which was intended to identify which moments are considered key for hand-washing by the respondents, the initial unprompted answers would often be met with confusion ("it is hard to say") or would be too abstract ("all the time" or "whenever I feel I have to"). When possible answers were given as prompts, interviewees tended to always answer affirmatively. Considering the bias posed by the researcher's prompts, the extent to which hand-washing is actually taking place in all of the above mentioned instances is highly doubtful (Fig. 7.15). Moreover, most people claimed to only wash their hands with water and without the use of soap (48.1%). This percentage was very similar between the responses from urban and from rural areas. Of the people who said to be using some kind of soap for hand-washing (47.3%), many specified that they will only do so after particular situations, such as after cleaning the house or when their hands are looking very dirty. Observations from the field repeatedly indicated that the practice of rinsing hands with running tap water is indeed the most common hand-washing practice. It was also clear that soap was absent from the sinks of many households, public offices, restaurants and even schools and hospitals.

So far it has been shown that evaluations of impurity seem to be based primarily on what the human senses can detect. It is clear that the wider public does not have a good understanding of the epidemiological and microbiological aspects of "invisible" health risks. As a result, water treatment practices are not always accurate, water choices are often governed by confusion, sanitation practices remain widely unconnected to water risks, and hand-washing with soap is not yet understood as important and therefore embedded in people's everyday life.

7.3.3 Identifying, preventing and treating diarrhoea

When residents of rural and urban areas were asked about the symptoms of what they understand as diarrhoea, the vast majority were able to describe those symptoms in good detail (Fig 7.16), which indicates a personal and experiential awareness of the disease.

Figure 7.16: Distribution of answers regarding the symptoms of diarrhoea

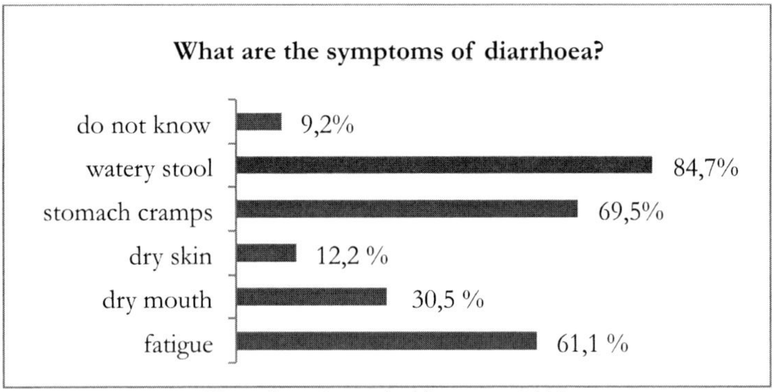

Data from household survey, 2011

More than half of the respondents revealed that they will suffer from diarrhoea at least 1 – 3 times every year. However, extracting precise information on the incidence of the disease was a hard task and many insisted that neither they (30%) nor their kids (26.7%) have ever experienced it (Fig 7.17).

Figure 7.17: Distribution of given answers regarding the annual frequency of diarrheal episodes, for the respondent and for the members of her/his family

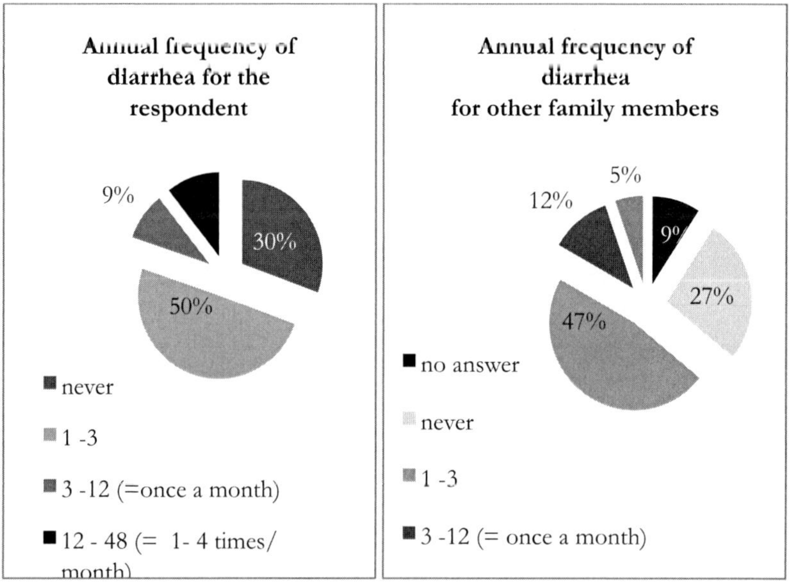

*For clarifications of the quality and validity of this set of data, see section 6.3. Data from household survey, 2011

As was discussed in previous chapters (particularly chapter 4), the Vietnamese have a tendency to self-medicate and not seek advice from public healthcare units unless they face health problems that they evaluate as serious (Fritzen, 2007: 1617, Nguyen Ha, 2011: 12). In cases where people think they require medical help, it is also likely that they will directly turn to a hospital and by-pass[167] the local healthcare system (MoH, 2010a), a phenomenon that was also recognised by health officials:

> "For serious diseases they will go to the hospital but for the normal ones, they will just visit the pharmacy or a private doctor…" (Top official in district Office of Health, Co Do, 18.07.11; personal interview)

---

[167] The term means that people are avoiding the commune - and district - level health care facilities and are rather seeking treatment in central hospitals, even for diseases that could be handled by local health units.

Findings from the household survey show that most people spend averagely 100,000 to 500,000 VND[168] every month for their health. The principal health expense for the majority of rural and urban residents is the purchase of medicine (74.8%). The health strategy of almost half of the respondents was to avoid health insurance (49.6%) and to buy medicine from a pharmacy or a local health clinic. For reasons already elaborated, the low rate of insured people and the tendency to circumvent medical consultation are seen as institutionally interconnected facts. In short, the connection between these two phenomena lies primarily with people's financial constraints; generally this prevents them from accessing healthcare and makes health insurance seem like a poor (short-term) investment. By taking the risk of remaining uninsured, people often opt for self-medication in the private sector.

Even if they are insured, Vietnamese often avoid public healthcare facilities because of the low trust towards the services that these facilities offer. Local clinics might be the easiest, closest and cheapest place one can turn to for expert medical advice, but they have been described as "...busy places where one has to queue and that are inconvenient" and where "the medicines are not as good as the ones you can get in the pharmacy"; this is compared to statements such as "going to the pharmacy is easy and fast" (Household representatives from Phong Dien (14.10.2011) and Cai Rang (18.10.11) districts; in-depth interviews). The widespread attitude of self-medication has also been reported for the case of diarrheal disease. Treatments for diarrhoea are often sought outside of the public healthcare system, unless the episode develops into a "serious" one:

> "Although the number of adult patients hospitalised with diarrhoea is not high, the actual number of people with acute diarrhoea in this hot season is much higher. That is because adults often self-treat the symptoms of diarrhoea. Patients visit the hospital only when the symptoms are severe, like high fever, vomiting, abrupt bowel movement, severe abdominal pain, or after self-treatment has brought no result" (Thanh Nien online, 2010).

Findings confirm this general tendency to visit the pharmacy as a first strategy for "normal" disease (Fig 7.18a). This was particularly common for the poor residents of Yen Binh area in urban Cai Rang. If the symptoms of illness do not recede, many respondents said that they would then turn to a public clinic or a private doctor. However, a significant percentage of people would continue with the same (first) strategy (Fig 7.18b) of self-medication.

---

168 Equal to 3.5 - 18 Euros

Figure 7.18: Distribution of answers considering initial and secondary strategies followed in the case of diarrhoea occurrence

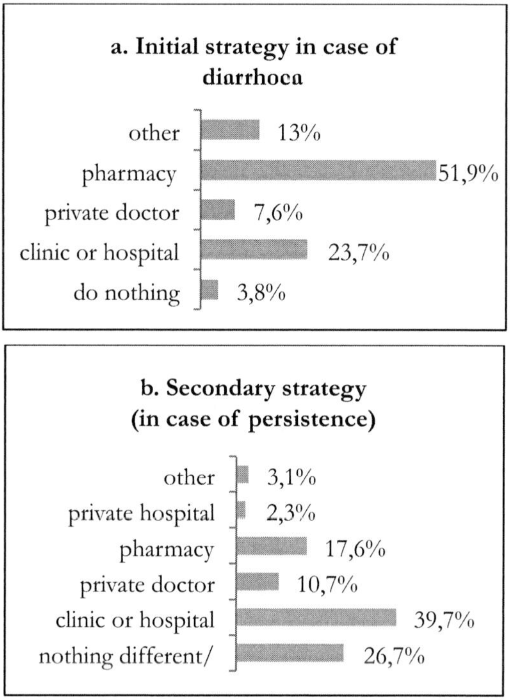

Data from the household survey, 2011

Many of the respondents view diarrhoea as an illness that is rather common and is not alarming unless it causes severe dehydration and thus threatens one's life. However, as common as it is regarded, some respondents were very reluctant in admitting their personal experiences with the disease. The attitudes of people when diarrhoea was discussed in personal reference to them revealed that this reluctance was due to a sort of stigmatisation that the disease carries. Many of the interviewed women would be embarrassed to discuss anything about the issue and they would even avoid using the word "diarrhoea" when referring to themselves, calling it rather a "belly pain" or "stomach ache". Some others would nervously laugh and completely avoid giving an answer, declaring complete ignorance about the disease. These reactions were obvious expressions of embarrassment. It is not clear, however, whether this embarrassment was indicating a tabooed perception of defecation (as a topic not fitting to the female profile or not proper for conversations that one has in public), or whether the disease itself carries some notion of disgrace related to inferiority, poverty and impurity.

Diarrheal disease is often publically discussed as the negative outcome of improper practices followed in a household, including mostly water and food related issues (following the central motto of "boil the water and cook your food"). The role of female actors is dominant in these spheres, as women are primarily responsible for work in the household, preparing food and keeping their children clean and safe. They have, therefore, certain responsibilities towards their families and also towards the state, which generally fit under the rubric of "healthy, cultural communes" and "happy families" (MoH, 2004). The hesitation of some interviewed women to admit the incidence of disease within their families is then also understood as an effort to safeguard their own reputation as mothers and housewives. Gammeltoft (1999: 134), in her study of women's health in Vietnam, explains how the human body needs to be understood as containing "both ethical and aesthetic aspects: it unites moral concerns with strivings for beauty and grace" (Ibid 1999:134).

Following the discourse of a number of health officials, some respondents also tended to discuss the disease as something happening only to "others", usually to the poor, the rural or generally those who are ignorant of proper hygienic practices[169]. Apart from moral or social considerations that might stand in the way of women admitting their own personal exposure to risks of diarrheal disease or to the experience of the disease, there is also the "optimistic bias" (Frewer et al., 1994) that people tend to apply to themselves (see section 6.2.2). As was seen above, water or food that is coming from within one's household is rarely considered by the members of that household as dangerous. Thus, the exposure to a health risk is automatically underestimated. Similarly, people might underestimate the severity of diarrheal episodes that they have gone through, categorising them as "gastro-intestinal problems" or "indigestion", but not as diarrhoea.

Nevertheless, not all of the respondents rushed to deny having any experience of the disease and some spoke openly about its high frequency and prevalence[170]. As one farmer commented, "no one can avoid diarrhoea; we can get it from anything" (Household representative P18, Phong Dien district; survey interview). Another elderly rural inhabitant frankly admitted, "diarrhoea is the

169 Sources: Household representatives (P42, P25, P39); survey interviews.

170 Sources: Household representatives (T18, P28, P18, N1); survey interviews.

number one health problem; I get it four times a month" (Household representative N1, Phong Dien district; survey interview).

However, many of the crucial preventive measures against diarrhoea proved unknown to, or not practiced by, many of the respondents (Fig 7.19). The message of "only drink boiled water" was a strong measure of prevention against diarrheal disease, equally known to rural and urban inhabitants (crosstabs). However, hand-washing was almost completely ignored as a preventive strategy, with only 6.1% of the respondents recognising its potential in protecting against diarrhoea. This disregard towards hand-washing was again equally present among rural and urban inhabitants. In-depth interviews showed that this reflects from the main messages circulated in health campaigns, which are reduced to the advice of "keeping your house environment clean, cooking food well and boil the water before drinking" (respondent HH2, rural commune; personal interview); these kinds of statements ignore hand-washing.

Figure 7.19: Distribution of answers regarding preventive measures against diarrheal disease

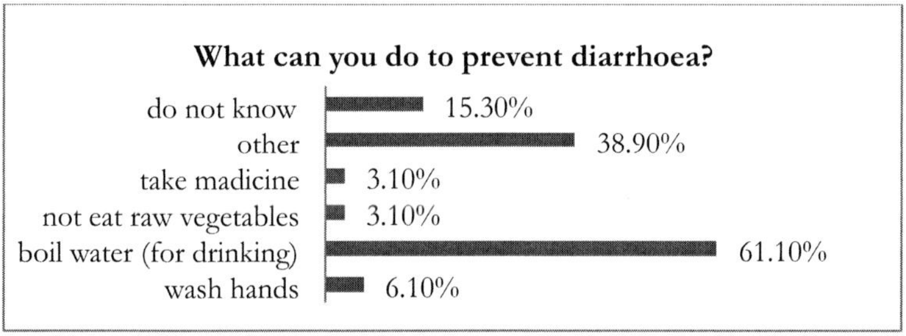

Data from household survey, 2011

Firstly, the findings reaffirm that there are serious shortcomings in the current health communication mechanism. They further prove how little importance hand-washing is given outside of school classes and the limited number of campaigns focused on children, underlining the serious lack of awareness about the connection between this practice (or lack thereof) and the spread of diarrheal disease. Secondly, the findings contradict claims about the rural and the poor being those particularly ignorant of disease-prevention measures; all sectors of the population were equally unaware of the usefulness of hand-washing. Moreover, other possible strategies that can significantly help in the control of diarrheal disease, such as vaccination, breast-feeding and hygienic food preparation, were completely absent from the given answers and indicate further gaps of awareness among the population.

Interestingly, a significant number of people gave answers that did not fall into any of the predefined answers. Most of the preventive strategies were described under the 'other' category (Fig. 7.19), as they were too diverse to be included in one category. These alternative preventive strategies included the consumption of certain beverages and foods, such as dark tea or coffee with lemon, small quantities of aged mangosteen alcohol, young green guava leaves chewed with salt and ginger tea. Often enough, the same strategies that were mentioned as preventive would also be identified as curative. The blurred line between the concept of prevention and cure might have also been a reason why many people could not readily identify everyday practices contributing to disease prevention (15.3%). Some respondents claimed that the prevention of diseases such as diarrhoea requires a consistent schedule of sleeping and eating. Others believed that avoiding fruit and vegetables that have been grown with pesticides and fertilisers could protect them from cholera. The use of salted water for washing vegetables (preventive) and the consumption of coconut water with salt (curative) were the only two mentioned 'other' preventive practices that had some connection to (traditional) medical explanations of disease.

When people were specifically asked about the means of treating diarrhoea when it occurs, most of them said they follow medical advice (35.9%) or take medicine (33.6%) without specifying whether this was from the public or the private sector (Fig 7.20).

Figure 7.20: Percentages of answers on the treatments of diarrheal disease

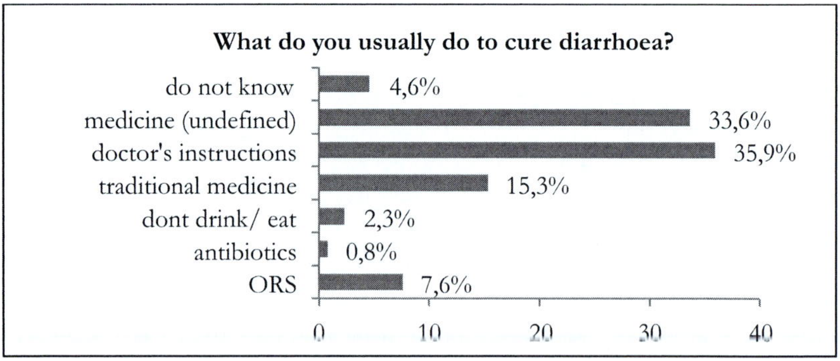

Data from household survey, 2011

The percentage of people recognising the usefulness of oral re-hydration solutions was disappointingly low (8%) and was a further indication of the low prioritisation that the CDD program nowadays receives. When people were specifically asked about the type of medicine that they are prescribed for diarrhoea, some mentioned ORESON (type of oral re-hydration solution) or SMECTA and charcoal pills (types of intestinal absorbents) for fighting the symptoms of diarrhoea. Others, however, presented medicine that is suitable for problems of indigestion, heartburn, stomach ulcers or gastritis[171].

Inappropriate and/or unadvised medication accentuates the problem of controlling the disease and can potentially lead to the disease's prolongation. Overall, the results underline the crucial role of the medical staff as well as the pharmacists in prescribing and selling medication that is adequate to cure (and control) the disease. Last but not least, it was clear in the results that traditional medicine was sought by a significant percentage of the respondents (15.3%), even if this is not advocated in any official communication material regarding the disease.

7.4 Conclusions

Looking into the perceptions and the practices of everyday people around issues of water, sanitation, hygiene and diarrheal disease, the findings presented here demonstrate that there are connections between people's assessments of safe hygiene, their cultural and social norms and their socio-economic capabilities. People strive to have clean water and they are very much concerned about their health and well-being. As findings show, however, the type of information and the resources that they have available might be limited or faulty and, thus, might not allow them to adopt the preventive behaviours that can protect them from disease.

Public perceptions of water safety were seen to vary in intricate ways in the case study areas. Local understandings did not always agree with assessments of water quality that rely on the measurement of pathogenic concentrations in the water. While many people would base their water safety evaluations on water quality information, considering factors such as the water's origin and its prior treatment in relation to its designated use, most of them would base their evaluations on the water's smell, taste and turbidity. Considering the high levels of

---

171 The commercial names of some of the medicaments presented as anti-diarrheal were: Gastra QK9, gastrogel, Kamingast-S, EDOZ, GD carbo, and AXOLOP (loperamide).

water pollution and the lack of water treatment systems in the region, such methods are increasingly risky, at least concerning diarrheal disease. Regarding sanitation, there was considerable confusion between notions of hygiene that were *felt* (personal senses) and those that were *known* (acquired information coming from institutions). Thus, open defecation was considered by some as healthier, while a latrine with a flush was considered by others as more hygienic. Not having a holistic understanding of the cyclic and interconnected processes of water use, wastewater disposal and sanitation, it was difficult for people to agree on what constitutes safe and hygienic sanitation and to relate their household practices with the health risks they are exposed to.

While a large portion of population depends on groundwater, rainwater and river water, many also maintain fishpond toilets or discharge sewage into the canals. Enhancing the knowledge of how water loses its quality and becomes unsafe for human use and consumption seems to be a missing link in improving people's water treatment and sanitation behaviours. However, traditional (sensed, experiential or felt) and new (informational, acquired, scientific) understandings of what constitutes healthy, hygienic and sanitary, are currently perceptually distant and sometimes contradicting, without being mutually exclusive. Taking this into account, any efforts to enhance knowledge on the prevention of diarrheal disease would have to use both these types of understandings and build on them to reconcile or clearly differentiate them in people's hygienic consciousness.

Generally, financial constraints were found to greatly hinder access to improved WSS, especially for the poorest. Even in cases when WSS improvements were feasible, however, the motivation for them was not always fuelled or accompanied by a health-related understanding of water safety and hygiene. The lack of clarity regarding these issues, as described above, paralleled the low awareness of the transmission pathways of diseases such as diarrhoea. As a consequence, disease prevention was a loosely understood concept. People could hardly attribute the prevention of diarrhoea to strategies other than "boiling water and cooking food well". Not being clear on the causes nor on the ways to prevent from diarrhoea, the public treated it as a taboo topic. Many were hesitant to even discuss it and often assigned diarrheal disease exclusively to poverty and backwardness. In order to maintain a discursive distance from the disease, there was a general tendency of people claiming that they follow certain hygienic behaviours (such as hand-washing, covering their water containers, having hygienic latrines), when in reality they were not. In a similar manner, while most recognised water and food as possible carriers of diarrheal disease, this was seen only to apply to water and food found outside one's household, which was related to *other* people's bad habits, dirty kitchens or careless behaviour with water.

The problems of bad hygiene and of disease were thus not perceived as clearly technical or microbiological, but were enmeshed in certain socio-economic categories. As one result, instead of feeling empowered and capable of controlling the disease in their communities, people appeared to be afraid of being associated with its "foulness" or being blamed for not following the publically advocated preventive measures. Diarrheal disease then becomes not only an indicator of a certain (low) social position, but also of (low) citizenship morals and (low) compliance to state regulations. Considering the notions of social morality that the state has attached to public health and prevention (discussed in chapter 6), these findings do not come as a surprise. The public opinions and attitudes that were expressed towards diarrheal disease also reflect claims about the "ignorant and indifferent poor" who do not care about their health, which state representatives repeated in order to justify the failures of the preventive health mechanism.

The results of the household survey showed that hygienic behaviours and prevention strategies can be inadequately practiced or misunderstood by both the poor and the better-off, as well as by those living in rural and in urban areas. This further underlines two major misconceptions that prevail in water and sanitation approaches in Vietnam and in other regions of the world. The first is that the expanded coverage of "improved" WSS equals improved public health understandings. As it was made clear, some people construct "hygienic" facilities without knowing how these might protect them from diarrhoea, while at the same time remaining uninformed about other preventive and curative measures, which can be even more effective in controlling the disease. The second misconception is that problems of disease can be lumped together with administrative definitions such as 'urban' or 'rural'. This chapter demonstrated that people's vulnerability to disease is shaped by inequalities of access to resources and services and that these inequalities go beyond administrative boundaries.

In a context of population movement between rapidly changing rural and urban areas, it would be of more value to unmask these administrative categories and to address problems in their socio-political complexity. Examining the topic of diarrheal disease indicates that there is the need to improve people's health literacy. In order to achieve that, health campaigns not only need to expand and multiply, but also to promote inclusiveness, participation and empowerment, instead of stigmatisation, shame and fear.

DISCUSSION AND CONCLUSIONS

CHAPTER 8

The central aim of this study has been to examine the constellation of institutional structures, cultural traits and socio-political dynamics that determine the risk of diarrheal disease in Vietnam's Mekong Delta. In order to do so, the study initially looked into the country's health institutions, which provide the setting in which the disease survives and spreads (chapter 4). Within the wider field of health risk management, attention was particularly paid to the implementation of strategies that are widely known to be effective in the control and prevention of diarrheal disease and that have been -at least on paper - adopted by the Vietnamese government (chapters 5 and 6). The analysis clearly demonstrated that there are major gaps between policy and practice and that implementation is ridden by inequalities and institutional weaknesses. This is not only evidenced by issues of access to safe water and hygienic sanitation, but also by the ways in which the state tries to shape hygiene-related behaviour in the population. The research then drew attention to how actors define and experience diarrheal disease, focusing on the strategies followed to deal with the disease, as well as on the prevailing ideas and perceptions about the disease, both in urban and rural settings (chapter 7). Combining institutional and anthropological findings, the gaps between policy and practice become apparent in the habits and the beliefs of the local population. Based on these findings, it is becoming clear that such discrepancies cannot be explained simply by the insufficient resources that are being used to remedy the disease's spread, but by the insufficient respect and unequal attention that is paid to the actual problems that people face and to their varying understandings of disease.

This chapter synthesises the empirical findings that were presented and discussed in previous chapters. It does so by revisiting the analytical categories that this study chose to examine and by commenting on how these findings contradict or supplement previous research on the topic. Subsequently, the analytical framework followed is reflected upon in order to trace its contribution to the field of political ecology. The chapter also highlights some possible areas of future research that have emerged in the course of this work. Finally, the chapter draws to a close by summarising the essence of this study's conclusions and by sketching a way forward for the broader field of public health.

8.1 The interplay of factors shaping the risk of disease: a synthesis of findings

Background information and primary data from the Mekong Delta indicated that diarrhoea remains an unresolved problem for thousands of people annually, many of whom are of a very young age. The population still suffers the same morbidity levels of enteric diarrheal disease as it did 30 years ago. While cholera and typhoid appear less often and with lower prevalence, diarrhoea has sustained a high incidence over the years (MoH, 2012b, Kelly-Hope et al., 2008). Given its preventable nature, questions about the disease have continually garnered attention and begged for context-specific answers explaining the real obstacles that stand on the way of its successful worldwide control.

The international health community has a vast amount of accumulated knowledge at hand in the form of principles and guidelines, which is available to Vietnamese policy-makers (MoH, 2009c). These high-level documents become referenced examples of national policy but are not being adopted in practice (see section 6.2). The inertia in policy is clearly demonstrated, for example, by the fact that the Rotavirus vaccination remains inaccessible for the masses and that the two crucial preventive strategies against diarrhoea (breast-feeding and hand-washing with soap) are still in great need of promotion. Evidence showed how the feeble or absent implementation of the state's declared policy objectives is contributing to the poor capacity of the population to embrace the recommended preventive measures. This weakness of the prevention policy was evident in the institutions that comprise the sector, with many of the actors in public health remaining ill-informed and therefore unable to effectively perform their personal and professional contributions in the fight against diarrheal disease (section 6.3.3).

Although Vietnam has a history of preventive health success (Marr, 1992), it currently faces serious health challenges, among which is the persistence of this preventable disease. Considering the significant economic growth that the country has been experiencing during the last decades (GSO, 2011b), which could provide support for the resolution of health issues affecting its population, the high morbidity rates of diarrhoea is indeed a peculiar issue. Scholars who have approached similarly unusually persistent health problems argue for the consideration and analysis of the various contextual synergistic factors which shape health problems (Briggs, 2003, Curtis and Riva, 2010). These factors often go beyond medical fields. They can either translate into direct health outcomes or can affect disease indirectly, appearing as inherent characteristics of the systems within which disease acts (Bloom et al., 2007, Morris, 2010). With this in mind, this study looked at the case of Can Tho City in Vietnam's

Mekong Delta, investigating the risk of diarrheal disease within four contextual and synergistic spheres: the personal, social, environmental and political.

8.1.1 *Health policy and the "normalisation" of diarrheal disease*

Access and attitudes towards public healthcare

Fundamental changes in the administrational and economic policy in the health sector has rendered public healthcare in Vietnam less accessible and less trusted than it perhaps was some decades ago. A significant decrease of central funding to health, which now barely covers 38.5% of national health expenses, has impacted the local units of the commune and hamlet clinics, which are increasingly depending on a trickle down from provincial funding. Even though the state has promised support to local health units as a national objective (MoH, 2007b), this is not being fully realised. In many localities, clinics are deteriorating, with this phenomenon being accompanied by a tendency to self-medicate and to avoid interaction with the healthcare mechanism at the local level. This weakened access to public health units – or the weakened "effective availability", as Roberts et al (2003) describe it, becomes more evident when looking at the trends in participation in the public health insurance scheme (which guarantees access to public healthcare). Namely, every time the health insurance becomes obligatory for more fragments of the population, the rate of insured people rises. However, almost all of the people who are not yet obliged to insure themselves (farmers, self-employed) choose not to pay for public health insurance (section 4.2.2).

When the public health system is not preferred, cure-seeking behaviours lean towards the private sector. However, private services are mainly concentrated in the urban regions and can range widely in quality and cost. With 27% of the country's population living in poverty (World Bank (WB), 2013) and with the inhabitants of remote rural regions disproportionately impacted by poverty (GSO, 2013), access to basic health care of one's choosing is evidently not easy. The current situation of access to healthcare certainly reflects wider socio-economic inequalities (section 4.2.3). The deterioration of primary healthcare units leaves the poor with no better option for low cost healthcare than self-medication. The findings of the household survey and of the in-depth interviews with inhabitants in Can Tho (section 7.3.3), confirmed that diarrheal disease falls into the category of diseases, for which the public does not consider it necessary to seek professional medical advice, unless they reach severe stages (Thanh Nien online, 2010). Moreover, findings from the household survey showed that it is especially the poor from the urban areas that tend to self-medicate and to avoid interaction with doctors when they, or their children, get diarrhoea. Barriers of access to public healthcare were seen to exist also in higher-level healthcare. Contrary to local clinics, the demand for services in the central specialised hospitals is high. This over-demand for treatment is, however, not addressed in a transparent and equitable way. Literature has repeatedly pointed to the frequent phenomenon of under-the-table payments, double standard treatments and widespread corruption, which have come to be everyday experiences at high-level healthcare units (Ha Mi, 2013).

Allowing decentralisation to diminish the quality of local units, on one hand, and tolerating the frequent financial abuse of patients, on the other, the Vietnamese state appears both unwilling and unable to safeguard healthcare access for the majority of people. Through opening up to the private sector and the toleration of an ill-regulated sector, the government has largely transferred its health-related responsibilities to the individual citizens, rendering healthcare dependent on one's willingness and ability to pay. Foley (2009: 60) finds that this is a common trend globally, as "international health priorities moved away from primary health care strategies and from their implicit assertion that universal health care is a basic human right". As the author continues, the experience of decentralised healthcare arrangement in Senegal has, similar to Vietnam, "meant the transfer of responsibility [to the city] with no transfer of means" (Ibid. 2009:71). Considering the low utilisation of healthcare services and the great number of uninsured people, empirical results showed that the healthcare system in Vietnam faces three major challenges in relation to diarrheal disease:

- widespread unadvised self-medication which relies primarily on the opinion of usually untrained pharmacists
- large portions of the sick population escape the reporting mechanism, because disease is being treated at home or via private practitioners
- the public health insurance and the healthcare system is being weakened financially, with the funds that are procured being circulated in an ineffective manner that is open to abuse (i.e. many people are not insured and much of the health spending is not going to public healthcare)

With diseases like diarrhoea that can be easily controlled only when an adequate diagnosis is administered in a timely manner, a lack of accessible and affordable primary healthcare is raising the possibility of disease aggravation and spread. At the same time, the regulatory framework concerning the provision of medication is weak and the retail of pharmaceuticals often takes place outside of legal provisions, hardly ever following a practitioner's prescription (section

4.3.2). Moreover, the decrease in utilisation of primary healthcare clinics compromises the potential for these units to carry out grassroots preventive health activities, a responsibility which is especially and exclusively assigned to them (MoH, 2007b, CERWASS, 2003).

What needs to be emphasized is that people's behaviours are not independent from the health system and the inequalities embedded in that system. The public sees the healthcare mechanism as one that is expensive, offering low service quality and having low capacity. This seems to be largely the reason why the Vietnamese public has developed an aversion to it. This aversion is effectively lowering people's expectations regarding their healthcare rights, since they exercise those rights increasingly only in the case of "serious" illness. This implies that the transfer of responsibility for health has not just shifted from the central state to the local health authorities, as mentioned before (Foley, 2009), but rather has shifted all the way down to the citizens. Individuals are now left to make the evaluation of how much money is worth spending on health, or, in other words, when is disease worth the trouble of seeking medical advice and treatment. The old proverb of "sức khỏe là vàng" - meaning "health is gold" - indicates how much the Vietnamese people value good health. The latest developments affecting the functioning of health institutions, however, has unfortunately provided for a more updated interpretation of the above quote: "health depends on wealth".

Interpretations of "normal" diarrhoea

Looking at the case of diarrhoea, the analysis demonstrates how a certain "normalisation" of the disease has been reached, not only through the public discourse in circulation and the healthcare policy being implemented, which tend to underestimate its spread and impact, but also through people's behaviour in response to its frequent incidence. Respondents often referred to diarrhoea as an "everyday" and "normal" disease. In-depth conversations showed that this "normality" refers to their familiarity with the disease, as it happens frequently and to everyone. Despite this familiarity, findings did not indicate that the public has a sound awareness about the recommended practices for its cure and prevention (section 7.4.3). Health cadres and state representatives in local offices spoke of the disease's "normality" in different terms. Their line of argument was often referenced the disease's low mortality rates in order to suggest that diarrhoea is a "normal" disease, from which people can easily recover (section 6.2.1). This claim was also used to justify its relative depriorisation in national health policy. Therefore, despite the disease's frequent occurrence, it is presented officially as a trivial issue that the preventive health system of the country is successfully dealing with.

Diarrheal disease is "normalised" also in another, more technical way, through its system of reporting and monitoring (section 4.3.2). A certain incidence is not considered as a diarrhoea epidemic unless it surpasses a baseline of cases in the population. This baseline, however, is based on the average incidence of the disease during the last 5 years, meaning that high morbidity levels of the disease will not appear as an outbreak if these levels have been maintained for years. At the same time, the public healthcare system does not report patients with diarrhoea unless they exhibit acute symptoms (indicating cholera or typhoid); thus the reporting mechanism itself is not capturing the actual baseline that is used for epidemic assessments. The contradictory and arbitrary reporting that has become standard in the health sector is further blurring the picture of the problem. Therefore, the extent of diarrheal disease spread and its significance for epidemiological and broader health prevention assessments remains unclear. As Trostle (2005) underlines in her anthropological assessment of diarrhoea and cholera, "when ill health is seen as normal, this itself can influence health service use and disease epidemiology".

Overall, although diarrheal disease is discussed and perceived as "normal" by many people, its normality differs according to the generators of such discourse. The disease was discussed as normal by many people living in poverty, who "don't know what to do to avoid diarrhoea" since "access to clean water is hard" and who, therefore, "can't avoid it"[172]; this all attests to their feelings of helplessness towards a health problem that they cannot address. This contradicts the type of normality that is constructed by many health cadres, who present diarrhoea as being under control, with the occurring cases being minor and not serious. This is not only underestimating the actual number of patients, but also disregards the health burden of those frequently suffering from diarrhoea and, in particular, the consequences it can have on child development, the susceptibility to other diseases, and people's day-to-day sense of being healthy. Literature suggests that an early assessment of a patient's de-hydration stage by an expert is of immense importance and that the inappropriate medication (i.e. antibiotics) can seriously inhibit a patient's recovery (Thapar and Sanderson, 2004). As was mentioned before, the cure-seeking paths for diarrhoea in the study region do not often include a medical diagnosis or the adequate rehydration treatments. Moreover, nutrition deficits are common among children in

---

172 Excerpts from the interviews held with household respondents in the urban and rural study areas in Can Tho City.

the region of the Delta and were found to be as high as 29% (stunted children) in Can Tho City (PHC Can Tho City, 2011a). Considering the repeated episodes of "normal" diarrhoea that often go unadvised, this points to a health issue particularly serious for the country's young, which appears to be deferred to the future by remaining under-addressed.

Misleading indicators of water-related health success

The reasons behind the retreat in national efforts to address diarrheal disease preventively and curatively are connected to the type of targets that are set in a global level. Many development organisations value health as a central humanitarian goal and try to evaluate it through selected indicators. The health-specific Millennium Development Goals, for instance, emphasize the control of HIV, malaria and "other diseases", focusing specifically on the reduction of children mortality rates (WHO, 2012e). In Vietnam, much of the official discourse and practice were aligned with such global health targets. Indeed, the country has managed to control malaria and is placing significant efforts into the prevention of AIDS, improving maternal health and increasing the number of healthcare establishments. Thus, the projected image of the country for international evaluators is largely one of good public health policy. As mentioned before, most of the reported cases of diarrhoea are not fatal, thus the disease does not appear as much of a threat to people's lives, unlike AIDS or pneumonia (WHO, 2012c). Nevertheless, it is also true that the annual incidence of diarrhoea - in both children and adults - is much higher in Vietnam than the rates of the above mentioned diseases. Diarrhoea constitutes a health hindrance for a very significant portion of the local population, but it is rather silent as an indicator of health or public health policy.

The target of fighting diarrheal disease does not prominently figure in the global health policy agenda, where it is addressed primarily through targets in the field of water supply and sanitation. This field has gained a central position in the efforts to eradicate all types of waterborne and water-related disease, as much in Vietnam as elsewhere. The discussion on indicators of "improved" facilities ranges from the subjects of disease eradication to rural development, women's empowerment and environmental sustainability. It was made evident however that, in the case of Vietnam, the presented success in WSS development masks the actual health objective of eradicating disease, which is not being achieved. Indeed, such indicators continue to only be concerned with the number of hygienic facilities constructed, subsuming many assumptions on the local distribution mechanisms, as well as on the behavioural patterns with regard to the use and maintenance of such facilities. Similar to what has been observed in other contexts (Movik and Mehta, 2010, Bain et al., 2012), the indicators that are used to describe access to clean water and sanitation in Vietnam were not able to capture the spatial, economic and social inequalities in the sector. Moreover, standardised indicators do not often describe local water-cultures, being thus rather uninformative about the actual effect that WSS expansion has in alleviating the risk of disease (chapter 5).

A closer look at water and sanitation realities has illuminated how the part of the population that is likely to be consuming contaminated water and to be living around unsanitary environments is much larger than what national statistics suggest. In Can Tho City, the percentage of people with access to "hygienic" water , according to the local reporting agency, mounted to 71.5% in 2011 (CERWASS, 2011a). The definition of 'hygienic water' can include rainwater, well water and river water, as long as "adequate" treatments are applied to this water in the household level (CERWASS, 2011b). The results of the household survey showed, however, that most well-water and rainwater was not being disinfected before consumption (45% of users stated that they do not boil this type of water and 44% do not filter it either). This indicates, moreover, that less than half of rural households had access to piped supply and that many people depended on the purchase of bottled water for their drinking needs. The exposure of the population to water that is polluted was also evident in the number of unsanitary toilets that were found in the study areas. More than 30% of the respondents practiced open defecation and the phenomenon of latrines discharging sewage directly into the river was also not rare (section 7.3.1).

Notwithstanding the advantages of expanded water supply networks, a vast majority of people in Can Tho continue to use water that can only be free of pathogens if it goes through further treatment at the household level (CERWASS, 2011a). This percentage reached 60% in the case study areas, assuming that the centrally supplied water does not need further treatment (section 5.2.3). The results of the household survey further show that the importance of water treatment is still not fully appreciated by the wider public. Both in practice and in theory, more than half of the interviewees said that they base their drinking water choices on factors other than its measured quality or prior treatment (section 7.3.2). Moreover, no more than 42% of the respondents considered prior treatment the basis of their assessments for water safety. If these claims reflect how and why people treat their water (or not), it becomes clear that people consume water of very different quality than what is assumed when simply looking at the parameter of access to water from a "hygienic" water source.

Apart from the false impression about the actual situation of water safety, the fixation of the Vietnamese bureaucracy with counting constructions, producing numbers and publishing reports (Waibel, 2010) has affected the way that local health workers operate. Namely, the duties and interests of preventive health authorities have been monopolised by the expansion of WSS and shifted away from "software" approaches like health education (section 6.3.3), an area in which the health system has not developed concrete indicators.

The trust placed in what indicators supposedly indicate was also seen to guide policy-making and priority-setting within the sector of WSS. In Can Tho, the expansion of "improved" water access appeared to be moving apace, but only to 43% of the population had access to improved sanitation facilities (CERWASS, 2011a). This reflects the nationally reported trend of a satisfactory expansion of water supply but a weak expansion of sanitation. As a result, attention - both nationally and regionally - turned towards the expansion of "hygienic" toilets and away from facilitating safe water access for the people still lacking it. This turn was made clear, not only through the guidelines circulated and the content of communicative activities, but also in the allocation of funding. The regional budget for micro-credit loans and subsidies in Can Tho were almost entirely directed to the sector of sanitation. These are the two main programs for supporting the poor in their efforts to achieve safe water supply and sanitation and for promoting the building of healthy communities. A close questioning of how these programs have materialised in Can Tho City showed that they are interdependent, such that the beneficiaries of one program are typically the beneficiaries of the other. Essentially, subsidies are only given to people who can undertake a microcredit loan. Thus it became clear that many people living in poverty are being excluded from both because their trustworthiness in repaying a loan is low. Considering the above factors, it appears that, in sum, the prevention of disease seems to boil down to the promotion of sanitary constructions, which in turn are not accessible to those that need support the most.

In the sector of WSS, it is important to note the contradiction between what people are experiencing and what the state reports and projects. While statistics of "improved" WSS indicators are climbing, the details that form the picture of water supply and sanitation in the region constitute a somewhat dirtier reality, which the Vietnamese state does not want to bring attention to. Although connections do exist between the presence of sanitary facilities and improved human health, what seems to be the common denominator between the sectors of WSS and health in Vietnam is the drive to satisfy indicators of development, such as increased coverage and lowered mortality rates. The preventive approach focuses on aspects that help in meeting such global targets and thus, probably, in attracting international funding. However, it often ends up having very little to do with the everyday health problems that people face. What seems to guide policy and prioritisation of proclaimed health targets in the country (MoH, 2007b) is the projection of a "healthy image" but not the cultivation of a healthy population. In the course of this process, the initial purpose of supporting health education, which is to promote healthy practices and prevent disease (instead of simply counting less deaths), appears to have been forgotten. The discursive "normalisation" of a frequently experienced disease is a good example of how this takes place. The promotion of water and sanitation facilities, irrespective of whether these change the quality of water people consume or the environmental sanitation that they experience, is another example.

8.1.2 Constructing sick identities of poverty and rurality

Considering the limited access of the poor to healthcare and the constraints they face in reaching programs of support for water and sanitation improvements, their vulnerability to diarrheal disease is relatively high (sections 5.3.2 and 5.4). Some correlation between poverty and diarrheal disease was also noticed through the study of health records, where the poorest regions of the country demonstrated the highest incidences (MoH, 2012b). This correlation was, however, not so clear at the scales of the province and the district, indicating that there is more complexity involved in the distribution of health risks than what macro-level statistics of poverty and health can show (section 4.3.1). Nevertheless, the association of poverty with diarrhoea has often been used by state representatives as a way of justifying the disease's persisting incidence. Public health failures are often presented as a result of improper hygienic behaviour from the side of the poor; in this way, they dissociate poor health outcomes from the way policy has been designed and implemented.

When the interviewed residents of Can Tho talked about how frequently they experience diarrhoea, there was no significant difference between residents in poor and non-poor households. Nevertheless, considering the cultural and moral constraints that seemed to characterize the issue, the validity of the given answers might be of question. Most interestingly, however, was that the awareness of practices that can prevent the disease appeared to be at *equally* low levels among all the respondents, indicating a rather widespread misunderstanding; this is, unsurprisingly, bound be reflected in people's behaviour across the socio-economic spectrum (section 7.4.3). The distinction between poor and not poor, in relation to their (un)informed hygiene behaviour, is therefore not supported by the findings.

A common contention, both implicitly and explicitly, supported by state officials in Can Tho in their effort to explain why the poor are more vulnerable to diarrhoea, was that "the poor don't care about their health" (Top official in district PHC, Binh Thuy, 12.07.11; personal interview). This claimed indifference of people towards their health was then further discussed as being exemplified in their use of river water, their practice of open defecation and their living in dirty environments. The study's empirical results widely contradict this claim. People from the poorest households attested to their dissatisfaction with their current sanitary situation, and their inability to change it due to financial constraints (Table 7.4). Similarly, the problems that people face in accessing water networks were emphasized in their responses, with only three out of the 131 respondents saying they would opt for drinking river water (and then only in the absence of any other alternatives). What health officials did not discuss is that, more often than not, people living in poverty do not have a choice about water supply and sanitation. Part of the reason why is the noticeable paradox of pro-poor policies (such as subsidies and micro-credit loans) that rarely actually reaching the poor.

As Krause (2008) explains, the two ideational forms of institutions that govern access to WSS are "free markets that allocate services according to the price mechanism and state organisations that allocate services according to a political logic". Evidence from the Delta confirms mostly the dependence on the rules of a free market, as the sanitary sewage disposal necessitates a personal investment in the construction of a septic tank (necessitated by the lack of public sewage collection and treatment network). Likewise, the availability of drinking water is currently dominated by the purchase of bottled water (42%) or a connection to an urban water company (38%)[173], the costs of which can be rather off-putting for the poor. Krause (2008) continues in arguing that "the poor are handicapped with respect to both allocation mechanisms because of their low purchasing power and because of their political voicelessness and powerlessness". This accurately describes what is taking place also in Vietnam, seeing how the poor minorities are not only unable to "buy" services, but are also excluded from the programs meant to assist them, due to their lack of assets, their resultant financial unreliability and their weak political leverage. The unions and the credit groups that exist in Vietnam can serve as mediators in the process of microcredit and thus help people to access capital but many people

[173] These percentages are from the results of the household survey and correspond to the rainy season. For detailed graphs showing the distribution of answers, see section 5.2.2.

said that it is not easy to be actively involved in such groups, as it demands both time and money (Waibel and Glück, 2013). In this way, the whole mechanism of pro-poor policy implementation leaves the very poor "outside of the game" (section 5.3.2). Joshi et al. (2011) have also discussed this pattern in Bangladesh, Kenya and India, where the very poor are being left out of sanitation programs and where politics underpin the decisions of where (and to whom) subsidies are directed.

The UNDP reports that in Vietnam, "remoteness (or geographical inaccessibility) has more to do with the decisions about the allocation of water supply systems than has poverty, although of course these are often linked" (MONRE and UNDP, 2008). In the region of the Delta it was indeed observed that regions with high poverty indicators are also those predominantly agricultural and remote (GSO, 2013). This was also the case when comparing districts and communes within Can Tho City (DSO Phong Dien, 2010, DSO of Cai Rang, 2010, Statistical Office of Can Tho City, 2011). Due to such demographic realities, many state cadres would conflate the category of "the poor" with that of "the people living in rural areas". This happens despite the outdated nature of the criteria used for national poverty indicators (World Bank (WB), 2013) and an even rougher and less transparent process for documenting the poor at the local levels (section 4.2.2). When these two groups are conflated, the outcomes of policies that target rural areas, such as the development of water supply and sanitation (MARD and MoC, 2000) are often presented as success stories of poverty alleviation. This does not only disregard the constraints that the rural poor actually face in accessing these beneficial programs (as discussed above), but also takes attention away from the poor of the urban areas.

In relation to diarrheal disease and the water sector, the urban poor are a disproportionately affected cohort. There are fewer alternatives available for water and sanitation in the urban areas because urban planning and design is pushing inland the location of housing and thereby stripping people of the potential of having easy access to surface water sources. Urban living presupposes the connection to a centralised water supply network or the ability to own a private well. It also demands a sanitary toilet that safely collects and stores sewage, since fishponds are rare and river canals are not next to every household. This model might indeed be one of good hygiene and friendlier to the environment but, nevertheless, it leaves no room for divergence to cheaper solutions. Empirical findings confirmed that indeed most of the urban population does not rely on alternative water sources, with 82% having access to piped water supply and 73% owning a latrine. The survey also indicated that there is a minority of urban poor who have no access to such facilities and who live in particularly unhygienic conditions.

As a consequence of the lack of programs to support hygienic WSS and, in combination with the high cost of owning land in urban areas, the requirements of the urban living model are, for some, very hard to afford. In search of conditions that provide a home at low cost (floating constructions that do not need the purchase of land) and cheaper alternatives of water and sanitation (access to river water and open defecation), many of the urban poor are "occupying" the edges of rivers and canals. The accumulated water pollution that results from their unhygienic practices, as well as from the surrounding activities of a dense urban population, is putting their health at risk. What emerges as an even more serious concern regarding the urban population and especially those with the highest exposure to the risk of disease is thus their low level of hygiene awareness. However, since urban areas are considered advanced in terms of WSS, they are also considered as low-risk areas concerning diarrhoea. As a result, they are excluded from the dissemination of educational material and activities that could potentially increase awareness about the prevention and control of diarrhoea. Characteristically, the central district of Ninh Kieu was completely missing from the agenda of health education activities, even though the number of documented cases of diarrhoea was higher there than in any of the other districts in the city.

Mylott (2009) has noticed that "public policies are often aimed exclusively at either urban or rural areas", emphasizing how this jeopardises the equitable distribution of their interventions. Looking at how the content of health education activities is too often connected to rural WSS and thus, organisations like CERWASS, indeed indicates why the aim of those activities to distribute specific health-related messages is being washed away. Mylott suggests that "for public policies to be effective in improving the economic, social and structural realities of urban and rural areas, they must address the entire region, and work to strengthen the ties between urban and rural areas" (Mylott, 2009: 32). Dichotomising society into urban and rural groups, each of them portrayed as inherently having either one or the other of a variety of characteristics (such as poverty, education, disease, infrastructure, etc.), contributes to oversimplifying the complexity of the characteristics that they share.

The risk of diarrheal disease, for example, is shaped by factors that go beyond rural and urban borders. Apart from WSS infrastructure or the access to healthcare and health information, the risk of disease can be greatly influenced by food safety, household hygiene and environmental sanitation (Heller et al.,

2003). Many of the institutional constraints and failures in relation to these issues were not geographically defined (chapter 6) and similarly, people from both rural and urban areas equally fall short in recognising and following disease-specific strategies of prevention, even basic hand-washing (section 7.4). As the findings demonstrate, the risk of diarrheal disease is equally distributed within and across regions. The discursive pinning of diarrheal disease to remote, rural and poor places not only incriminates the groups that inhabit those places, but also ignores the scope of the population that is actually vulnerable to the disease.

8.1.3 Perceptions and practices through an epidemiology of health messages

Public senses and understandings of hygiene

Much of the discourse about what is hindering progress in improving public health, particularly in the prevention of diarrheal disease, tends to single out the practices and strategies followed by individuals at the household level (UNICEF and WHO, 2009). This was largely acknowledged by health cadres and professionals for the region of the Delta and for the whole of Vietnam. Research indicated that there is indeed a lack of concrete public understanding of the epidemiological causes of disease, as well as a high level of confusion around the potential health consequences of unhygienic behaviour (section 7.4).

Much of the officially-generated discourse in the study region fails to provide a convincing explanation of why people continue to behave in ways that endanger their health, instead only referring to financial constraints, ignorance and indifference to the risk of disease. As discussed above, the socio-economic categories of poverty and rurality are often linked to the above characteristics. The low coverage of hygienic water and sanitation facilities and the low health insurance rates among households that belong to these categories (CERWASS, 2011a, Tran Van Tien et al., 2011) are often the indicators used by state representatives to make such claims. The difficulties that people face in adopting nationally advocated health-improving behaviours are, however, rarely discussed as a failure of the state to effectively promote and facilitate such behaviours. Certainly the shortage of financial means can be a significant hindrance in the uptake of healthy and preventive strategies, as these normally involve some costs (medicine, clean water, disinfection tablets, wood or electricity, storage jugs, etc.). However, from the analysis of the communication methods that are used in public health education, it seems that it is also the content and the quality of the advice being circulated that interferes with people's ability to take preventive action.

The emphasis which is given to the message of "boil your water and cook your food well", for example, has had a clear impact on how people act with regard to water safety (61% recognised boiling water as the most important preventive measure against diarrheal disease). However prevalent and inculcated in society this practice seems to be, its importance in eliminating gastrointestinal pathogens is still very loosely understood by the public. This was demonstrated foremost by the poorly consolidated ways in which respondents linked the concepts of water treatment, water consumption and the incidence of disease. Despite recognising the need to "boil water", each person would conceive of disease-transmission processes differently; some would see the connection with water quality while some would not. It was clear that most respondents lacked a general understanding of the nature of pathogens and on what governs their survival and spread. Local health communicators, being the main carriers of preventive information, should themselves acquire such knowledge and be able to effectively transmit it to the public. The limited extent and low quality of the training that they receive is likely a contributor to the public's misunderstandings of the epidemiological causes of diarrheal disease (section 7.3).

The analysis showed that the concept of 'hygienic water' is often encountered with confused definitions and contradicting usage from various state cadres in water and health related posts (section 5.2.2). A closer look at the prevailing expert discourse at each administrative level showed that the ability to connect and communicate the various aspects that shape the disease's spread is mostly found at higher-level institutes that specialise in health. During the "journey" of messages from national-level experts to local communicators, through the training-of-trainers process, much of the valuable information regarding the ecology and epidemiology of disease is lost (section 6.3.2). Eventually, the messages that reach the public in the districts and communes are rather limited and lacking in explanation (section 6.3.3). The majority of the materials used to inform people about the prevention of diarrhoea, for example, mainly listing "good" and "bad" behaviours and focus on the practice of drinking boiled water and eating cooked food.

Apart from communication capacity limitations and weaknesses in content, the sector of public health is ridden by other more complex institutional obstacles. The thematic binding of diarrheal diseases with issues of water supply and sanitation has rendered disease-related education simply a part of promoting CERWASS water connections and hygienic latrines for rural areas. As a consequence, findings have indicated that the practice of boiling water has become perceptually connected to the consumption of water from a piped supply (either from CERWASS or CTWSC). People indeed boil their tap water (92%)

but many are not aware of the need to do so also with water from other sources (section 7.2.2). Evidently, the health benefits of disinfecting water are thus not fully communicated nor understood by the public. As a result, people either follow the prescribed route (getting access to piped water which they boil), or diverge completely from it (using other sources and often not treating them adequately). Considering that alternatives for disinfecting water - other than boiling - are not popular, this association between tap water and the necessity for boiling, which is cultivated through the communication mechanism, seems to leave people confused about whether and how they can truly achieve a safe water supply if they cannot connect to a piped water network. This scenario clearly demonstrates why downgrading health education and compartmentalising its messages contributes to the fact that the preventive information being circulated hardly ever serves as a strong factor of behavioural change.

This confusion that exists can also be seen in the way the practice of water chlorination is encountered by rural and urban inhabitants (section 7.2.2). Water provided by CERWASS or a central water company is already chlorinated. This gives water a smell which people describe as "chemical" and "unpleasant". However, chlorination is widely recognised and accepted as a treatment that disinfects water. Smell, as an indicator of safety that is rooted in gut reactions of disgust or unfamiliarity (section 7.4.2), seems to somehow contradict the institutional claims about chlorination's harmless purifying effect. As a result, if given a choice, some people prefer to drink rainwater, which is perceived as more refreshing and tasty. However, rainwater was often found not to meet national criteria of safety (section 5.2.3) due, variously, to inadequacies in the practices of collection, storage and treatment; this phenomenon, in particular, became clear in the findings of the household survey (section 7.1.1). Traditionally, reactions of disgust to smell or taste have evolved out of rudimentary hygiene adaptations for detecting water quality and managing risk (Curtis et al., 2011). In this sense, people might find themselves in a dilemma between what they know from personal experience and social interaction ('a chemical smell indicates danger to my health') and what they trust and/or experience as true ('chlorinated water protects me from waterborne disease').

A closer look at the criteria with which people make assessments of water safety revealed that the personal senses (smell, taste, clarity) are trusted more than information about the kind of treatment that water has undergone. The reliance on personal judgments and emotive senses of cleanliness were also seen to relate to hygienic practices. Hand washing with soap, for example, was said to be mostly practiced when "hands are visibly dirty" (84%). This concurs with findings from Kenya (Aunger et al., 2010), about how feelings of disgust and the sense of social affiliation (instead of knowledge on the spread of pathogens) both acted as central motivators for hand-washing with soap. These sensed (rather than understood) notions of purity and safety were seen to also govern the choices of those who expressed a preference for practicing open defecation. The reasons claimed for preferring defecation in the open were all related to the sense of smell and air circulation. People said that when defecating in open air, they do not feel "invaded" by the odour of faeces which is unpleasant and feels suffocating (section 7.4.2). Many of them would support that the presence of a fishpond toilet in close proximity to their household is not a problem, as long as the disturbing smells do not reach them.

The percentage of people who practiced open defecation in fishpond toilets by preference was, however, not high (9.9%). It is observed in national and local statistics that the uptake of septic-tank sanitation has been quite fast in the Vietnam (section 5.1.2). Almost all of the survey respondents reacted very positively to the idea of hygienic toilets and expressed their desire to have one (70.2%). The reasons for wanting a latrine varied. Some people recognised its sanitary benefits, but some simply wanted the convenience of having a private toilet in their house or they felt compelled to comply with state guidelines (MARD, 2003, CERWASS, 2011c). Nevertheless, the phenomenon of badly maintained or improper latrine constructions was very common in the study area, demonstrating that even if in theory people want to have a "hygienic" latrine, they often fail to do so in practice. Apart from the financial constraints of building a properly hygienic toilet, this contradiction seems also to owe also to the confusion regarding what exactly qualifies as a hygienic toilet and, by extension, what makes hygienic latrines safer for a household and for a community (section 7.3.2). Seeing the fragmentation with which issues of environmental sanitation are managed and communicated by the state (section 6.2.5), it does not come as a surprise that people's understandings of personal and community hygiene are rather blurred.

As Kasperson and Kasperson (2005) contend, the credibility of information about risk is closely related to the trust towards the institutions that produce and circulate this information. This would point to the unreliability of the state's mechanism for guaranteeing that treated and regulated water sources (bottled water, water from piped-supply networks) are actually safe for drinking. Indeed, complaints and doubts about the quality of such water were commonly expressed by the interviewees. Moreover, it is perhaps the gap that exists between common understandings of water safety and the communicated messages that reach people (one based personal feelings and senses, while the other on expert information on concepts such as pathogens, purification, concentration etc.), which also contributes to blurred and conflicting understandings related to the risk of diarrheal disease.

Perceived and protected borders of safe households

Another set of categories that people applied in parallel to the concept of hygiene was the differentiation between the *inside* and the *outside* of one's household (sections 7.4.1 and 7.4.3). The household is considered a fortress, within which cleanliness and safety are both rarely doubted. It was noteworthy how during the interviews, female respondents who were discussing the risk of diarrheal disease would often accompany their answers with motions signifying the distance between the disease-causing agents and their own proximate living environment. This would include for example the turning of the eyes, or the body, towards the door or the yard, pointing to the general "outside" where harmful water or food can be found. Thus, in a sense, the source and the risk of diarrheal disease was conceptually dissociated from the space of the household by its members.

Along the same lines, Knudsen et al. (2008) found that farmers in a peri-urban area near Hanoi identified "dirt" as a disease-causing agent that should not enter the house, but such worries did not exist when they talked about their working time in the field, during which they would happily use excreta as fertiliser. Specifically referring to the example of food safety, Bennett et al. (2010: 42) explain how this denial of risk is something common as people have a general tendency "to rate their own behaviours and situations as less risky than they actually are". This denial, however, was not present when people described their experiences with food bought along the street, beverages that they were served in restaurants, and water that they drank in other households. Thus, the denying claims were not directed towards their individual actions and personal judgment, as they admittedly do fall victim to unhygienic products, but towards what takes place in their household. Vietnam is a communist society where the unit of the family is largely emphasized as the basis of social integrity and organisation (MoH, 2004, Waibel and Glück, 2013). Consequently, a tendency to protect one's reputation and social identity is understandably very much related to the projected image of the household.

In agreement with previous findings from the region of the Delta (Herbst et al., 2009), many observations confirmed that taking care of the household's order and hygiene, particularly in relation to the preparation of food, is principally a woman's preoccupation. The difficulty in perceiving - or admitting - that food and water from one's kitchen could be unhygienic, reflects how health in the household is a display of the "face" of a family, an indicator of societal order and dignity. Considering the discursive association of diarrhoea to poverty and backwardness by many state officials, the difficulty of openly admitting the diseases' prevalence in one's family is also understood as one way to protect the household's socio-economic image. Gammeltoft (1999) notices how Vietnamese women carry a sense of responsibility towards their households, similar to the inherent need of protecting one's body from harm. This type of moral responsibility is one of many strong connections that exist between the individual and social body:

> "Just as bodies have insides which need protection from harmful winds and other outside pathogenic influences, families have insides which need protection from the public gaze and malicious gossip... Bodies and families mutually influence and depend upon each other: as strong and stable bodies are a precondition for the strength and stability of families, so do the health and strength of the bodies depend on families being happy and harmonious" (Gammeltoft, 1999: 132).

The hygiene of the general *outside*, on the other hand, is seen by the respondents to be governed by a set of rules and conditions, which function in scales larger than the family and beyond the control of one woman. The mistrust towards these rules connects back to the credibility of state institutions and their capacity to control water quality and food safety. The perceptions about what constitutes safe, where disease prevails, and how it is transmitted were similar between urban and rural inhabitants from various educational backgrounds and of different income levels. This shows that, despite how different vulnerabilities might relate to the consideration of their socio-economic position, many people's beliefs and attitudes towards the risk of disease are shared, shaped by the same discourses, whether contemporary or historically rooted. The subtle particularities that were noticed regarding the perceptions of the cyclic processes of food, faecal matter, and disease and the human body, are parallel to what Jewitt (2011) refers to of as 'hygienic beliefs' that shape people's practices of sanitation. Similar to the analysis of Douglas (2002), the perception of purity and dirt appeared to be very much related to the contextual social and cultural backgrounds that background them in the Mekong Delta.

Weakening health communication by narrowing its content

Culture and society constitute a historical platform upon which more volatile socio-economic factors and conditions act to define the choices and behaviours of people in relation to health and disease. However, societies and cultures are also undergoing change, even if the pace is variable in different contexts. In consideration of this ongoing transformation and evolution of societies and cultures, it is fair to expect that people's perceptions and practices with regard to disease will be neither static nor monolithic. However, the rate at which people's beliefs and understandings develop is not always in concert with the rate of change that is taking place in environmental, socio-economic and political spheres. The public health education system in Vietnam is suffering from a public health discourse which not only lacks scientific clarity but also does not take into account the traditional beliefs and practices through which disease becomes relevant and meaningful to local people.

Phenomena such as the severe and ongoing pollution of surface waters, the increasing population in urban areas, and the increasing price of water delivery, are all taking place concurrently and are combining to affect people's vulnerability to disease. Local policies are also changing, often in response to global development paradigms, which shape programs of intervention for improved sanitation or regulation of public healthcare access. Such changes, internationally and locally, do not always appear to take into account the distribution and the growth of vulnerabilities towards, in this case, disease. The capacity to adapt to such contextual changes seems to be particularly hard for those living in remote areas, for the ethnic minorities, for the landless and the poor. The risk of disease might thus be increasing at a pace faster than what support policies require in order to develop and to reach everyone, especially those mostly vulnerable. Considering the pressure that the above changes are having on the people of the Mekong Delta, and considering also the existence and persistence of beliefs and practices that exacerbate the spread of disease, a health education mechanism would help in bridging knowledge gaps by addressing contradicting perceptions between local values and will expand the range of options for achieving consistently safer behaviours. One of the difficulties in achieving a dynamic, empowering and adaptive public health education system was its current inability to integrate and preserve useful knowledge in its content. The term "useful knowledge" is here meant to encompass both scientific and lay understandings, both biomedical and traditional principles of medicine, both factual and socio-cultural meanings of disease.

The fact that people maintain categories of health and hygiene that might be rooted in local culture but do not correspond to current conditions is a largely disregarded issue despite the fact that it has clear implications for health outcomes. The content of the communication approaches for healthier WASH behaviours in Vietnam seems to leave out lay knowledge and everyday practices. Instead of bridging, comparing and reconciling understandings, the efforts aim only to introduce new knowledge to replace the old. When people's habits and understandings are not adequately addressed in health education programs, it is likely that state-produced messages will be discarded by the public as irrelevant or misleading. Considering also that people do not always see the health benefits of following the state's advice, either because it is too narrow to have an effect, or because it is not justified properly, placing trust in this advice is is less likely. Health education on diarrheal disease would therefore perhaps stand a better chance of being successful if it was able to include and address the real-world aspects of the problem. In the end, trust and respect always go both ways.

The way interviewees described the causes of diarrhoea and the preventive strategies they employ differed depending on the institutional unit where interviews were held. From single household members to community leaders and representatives of the Ministry of Health, views and beliefs were communicated using elements from both the scientific and the lay fields of knowledge, with mixed levels of clarity and accuracy. The analysis demonstrated that this knowledge is compartmentalised along administrative levels and dichotomised according to the positioning of the interviewees along civil-to-state lines. The content of the interviews is illustrative of a gap between how experts from national research institutes and offices explain the presence of diarrheal disease and the presence of these explanations in the discourse produced by local-level counterparts. High-level health representatives are not only more informed regarding the scientific knowledge that exists on the topic, but are also more capable of linking problems of disease to the socio-economic and institutional context in the country. Consequently, they appear to better understand the salient and the underlying factors that shape disease (section 6.3.3). Health workers and cadres from the grassroots, on the other hand, appear rather unable to provide elaborate explanations and arguments about how to reduce the risk of diarrhoea.

As was addressed in above, it is natural to connect this superior ability to understand and elaborate on the issue of disease with the higher education requirements of staff at upper administrative levels. However, there is an important underlying to take into account when interpreting the content of discourse provided by state representatives: there exists a strict notion of hierarchy and central-level control in the Vietnamese system of administration - which has its roots in Confucianism - and which penetrates aspects of social and political life (Kerkvliet, 2001). The staff of the Ministry, for example, rank higher in this hierarchy and are therefore less vulnerable to castigation when expressing their honest - but critical - opinion on a topic such as the socio political drivers of disease. Unlike the cadres in commune or district levels, which are always subject to control and surveillance from higher-level authorities, ministerial staff is not reluctant to correlate the incidence of disease with the bad implementation of policy and with phenomena such as the privatisation of health services or rapid urbanisation.

The effect that this can have on the discourse on disease being circulated is the hesitation of local cadres to discuss the connections that exist, for example, between the quality of primary healthcare, price of medicine, ownership of land, participation in community education programs, and the incidence of disease. This is because more explanation and elaboration on the problem will inevitably imply - or explicitly refer to - shortcomings of party-formulated policy and party-driven practice. In summary, apart from educational weaknesses, the lack of connecting discourse on the issue of disease at the local levels might also be due to the silenced opinions of cadres whose position and 'party loyalty' are more strictly expressed in the stance they take towards governmental decisions and policies. Even within the context of a one-party state, where grassroots critique is often discouraged and in which the Vietnamese have learnt to exist and manoeuvre, the question of what governs the "epidemiology" of health messages remains. Following Nichter and Nichter (1996b), the question becomes Why do certain messages - even in their discursive simplicity and critical "dryness" - survive while others are lost in the process of public communication and health education?

Through the analysis above, it has been illustrated that there exist alternative understandings about the risk of diarrheal disease which are either based on traditional medicine principles or lay knowledge. The example of how people assess the safety of water using sensory information is illustrative of how important addressing this is in order to understand why unhealthy practices persist. In a related example, many survey respondents thought of traditional medicine as the best cure (15.3%) for diarrheal disease, even though official guidelines strongly recommend the use of Oral Rehydration Solutions (ORS) combined with sufficient intake of nutritious food and clean water (MoH, 2009c). Some people also believed that food intake should be minimised in case of diarrhoea (2.3%) and a few (7.6%) recognised ORS as the appropriate treatment measure (section 7.3.3). Many people suggested that preventing a disease is a matter of maintaining a healthy balance of sleep, and the intake of "hot" and "cold" foods in relation to the outside weather or to other external conditions (section 7.4.3). Irrespective of how accurate or effective, these are also ways in which people understand their bodies and their health. As already discussed, instead of addressing such beliefs, the materials produced to promote safer and healthier practices seem to widely disregard them.

The widespread presence of traditional Vietnamese medicine in the national healthcare and medical education sector has not hindered the expansion and development of biomedical approaches (Wahlberg, 2006), a phenomenon which is evident in the remarkable expansion of biomedicine in Vietnam and the wide use of western medicine by Vietnamese people (chapter 4). Despite its long history, traditional medicine has been largely absent from the preventive health discourse, perhaps being viewed as irrelevant, or as a hindrance to the adoption of globally prescribed disease eradication measures. As with many other types of policies that are imported and implanted - rather than incorporated - into local context, public health campaigns related to the prevention of diarrhoea were also found to be rather blind to the cultural and social realities of much the population. It might be hard to translate microbes, antibiotics or toxic chemical substances into traditional categories of health and equally difficult to translate local language into medical diagnosis in order to understand the meanings that people frequently ascribe to disease. However, at least attempting this seems to be rather necessary if health prevention campaigns aim to become interesting and relevant to the people whose health is at stake. The research of Nichter and Nichter (1996b) on the anthropology of international health concludes that for health communication to be "infective" it has to start from the facts and metaphors people understand and relate to:

> "In the field of health education far more time, energy, and resources have been expended identifying what a population does not know or do, than in assessing what a population does know and the way in which it is known. What is often neglected is a consideration of those concepts of health and images of body processes which underlie the layperson's health practices. Due to this lack of appreciation of tacit knowledge and the cultural common sense (and empirical observations) upon which it is based, cultural resources are often underutilized by health educators [....] There seemed to be a tacit assumption on the part of health trainers that once health workers were supplied information, they could then pass it on to villagers in a suitable manner." (Nichter and Nichter, 1996b: 407)

With a strict top-down approach to the selection and communication of preventive health messages, the Vietnamese state appears to care and be knowledgeable about the health issues that trouble its citizens. At the same time, however, the state does not allow for an active bottom-up enrichment of these topics by not allowing an active dialogue on the policies followed in the field of preventive medicine, as the following section will discuss in more detail. In that sense, much of what people *do* know gets dismissed, with the only goal being to transmit what people do *not* know. Unlike what the public health mechanism implicitly tries to suggest, different kinds of knowledge do not necessarily contradict each other; often they can be used collaboratively to address the risk of disease, particularly if they go through an inclusive process of discussion and debate. Through this process of inclusion, new concepts that were before unknown or uncommon, but potentially beneficial, can be better understood and more easily accepted and remembered.

Beliefs and practices about disease prevention are versatile and co-evolving with the social, cultural and natural environments within which they are used and (re)invented. In the context of fast-paced change, however, some ideas and beliefs might clash and eventually distort people's vulnerability to risks. This is either because old risks change or new types of risks arise. It is precisely the space where ideas and beliefs about disease clash and call for reinvention that presents an opening for health communication strategy to play a significant role. In Vietnam, this space was often found to be shadowed by a top-down communication approach that is woefully behind in content and methods of implementation. Bennet et al. (2010) refer to the "shadow" spaces which surround such contested and debated issues of risk, underlining how these spaces are often dominated by technical experts who are not paying attention to local context and not involving the public. The authors stress and warn that, no matter the expertise that this type of discourse might contain, "all forms of knowledge construction have their limitations when taken out of the specific context in which knowledge was created" (Bennett et al., 2010: 34). This accurately describes how the tailoring of preventive health policies in the study region stops at the highest administrative levels and does not manage to reflect the specific problems and needs of the localities. As Waibel et al. (2012: 191) have described for the water sector in general, "the devolution of decision-making powers and management responsibilities stops at the provincial level, hindering the development of solutions appropriate for local conditions at the district and commune level".

8.1.4 The politics of health risk communication

Crippled participation in a disempowering health education

One way in which the public is excluded from health education activities in the study region is through the formal and informal rules that govern the participation in the training classes of the commune level. Formally, the state supports the dissemination of information through training classes and educational material and by assigning provincial experts to guide this process and pass information down to the localities (section 6.3.2). The law governing these processes does not specify how and for whom health education will happen, but generally points to its potential and to the need for the trickle-down of information from the experts to the public (MoH, 2007b, CERWASS, 2003).

Observations and interviews within the communes and wards showed that health education activities are scarce and rarely ever take place twice in the same commune (section 6.3.2). This makes it hard for people who participate in these classes to come back and give feedback on the strategies they were recommended and on the advice which they might have followed. It is not only the scarcity, but also the methodology that characterizes these classes, that does not encourage feedback and participation from the audience (health education activity O Mon, 05.08.11; personal attendance). Moreover, the audience is limited to 50 attendants and was seen to only include state cadres, public office employees and representatives of unions. In other words, the opportunity to be part of the education process is restricted to a rather select number of people, who are directly or indirectly connected to the Party. Considering the moral commitment of the participants to faithfully serve the government, complaint or questioning of the given information and the prescribed advice is unlikely.

The participants of these classes were referred to as local communicators. They are the considered human "loudspeakers" who carry the responsibility of spreading the health-related information they receive to everyone in their community, mainly through group gatherings and household visits. Despite this mini-narrative about their role and activities, which was repeated by many state officials, it was made clear that local cadres who visit households do not discuss issues of health, but rather run checks about whether certain practices are followed. The list of activities that is being checked mostly includes issues of water and sanitation and is principally focused on the presence of facilities defined as "hygienic" (section 5.3.1). The latter is considered a preventive measure against diarrhoea and as an indicator of awareness about it. Health education for the wider public becomes, in the case of a waterborne disease like diarrhoea, merely a test of how much people have invested in the prescribed water and sanitation solutions and a reminder of the state's expectations for them to make such investments.

This issue goes back to how much the two topics of disease and of household water infrastructure are discursively interwoven. Institutionally, this also goes back to the national fixation on such indicators and the related production of statistics, which will accordingly boost the country's image with regard to global developmental goals. However, it also illuminates how the hierarchical attitude of the state is maintained and it represents itself to the citizens, even at the very local levels. Namely, even if local cadres are close to and literally part of the communities, they preserve an approach of supervision rather than trying to engage in a constructive dialogue with the citizens around health. This way of understanding participation is not new to the Vietnamese state. As it has been discussed by Waibel et al. (2012: 173), the political system in the country depends on the assumption that people's concerns, needs and ideas are fully understood and represented by the selected cadres and therefore, once this determination has been made, the activities of those cadres are not to be called into question.

This ingrained political assumption reflects how health campaigns are executed, with the public being only a receiver of information, advice and concrete guidelines. Then negotiation of this advice is not given any public space. On the contrary, the public is subjected to control with regard to proper implementation. The whole process has ironically adopted the name of "health information, education and communication activities". Studies of risk communication and risk understanding have widely discussed how the perceptions and the practices of people are highly dependent on the level of involvement they have in risk education activities (Kasperson and Kasperson, 2005: 22ff). Based on this, the behavioural factors that shape the risk of diarrheal disease in Vietnam are more than likely connected to the public's inadequate exposure to, and involvement in, such activities. What has been described by state representatives as improper health behaviours of "stubborn", "backwards" or "ignorant" people (section 6.3.4) is then better understood as the uninformed behaviours of excluded, ignored and marginalised people. Apart from public health objectives not being achieved, the non-involvement of the public is hindering the many empowering effects that health education can have (Nutbeam, 2000). Policing health behaviours but not being able to offer the knowledge that people need in order to formulate their own informed judgments and strategies, is leaving them insecure, uncertain and often unable to act to the benefit of their own health. Echoing Bandura (2004), health education is a lens on the practices of social systems. If participation is not encouraged in society, health education can hardly ever be successful.

Public non-compliance in the face of a dominant state

The impact of health campaigns is largely dependent on how the public encounters, embraces, adjusts or rejects the supplied messages (Nichter, 1996c). The results of this study show that even if many people are aware of what the state wants them to do, they cannot - or simply will not - follow state guidelines or advice. This becomes clear in the example of sanitation, with a share of more than 20% people who practice open defecation reported nationwide (JMP Vietnam, 2012b), and similar proportion (25%) in Can Tho City (CERWASS,

2011a). Despite the prohibition of the fishpond toilet and the strong promotion of hygienic facilities, there are still many families who "insist" on this practice. The household survey actually showed that the percentage of people practicing open defecation is as high as 45% (section 7.3.3). As was noted before, this statistic is not only indicative of institutional shortcomings but is often the result of an underprivileged socio-economic position. People might insist on open defecation and ignore the advice for sanitation, but this can also be understood as the result of "suffocating" and badly maintained toilets which are a result of restricted access to microcredit for improvement, expensive construction requirements, or the lack of proper justification from a hygienic view. Similarly, the practice of hand-washing with soap might seem incomprehensible if one is unaware of how pathogenic transmission through the hands takes place, and also if soap and clean water is a considerable expense for a family. This type of non-compliance is thus a result of financial difficulties and of a lack of access to support resources and information.

Kerkvliet (2003 cited in Waibel et al. 2012: 173) speaks of this discrepancy between what the state commands and what people actually do, pointing to the bottom-up process of decollectivising agriculture in Vietnam during the 1980s. In the sector of agriculture discussed by Kerkvliet (2003), people have a good grasp of the practical benefits they need to subtly negotiate on, which is apparent when they do not following centrally prescribed *practices* and instead prefer other forms of *action*. Issues of health, however, contain a lot of abstract, unknown, ungraspable and unexplained risk. Some people's ideas and opinions about how to safeguard their health have their roots in traditional and herbal medicine, others are acquired through experiential learning and many are, of course, based on acquired medical understandings. As findings showed, the public's health perceptions are often an amalgam of the above sources and, more often than not, result in contradicting health behaviours. The persisting incidence of many infectious diseases, diarrhoea included (section 4.3.1), indicates that few people manage to protect themselves from this type of risk. Half of the respondents in the household survey admitted that they suffer from diarrhoea at least 3 times per year (section 7.3). With only 15% of people able to readily recognise the risk of waterborne disease and only 6.1% presenting hand-washing as a known measure of prevention, the need for behavioural adaptation and change does not seem to be fully realised by the local communities of the region. Unlike the case of agricultural decollectivisation, where people took action for their own vision of agricultural life and practice (Kerkvliet, 2003), the non-compliant practices of hygiene and sanitation do not appear as a conscious form of resistance. Instead of leading to some commonly desired outcome, the behaviours that are often followed perpetuate the loose control of the disease's spread and boomerang against the health of local people.

The figure of a dominant state is, however, seen to play a role in shaping health behaviours. Although in some cases the state has successfully promoted healthy behaviours, in many other cases it has resulted in superficially compliant but ineffective behaviours, or clearly incompliant and still risky ones. In Vietnam, the communication of health risks has a commanding character with a top-down and didactic tone, reinforcing the idea of the central state's unquestionable expertise. This was demonstrated in how "do's" and "don'ts" constitute the only form of communicated health related information, especially at the level of the district and below, and within the circulated educational material (section 6.3.3). Bennett et al. (2010: 32) have spoken of this mistaken tendency "to summon up the *deficit model* [174] of an ignorant and ill-informed public" and stress how this approach "fails to understand the basis of public concerns and provokes feelings of antagonism and rejection". In other words, when the form of advice assumes public ignorance, it will probably be rejected by a public that does not want to be identified as ignorant. This relates also to the "optimistic bias" (Frewer et al., 1994) people tend to have, which leads to the assumption that one's own behaviour is not risky and that information about disease risk is directed at "others", who are not knowledgeable and not aware (this was discussed in relation to food safety, section 6.2.2). This can explain why people do not follow state advice, even if it is within their ability to do so. Survey data shows, for example, that many of the average-income households are not adequately following recommended water treatment practices and that very few respondents actually practice hand-washing with soap, even though many were aware of both these practices as health-promoting behaviours.

In this light, it is better understood why any health-related information and advice needs to be framed in a way that will respect the views, the knowledge and the socio-cultural realities of the people whose problems it aims to address. Dismissing people's abilities to protect themselves by trying to replace their understandings with new concepts that are loosely understood and unfamiliar, is a strategy doomed to fail. As Bennet et al. (2010) further note, "people do not need information for information's sake, but as a means of taking responsibility for personal choices, improving their own or their family's wellbeing or supporting their role in society" (Moore 2002 cited in Bennett et al., 2010: 149). The marriage of new knowledge with pre-existing perceptions is, as already discussed, a process which can build trust and facilitate educational empower-

[174] Bennett et al. (2010) are here citing Irwin and Wynne (1996).

ment with relation to health. In line with the above, Nichter (1996c) notes that the difference between empowerment (active demand) and imposition (passive acceptance) can define whether healthy practices are adopted or not:

> "It is only when vaccinations are recognized as a perceived need and demanded by the 'community' that they become community development resources in a 'comprehensive primary health care' sense" (Rifkin and Walt 1986 cited in Nichter, 1996c).

The state-society nexus in Vietnam has special characteristics which render the compliance with state policy a socially complicated process. Gammeltoft has linked health to Confucianism, which she refers to as the "intellectual and ideological backbone of Vietnam" (Nguyen Khac Vien cited in Gammeltoft, 1999: 134). The author (Gammeltoft, 1999) sees health understandings and practices as social behaviours related to the hierarchical balances kept between the individual, the family and society. This linkage was indeed observed, firstly in the written preventive health guidelines, which are often presented as moral obligations towards the community or the country (section 6.3.1) and secondly through the defensive responses of people (mainly women), who assertively protected their household's and their own reputation when discussing hygiene behaviour and the (lack of) disease risk in the household (section 8.1.3). The compliance to norms and guidelines was thus often on the basis of keeping an image of good citizenship and representing a healthy community.

The attitudes of respondents reflected how these moral notions have created an imperative for healthy behaviour, with most people being hesitant to declare non-compliance with state-provided advice in the presence of state officials. Respondents would rush to declare that they have a "hygienic latrine", they drink "boiled water" and eat "well-cooked food", even if that was not the case. As findings indicate, the mere recognition of advocated messages does not imply that an understanding exists of the links between these practices and the spread of disease. Rheinländer et al. (2010) similarly observe that "the drive for sanitation and hygiene can be not due to biomedical knowledge but more to show social class or cultural compliance". Nevertheless, it is precisely when people superficially try to show their compliance without being clear on how to achieve healthier lives, that public health measures expose a flawed implementation. This was seen in the example of latrines that are labelled as hygienic, but discharge untreated sewage into the river (section 7.2.1) and in the case of households which are connected to the water network, but also consume other types of untreated water (section 7.1.2).

Policy and politics shaping the distribution of health risks

As was discussed above, respondents might be pushed to report compliance with advocated measures because of their feelings of responsibility towards the state and moral obligation to good citizenship. The same kind of tendency to declare compliance and progress towards achieving national targets was also observed from offices of the local state. This was not only through the contradicting claims of representatives from these offices, but also through their produced reports. An example here would be the over-reporting of the expansion of "hygienic" water and sanitation by district level authorities (section 5.4). In making reporting, instead of effective implementation, their primary concern, Beresdorf (2008) notes that "local authorities are largely responsible to their superior levels rather than to the people".

This strive to comply in the eyes of superiors seems to be, at least in the WSS sector, primarily a matter of attracting funding. It was made explicit by informants that the distribution of provincial funding in the sector of WSS depends on each province's declared public demand for construction (i.e. number of people willing to invest) and on the province's previous performance in attracting funding and in realising "hygienic" constructions (section 5.3.2). The generated discourse on the demand and the implementation success of WSS, therefore, serves not only as a moral achievement and an expression of loyalty to the Party, but also as a way of attracting funding. In this context, the tendency to over-report compliance in the sector becomes a matter of provincial competition for resources. The examination of these processes in the study region flagged accounting discrepancies and indicated a serious misappropriation of funds (section 5.3.2). For example, while the Vietnamese Social Policy Bank gave out about 27 billion VND for the purposes of WSS micro-credit loans in 2010-2011, the newly constructed facilities reported by CERWASS would have only cost a maximum of 12 billion VND (VBSP, 2011, CERWASS, 2010, CERWASS, 2011a). This leaves a tremendous amount of 15 billion VND unaccounted for, either as a result of administrative mishandling or because beneficiaries used the money for purposes other than investing in WSS. Irrespectively of how or by whom these funds were spent, it is clear that the lack of transparency in the distribution compromises the potential of such policies to deal with disease, unhealthy environments and poverty.

Another issue that arises in the sector - apart from the inability of the poor to benefit from credit that goes unaccounted for - is the overemphasis on measures that require capital investment (i.e. sanitary constructions) over those that mostly require an effective and inclusive communication between experts and the public (education on how people can prevent and cure disease more efficiently). Reis (2012: 190ff) has indicated that prioritising sanitation over alternative water options is underpinned by the personal interests of local bureaucracies. Taking into account also that "software" measures are being overshadowed by "hardware" solutions, the latter of which promise more funding for the provinces, the political nature of preventive health policy begins to surface. Part and parcel to such phenomena appears to be the increased level of bureaucratic corruption that operates in Vietnam under what Gillespie (2001) terms "fuzzy" legality. As Gillespie (2001) explains, despite the efforts of the state to promote legal conformity and control corruption, the power of cultural ideologies often seems to overcome the law by reinterpreting its purpose and ultimately ignoring it. Much of the Vietnamese bureaucracy is operating under what the author terms a 'socialist legality' which "only incidentally promotes legal conformity" (Gillespie, 2001: 24). Waibel et al. (2012: 173) have noted how the gaps between policy and practice in the wider water sector are not simply due to economic or capacity constraints, but as a result of intricate political and managerial paradigms followed in the country. In agreement with their findings, the unequal emphasis on "hardware" versus "software" solutions seems to be much more than an issue of insufficient funds or a lack of expertise in communication.

The political nature of disease begins to emerge when considering the processes that will define risk. The selection of appropriate responses and prevention strategies requires recognition of the exact factors that constitute the risk of disease. These processes are dependent on social and political structures. Moreover, in order to address a risk, there needs to be an agreement on the evaluation of its gravity. For these reasons, risk in general is often seen as entirely socially constructed (Bennett et al., 2011: 18). In Vietnam, public discussion and bottom-up participation was not seen to be encouraged. The domain of disease prevention, through disease risk recognition and formulation of strategies, was seen to be exclusively occupied by the central state. In return, the priorities of the state are largely influenced by international development requirements and defined indicators in the sectors of water and health. Examined though the example of water supply and sanitation, part of the reason why the country tries to tune its efforts to international demands appears to be the fact that, in this way, development points are gained and more investment flows in. This way of designing risk policy, of recognising the factors that constitute this risk and of formulating strategies to address it, is not driven by local needs. It does not allow for genuine feedback about whether the strategies followed actually benefit the health and the life of the majority. The reported "hygienic" latrine becomes a symbol of progress and compliance, but not a means of achieving disease-free communities. Similarly, the high coverage of piped water supply (JMP Vietnam, 2012a, CERWASS, 2011a) ticks international development boxes for rural development, while the actual drinking water needs of the majority are met through the purchase of bottled water or through the consumption of polluted water sources (section 7.1.1).

The political side of disease and of health communication goes beyond questions of how capable or functional the governing bodies of the sector are. As Lupton (1994 cited in Geist and Gates, 1996) has warned, "until health communication takes cognizance of recent developments in social and political theory, media and cultural studies, discourse analysis, and their application to communication in the health setting, it is destined to remain a derivative paternalistic and narrowly focused version of health education". Findings from the Delta show how the process of defining a health risk is inherently political, as it empowers the state to be the only knowledge carrier, the solution provider and the entity to which people must be amenable to. The analysis points to the fact that attaching moral and ideological content to public health messages might enhance the implementation of the advocated measures to an extent, but most importantly, it weakens the potential of empowering people with knowledge. As a result, the ability of these messages to yield sustainably informed practices is also weakened. Moreover, when lacking such empowering knowledge, people are also less likely to express concern about their current situation. Reis (2012: 212) has questioned the potential for people to react against the root causes their non-accessibility to clean water when "the awareness about health risks connected with drinking polluted water is not very distinct among the rural population, even if many feel uncomfortable with drinking river water" and when "the problem of polluted water is not assigned to failures of state management [...] but to economic development involving the arrival of pesticides, fish farming and factories" (Ibid. 2012: 211). It is perhaps an underlying interest of the state not to overemphasize the issue of waterborne disease, as this would reveal the large and unequal distribution of such risks, which are largely a result of party politics and local administration decisions.

It is becoming clearer why the distribution of health risks is not only a highly complicated matter, but mostly a political one. Bambra et al. (2005) attest to the political nature of health, noting that "like any other resource or commodity under a neo-liberal economic system, some social groups have more of it than others". In the case of diarrheal disease in Can Tho City, such correlations between sickness and poverty were not made clear through the empirical examination of disease incidence. However, it was shown that access to healthcare is almost entirely commodified and thus subject to people's financial capacities (chapter 4). This has rendered the poor over-exposed to potentially disastrous health costs and has cultivated a view of healthcare as a sort of a luxury or last resort only to be sought in case of "serious" disease (section 7.4.3). The constraints in accessing clean water, sanitation facilities and sanitary environments faced by those living in poverty further support this claim.

Bambra et al. (2005) continue their claim that "health is political because its social determinants are amenable to political interventions and are thereby dependent on political action (or more usually, inaction)". Sectors like food safety, Rotavirus vaccinations and the control of malnutrition have all been proven crucial for the management of diarrheal disease risk. In order to be able to substantially contribute to the strengthening and the accessibility of these sectors, however, requires political will, prioritisation and transparency. As witnessed in Vietnam, such measures largely remain on paper only (MoH, 2009c). Instead of being prioritised, they are rather downplayed by policies which guarantee the circulation of funds within the Vietnamese public administration (section 6.2). As the authors (Bambra et al., 2005) conclude, "health is political because power is exercised over it as part of a wider economic, social and political system".

Indeed, human health is a field where the fear and the faith of people are both magnified. Health is a personal but also a public domain that is imbued with uncertainty due to the coexistence of many knowns and unknowns. This uncertainty might increase when people feel disempowered to control its outcomes. Due to this uncertainty, the discourse around health risk is a vivid field, within which opinions are shaped and power is negotiated. In Vietnam, this field is dominated by the state and the power that comes with access to this field is used to re-empower the state. Through the platform of health education, social moralisation is reproduced. Knitting a web that ties together ideas of public health and state ideology, the VCP strives to reinforce its legitimacy. Through the disguise of bureaucratic procedures and meaningless reporting as health-promoting activities, the "success story" of adequately addressing water and health issues seems to be kept alive for the purpose of attracting international funding. At the same time, however, the implementation of even the most basic elements of diarrheal disease prevention falls short.

8.2 A political ecology of disease: theoretical implications

With diarrheal disease as a central research topic and point of departure, this study paid particular attention to water as the encompassing element defining this disease. The principal theoretical connections with the field of political ecology have thus been the access to resources and of the interaction that takes place between societies and the natural environment. The analysis demonstrated why people's access to safe water, a basic human right, is anything but a simple issue. In order to examine this in a holistic manner, the study's theoretical grounding expanded outside the borders of a 'political ecology of water' and explored a more specific and more inclusive, 'political ecology of disease'.

Whereas environmental issues, like resource scarcities and natural disasters, have often been analysed by political ecologists who tend to reveal their social and political nature (Otero et al., 2010, Kaika, 2003), the same can hardly be said about the health outcomes of those issues, such as disease and epidemics (but see: Turshen, 1977, Mayer, 1996a, King, 2010). By focusing on the related health problem, rather than on the problem of water management, a political ecology of disease includes aspects of public health governance, and goes deeper into the question of how the population is affected - within the scope of natural resources management. As Richmond et al. (2005: 352, my emphasis) contend, "political ecology identifies the dimensions of a politicized environment and focuses explicitly on the role of power relations as a source of environmental debate [...] yet seldom addresses *how* the health of populations is affected". There is a difference between the questions of *what* kind of environmental health problems can be created and *why* this happens and the question of *how* such a health issue is shaped and expresses itself. The difference lies, primarily, in that in order to answer *how*, one has to employ methodologies that will turn attention to the people, to how they understand, document and represent health and to how they experience disease. One of the core novelties in the analytical approach followed here, is that it incorporates two different perspectives in the study of an environmental health problem: the institutional and the cultural.

Figure 8.1: The fields of study contributing to a political ecology of disease

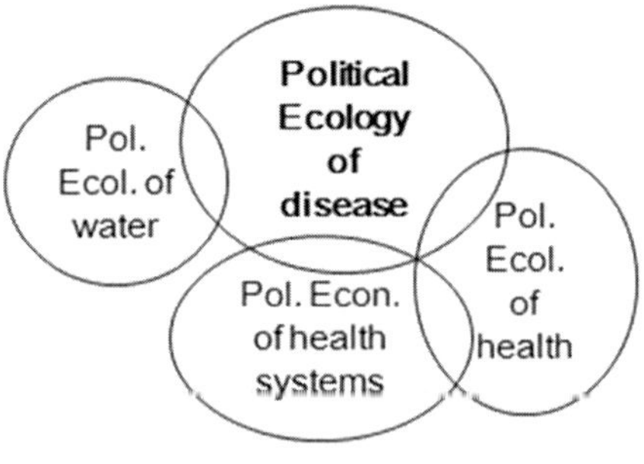

Author's elaboration, 2014

To begin with, in order to critically examine the institutions that govern disease, a political ecology of water resources needs to be complemented by a political ecology of *health* and of *healthcare* systems. A political ecology of health will examine how and why the risk of disease is distributed along different environmental and socio-economic terrains. A political ecology of healthcare will assess how the structure and function of health services affects the vulnerability of different individuals to disease risk. While studies in the political economy of health and disease are not lacking (Farmer, 2005, Foley, 2009), and especially not in the transitional context of Vietnam (Fritzen, 2007, Forsberg, 2011, Bloom, 1998), they have rarely offered an empirical coupling of critical views regarding both the issues of natural resources management and health governance (but see: Collins, 2001, Saravanan et al., 2011, Few and Tran, 2010). This study filled this lacuna, by focusing on the links between water pollution, water supply, sanitation and the spread of diarrheal disease, not only from a biophysical point of view but through their common institutional underpinnings. This is how the unique aspects of a political ecology of disease were allowed to emerge.

One of these aspects was the examination of the ways in which the country's formal institutions communicate the risk of the disease's spread. Prevention in health has gained recognition as "the best cure", but for public health preventive action to even begin, health risks need to be defined. In relation to this, the second analytical theme that arose through the political ecology of healthcare systems was how health risks in society are defined, re-defined and communicated within these systems. Interestingly, in the study of diarrheal disease, the definition of health risk entails discussions about water management, water pollution and water treatment. While management of these issues can be assigned solely to the realm of individual personal behaviour, which was often the case in Vietnam, they go beyond this to constitute major fields of public policy and related debates. There was therefore a critical transition, from asking questions of how and why environmental risks are *distributed,* to asking how and why they are *communicated* in the frame of public health policy. Surprisingly, many of the answers pointed back to the same essential elements of what guides policy and what characterizes the relationship between state and society in Vietnam. It was argued that diarrhoea has been rendered "normal" through the intricate discourse-building processes of the state, materialised through legal, professional and communicative practices, in order to define the acceptable limits of ill-health and healthcare quality, as well as of water quality, implementation of law and, more generally, of acceptable risks.

Despite the apparent uniformity with which the acceptability of risk is treated, risk does not seem to affect all people the same way due to structural inequalities and varying vulnerabilities. It is this basic notion of inequality that the politics of environmental risk and the politics of health risk communication have in common. Merging and comparing the distribution of risk to the communication of this risk, pointed to their common denominators. In Vietnam, these denominators have roots in the drive for modernity and relentless economic growth that the state follows (with the precondition that the current political structures will be sustained). Polluting waters is accepted if the economy requires it, and "hygienic" constructions are showcased as promoting health if this attracts international funding. In other words, it was made obvious through the study of a health risk how the "shadow" spaces in the debates about risk (Peeling et al. in Bennett et al., 2010) are used to reproduce a system of values where privileged elites maintain their privileges and the participation of the masses in defining policy is essentially hindered.

It is precisely the issue of participation that begged for an examination of human agency and the inclusion of culture. Participation can be roughly described as a process through which communities and civil society engage in dialogue with the state, with the results of this dialogue finding representation in the central offices of policy-making, or directly translating into practice at a local level. As Reis (2012) argues, policy should not simply be thought of as the push-factor for practice, but "as a metaphor and as a context where practice takes place" (Molle 2005 cited in Reis 2012: 9). If we consider institutions as social structures "made up of a collection of individuals or organisations, within which collectives exercise action or orientations" (Weerakody et al. 2009: 53 cited in Collyer, 2012: 46), then policy needs to be understood as shaping and being shaped by practice. Actions themselves can be institutionalised when they are habitualised and reciprocally typified (Burger and Luckmann 1984 cited in Collyer 2012: 46). In that sense, the practices performed and the ideas shaping these practices also count as indicators of participation. In order to examine such cultural practices and ideas in this analysis, the methods and the analytical categories of anthropology proved extremely useful. Through tracing patterns of behaviour that are culturally specific and are linked with people's beliefs, values and world-understandings, many of the shortcomings in public health were brought into the light. By questioning the extent to which culturally specific traits enter the field of policy or practice concerning diarrheal disease prevention, patterns of exclusion were revealed and reasons behind the failure of health education and disease prevention campaigns were further explained.

Though Bryant (1992) has long argued that "the role of ideology and culture in environmental change seems particularly important", political ecology has often dealt with culture as a "black box" in which certain behaviours and ideas are placed, in order to be later questioned in relation to the workings of socio-economic and political spheres. This, however, ignores how powerfully these behaviours and ideas demonstrate the transfer and the transformation of knowledge about both environmental and health-related issues. A single focus on formal institutions might lose sight of the different meanings people give to concepts such as nature and life, including water, food and the human body and which define their actions in relation to dynamics like the handling water in the household, children's nutrition and health-seeking behaviour. The actions of collectives or individuals are not homogeneous and are not independent of the institutions in which they act, but rather "highly-interactive and mutually constitutive" (Hall and Taylor, 1996). For this reason, when institutions and policies are studied through the lens of political ecology, an accounting for local context in an ethnographically informed way emerges as necessary. As Escobar argues,

> "We need new narratives of life and culture. These narratives will likely be hybrids of sorts; they will arise from the mediations that local cultures are able to effect on the discourse and practices of nature, capital, and modernity" (Escobar cited in Peet and Watts, 2002: 65)

Incorporating cultural questions, by studying local perceptions and beliefs about diarrheal disease, made it possible to distinguish the subtle ways in which people are eventually excluded from health understandings, how they are made more vulnerable to disease and most importantly, how they are disempowered in their to pursuit and claims for better health. Viewing this through the concept of an "epidemiology of communication" (Nichter, 1996b: 125), attention was drawn to the social and cultural environments where disease is encountered, tracing *how* and *why* knowledge around health circulates through different parts of society and what kinds of "black holes" exist that prevent it from reaching more people in a more effective way. This showed how the de-prioritisation of "everyday" diarrheal disease did not only take place because measures against its spread were not adopted. It also happened due to a continuous disregard for people's traditional beliefs, a dismissive attitude towards lay knowledge of health risks and a didactic and moralising approach to health education by the state. Moreover, the de-prioritisation of diarrhoea was a symptom of attaching meanings of backwardness, poverty and foulness to it, which allowed the disease to be used as a negative social category and turned it into a taboo issue. As such, it becomes more imperative for people to deny the disease than to publically address it.

Practically speaking, while political ecology looks at problems and asks for people to "change the system", pointing to the need for different processes of political participation, for a redistribution of the risks and benefits that emanate from the use of resources and for the inclusion of more voices in the definition of social values, critical anthropological views follow up on this, highlighting where change can beg: in the ideas and the practices of everyday life. The turning of attention to culture entails grappling with meanings, ideas and forms of knowledge that might be unfamiliar in western knowledge paradigms. However, in return, this entails the reward of better understanding human behaviour, which proves essential particularly in the field of development studies. Challenging categories of shame, disgust, safety, cleanliness and health, as they are understood in the context of a Vietnamese rural village or peri-urban area, helped to clarify elements of hygiene behaviour that heretofore had gone unexplained.

That people's understandings of how to prevent disease were still far from what the state has adopted as its official guidelines, pointed to the fact that much of the knowledge available on paper remains unrealised and thus not useful to local communities. It further demonstrated that the size of the chasm between 'what the state says' and 'what people do', owes also to the detachment of people's understandings and opinions from the state's nationally enforced policy. In a context where expressions of discontent are generally silenced, "everyday politics" (Kerkvliet, 2005) can be a form of public contestation. At the same time, the strictly hierarchical and regulated ways in which the one-party state communicates with its citizens, while not explicitly a means of exercising control, favour a Gramscian notion of hegemony, where force and consent are combined and "balance each other reciprocally, without force predominating excessively over consent" (Hoare and Nowell-Smith, 1971 cited in Karim, 2008). Critical anthropological views were able to reveal the indirect and subtle ways in which public disobedience, as well as state control, has been taking place.

What has been gained from this study's use of an analytical framework that centres on political ecology and embraces the critical approaches of medical anthropology? The usefulness of the resulting analytical framework was evident in its ability to outline the multiple spheres (cultural, social, environmental, and political) that encompass health risk and also to allow for intricate connections and interrelations between these spheres to arise. Institutional structures were placed under the same lens as ideational realms. This revealed not only that the outcome of public health policy cannot be explained without examining common understandings, but also that the prevailing discourse is significantly shaping the extent to which people can support and safeguard their health. The analysis further showed that in Vietnam, the formulation and implementation of that policy appear to be mostly serving the actors that have the power to negotiate them. In retrospect, it becomes clearer why studying the spread of disease strictly from an epidemiological point of view would have deprived it of valuable explanations related to human agency and social context. The integration of different analytical scales allowed for the discovery of their connecting thread, which is crucial in order to better understand disease and to address it.

Despite the attempt to be holistic in explanation, this study has faced limitations in discovering every aspect and answering every question in relation to the socio-political and cultural determinants of diarrheal disease in the Mekong Delta. Some of these issues with potential for future research within the fields of political ecology of disease and critical medical anthropology include:

- The evolution of cultural food habits and understandings of safe nutrition, as they correlate to the incidence of chronic disease (cardiovascular and cancer)
- The silent or unheard concerns of communities about health in the context of changing socio-ecological landscapes. The spaces that exist (or not) for such concerns to be turned into a movement for environmental health justice
- The role of global climatic change and local environmental degradation in bringing about mutation of epidemic-capable pathogens, and the consequences of this for human health, especially in the context of extreme and un-regulated consumption of antibiotics

8.3 From discourse to incidence

Indicators of disease incidence and mortality provide a measurable and logical way to assess health risks. However, through this type of assessment, risk is necessarily very narrowly defined. The analysis of discursive practices in societies that face such risks provides the basis on which to reflect on the processes that underpin risk definitions and thus, offers a better understanding of the risk itself. This work intended to point out that, just as development is not to be understood, defined or determined only through the field of western inspired economics, human health is also not to be understood, defined or determined only through biomedicine. By dissolving the images that have been painted through culturally and politically uninformed indicators of health and of development in general, the consequences of persisting inequalities will crystallise and the basis of inequality can be better understood.

In the case of Vietnam, it was shown how the projected image of a modernised and developed state which takes care of its citizens contradicts the reality of a degrading and increasingly unhealthy environment, with significant parts of the population being vulnerable and suffering from a disease that can be controlled. This now obvious contradiction, however, remains blurred within the country. The constructed discourse marginalises the poor and normalises suffering, while at the same time legitimising the state's abdication of its responsibility to provide basic healthcare and clean water; instead the state transfers these responsibilities to the people. The Vietnamese state has subtly, but methodically, designed its institutions in a way that they obey bureaucratic order and present proof of their prescribed activities even if in reality, much of the policy is hardly ever turned into meaningful practice.

In the example of health education, millions of VND are being spent annually with the objective to spread information and to foster public participation, but health education remains a limited process which, more than anything else, advocates the values and priorities of the Party and the government. The construction of an identity of a powerful nation where the state takes care of its citizens and is oriented on fulfilling their common desires, serves a dual purpose: it satisfies both the socialist imperative of one-party rule, which could not survive under widely-voiced public dissatisfaction, and also the requirements of international development agents which rarely examine the products of the country's meticulous bureaucracy in critical depth. In this context, it becomes clear why, in order to understand any complex problem, one would always need to look at the relationships of state and society, nature and culture, institutions and agency.

This leads to the second core insight of this study, which aims to provoke discussion about the potential of interdisciplinary approaches for the study of disease. The core message that this work transmits with regard to the epistemology of health is that scientific reality means very little if it cannot help real people. In other words, even if the factors that govern the distribution and the transformation of a health risk have indisputable biophysical attributes, what happens in the socio-political sphere where those attributes are to be encountered can also shape risks and health outcomes. It is for this reason that biomedical experts, public health practitioners and international think-tanks on health need to engage in a sincere dialogue with the humanities, including ethnographers, sociologists and political scientists. Although the methodologies and the epistemologies followed in these widely-defined fields might diverge immensely, they share a common interest of acting for the improvement of human health. If such a claim holds truth, then there is a lot to be gained from interdisciplinary thinking and sharing.

BIBLIOGRAPHY

Abt Associates Inc. 2011. Distribution of Aquatabs through Commune Health Collaborators in Can Tho, Vietnam. *In:* Ha Nguyen, et al. (eds.) *Safe Water Project implemented by PATH.*

ADB 2007. Water Sector Review Project: Subsector Water Supply and Sanitation. *In:* Trinh, X. L. (ed.) *ADB.TA.4903-VIE.* Hanoi: Asian Development Bank (ADB).

Aguilera-Klink, F., et al. 2000. The Social Construction of Scarcity. The Case of Water in Tenerife (Canary Islands). *Ecological Economics,* 34, 233-245.

Akala, W. J. 2006. The Silent Victims of HIV/Aids in Kenya:The Plight of Uninfected Children among Nomadic Pastoralists. *In:* Falola, T. & Heaton, M. M. (eds.) *Endangered Bodies: Women, Children, and Health in Africa.* Africa World Press.

Allen, A., et al. 2006. The Peri-Urban Water Poor: Citizens or Consumers? *Environment and Urbanization,* 18, 333-351.

Amsterdamska, O. 2005. Demarcating Epidemiology. *Science, Technology & Human Values,* 30, 17.

Anh, D. D., et al. 2011. Use of Oral Cholera Vaccines in an Outbreak in Vietnam: A Case Control Study. *PLoS Neglected Tropical Diseases,* 5, e1006.

Anh Tuan Nguyen, et al. 2009. Medicine Prices, Availability, and Affordability in Vietnam. *Southern Med Review,* 2, 2-9.

Aunger, R., et al. 2010. Three Kinds of Psychological Determinants for Hand-Washing Behaviour in Kenya. *Social science & medicine,* 70, 383-391.

Aven, T. & Renn, O. 2010. *Risk Management and Governance*, Springer.

Axelson, H., et al. 2009. Health Financing for the Poor Produces Promising Short-Term Effects on Utilization and out-of-Pocket Expenditure: Evidence from Vietnam. *International Journal for Equity in Health,* 8, 20.

Baer, H. A. 1996. Toward a Political Ecology of Health in Medical Anthropology. *Medical anthropology quarterly,* 10, 451-454.

Baer, H. A. & Singer, M. 2009. *Global Warming and the Political Ecology of Health: Emerging Crises and Systemic Solutions*, Left Coast Press, Inc.

Bain, R., et al. 2012. Improved but Not Becessarily Safe: Water Access and the Millennium Development Goals. *Global Water Forum*

Bakker, K., et al. 2008. Governance Failure: Rethinking the Institutional Dimensions of Urban Water Supply to Poor Households. *World Development,* 36, 1891-1915.

Bakker, K. J. 2000. Privatizing Water, Producing Scarcity: The Yorkshire Drought of 1995*. *Economic Geography,* 76, 4-27.

Bambra, C., et al. 2005. Towards a Politics of Health. *Health Promotion International,* 20, 187-193.

Bandura, A. 2004. Health Promotion by Social Cognitive Means. *Health Education & Behavior,* 31, 143-164.

Bartlett, S. 2003. Water, Sanitation and Urban Children: The Need to Go Beyond "Improved" Provision. *Environment and Urbanization,* 15, 57-70.

Benedikter, S. 2014. *The Vietnamese Hydrocracy and the Mekong Delta. Water Resources Development from State Socialism to Bureaucratic Capitalism,* Berlin, Münster, Wien, Zürich, London, Lit Verlag.

Bennett, P., et al. 2010. *Risk Communication and Public Health*, Oxford University Press.

Bennett, S., et al. 2011. Influencing Policy Change: The Experience of Health Think Tanks in Low-and Middle-Income Countries. *Health Policy and Planning.*

Beresford, M. 2008. Doi Moi in Review: The Challenges of Building Market Socialism in Vietnam. *Journal of Contemporary Asia,* 38, 221-243.

Black, R. E., et al. 1981. Enterotoxigenic Escherichia Coli Diarrhoea: Acquired Immunity and Transmission in an Endemic Area. *Bulletin of the World Health Organization,* 59, 263.

Blaikie, N. 2009. *Designing Social Research,* Cambridge UK/ Malden USA, Polity Press.

Blaikie, P. M. & Brookfield, H. C. 1987. *Land Degradation and Society*, Routledge Kegan & Paul.

Bloom, D. & Canning, D. 2003. The Health and Poverty of Nations: From Theory to Practice. *Journal of Human Development,* 4, 47-71.

Bloom, G. 1998. Primary Health Care Meets the Market in China and Vietnam. *Health Policy,* 44, 233-252.

Bloom, G., et al. 2007. Health in a Dynamic World. *STEPS Working Paper.* Brighton: STEPS Centre, University of Sussex.

Blum, D. & Feachem, R. G. 1983. Measuring the Impact of Water Supply and Sanitation Investments on Diarrhoeal Diseases: Problems of Methodology. *International journal of Epidemiology,* 12, 357-365.

Briggs, D. 2003. *Making a Difference: Indicators to Improve Children's Environmental Health*, World Health Organization.

Brocheux, P. 2012. Reflections on Vietnam *New Left Review*, 73-91.

Brooks, N. 2003. Vulnerability, Risk and Adaptation: A Conceptual Framework. *In:* Research, T. C. f. C. C. (ed.) *Working Paper.* University of Manchester.

Brown, M. 2006. Sexual Citizenship, Political Obligation and Disease Ecology in Gay Seattle. *Political Geography,* 25, 874-898.

Bryant, J. 1998a. Communism, Poverty, and Demographic Change in North Vietnam. *Population and Development Review*, 235-269.

Bryant, R. L. 1992. Political Ecology: An Emerging Research Agenda in Third-World Studies. *Political Geography,* 11, 12-36.

Bryant, R. L. 1998b. Power, Knowledge and Political Ecology in the Third World: A Review. *Progress in physical geography,* 22, 79.

Budds, J. 2013. Water, Power, and the Production of Neoliberalism in Chile, 1973 - 2005. *Environment and Planning D: Society and Space,* 31, 301-318.

Cairncross, S. 2003. Editorial: Water Supply and Sanitation:Some Misconceptions. *Tropical Medicine & International Health,* 8, 193-195.

Cairncross, S., et al. 2010a. Hygiene, Sanitation, and Water: What Needs to Be Done? *PLoS Medicine,* 7, e1000365.

Cairncross, S., et al. 2010b. Water, Sanitation and Hygiene for the Prevention of Diarrhoea. *International journal of Epidemiology,* 39, i193-i205.

Can Tho Regional Paediatrics Hospital 2011. Monthly Data on the Number of Diarrheal Disease Cases (2009, 2010 and 2011). Can Tho.

Carter, R. C., et al. 1999. The Impact and Sustainability of Community Water Supply and Sanitation Programmes in Developing Countries. *Water and Environment Journal,* 13, 292-296.

Center for Health Market Innovators. 2012. *Enhanced Diarrheal Disease Control in Vietnam* [Online]. Available: http://healthmarketinnovations.org/program/national-guidelines-for-enhanced-diarrheal-disease-control-in-vietnam [Accessed 13.02.13 2013].

Central Committee CPV & Communist Party of Vietnam 2001. Strategy for Socio-Economic Development 2001-2010. Hanoi.

Central Interdisciplinary Committee for Food Safety and Hygiene 2011. Plan on the Implementation of 'the Action Month' for Food Safety, Quality and Hygiene, for 2011. *In:* Health, D. o. (ed.). Can Tho.

CERWASS 2003. Guidelines on Information-Education-Communication (Iec) for Rural Water Supply and Environmental Sanitation. Hanoi: Ministry for Agriculture and Rural Development (MARD).

CERWASS 2010. Collecting Data on Water Supply and Sanitation for Households in Can Tho, by Commune. Can Tho: CERWASS.

CERWASS 2011a. Collecting Data on Water Supply and Sanitation for Households in Can Tho, by Commune. Can Tho: CERWASS.

CERWASS 2011b. Guidelines for Collecting Information on Hygienic Water and Sanitation. Can Tho: CERWASS.

CERWASS 2011c. Implementation of the Ntp for the 6 First Months of 2011, Plan for the Last 6 Months of 2011 and the Proposed Plan for 2012 Can Tho: CERWASS.

CERWASS 2011d. Instructions on How to Complete Data for the Survey on Sanitation. Can Tho: CERWASS.

CERWASS 2011e. Instructions on How to Complete Data for the Survey on Water Supply. Can Tho: CERWASS.

Chay Navuth. 2006. *Toward an Effective International Development Assistance. Grassroots Level Community in Cambodia.* PhD, Waseda University.

CHECC 2011. Monthly Reports of Iec Material Distribution in the Districts and Communes, for September, October and November 2011. Can Tho: Department of Health.

Cheschier, S. C. 2010. *The New Class in Vietnam.* PhD, Queen Mary, University of London.

Chiabi, A., et al. 2010. Current Approach in the Management of Diarrhea in Children: From Theory and Research to Practice and Pragmatism. *Clinics in Mother and Child Health,* 7.

CIA 2012. The World Factbook: Vietnam.

Clasen, T., et al. 2006. Interventions to Improve Water Quality for Preventing Diarrhoea. *Cochrane Database Syst Rev,* 3.

Clasen, T. F. & Cairncross, S. 2004. Editorial: Household Water Management: Refining the Dominant Paradigm. *Tropical Medicine & International Health,* 9, 187-191.

Clasen, T. F., et al. 2008. Microbiological Effectiveness and Cost of Boiling to Disinfect Drinking Water in Rural Vietnam. *Environmental science & technology,* 42, 4255-4260.

Coker, R. J., et al. 2011. Emerging Infectious Diseases in Southeast Asia: Regional Challenges to Control. *The Lancet,* 377, 599-609.

Collins, A. E. 2001. Health Ecology, Land Degradation and Development. *Land Degradation & Development,* 12, 237-250.

Collyer, F. 2012. *Mapping the Sociology of Health and Medicine: America, Britain and Australia Compared*, Palgrave Macmillan.

Confalonieri, U., et al. 2007. Human Health. *In:* Parry, M. L., et al. (eds.) *Climate Change 2007: Impacts, Adaptation and Vulnerability. Contribution of Working Group Ii to the Fourth Assessment Report of the Intergovernmental Panel on Climate Change.* Cambridge, UK.

Curtis, S. & Riva, M. 2010. Health Geographies I: Complexity Theory and Human Health. *Progress in Human Geography,* 34, 215

Curtis, V. & Cairncross, S. 2003. Effect of Washing Hands with Soap on Diarrhoea Risk in the Community: A Systematic Review. *The Lancet infectious diseases,* 3, 275-281.

Curtis, V., et al. 2000. Review: Domestic Hygiene and Diarrhoea - Pinpointing the Problem. *Tropical Medicine & International Health,* 5, 22-32.

Curtis, V., et al. 2011. Disgust as an Adaptive System for Disease Avoidance Behaviour. *Philosophical Transactions of the Royal Society B: Biological Sciences,* 366, 389-401.

Curtis, V. A., et al. 2009. Planned, Motivated and Habitual Hygiene Behaviour: An Eleven Country Review. *Health Education Research,* 24, 655-673.

Dam Viet Cuong. 2009. Current Situation of Health Insurance, Healthcare Utilization, and Health Expenditures in Hai Duong and Bac Giang Provinces - Findings from a Baseline Survey. Available: URL: http://en.hspi.org.vn/vclen/trang-chu [Accessed 13.09.12].

Dang Ngoc Chanh & Nguyen Ngo Thiep 2010. Surveying Rural Water Quality and Determining Pollution Factors Which Impact on Water Sources at Households in Three Provinces: Long an, an Giang and Hau Giang. Ho Chi MInh: Istitute of Hygiene and Public Health & University of Technology.

Daniels, D. L., et al. 1990. A Case-Control Study of the Impact of Improved Sanitation on Diarrhoea Morbidity in Lesotho. *Bulletin of the World Health Organization,* 68, 455.

Dao, H. T., et al. 2008. User Fees and Health Service Utilization in Vietnam: How to Protect the Poor? *Public health,* 122, 1068-1078.

Dat V. Duong, et al. 2004. Utilization of Delivery Services at the Primary Health Care Level in Rural Vietnam. *Social Science & Medicine,* 59, 2585-2595.

Dawson, D. 2005. Foodborne Protozoan Parasites. *International Journal of Food Microbiology,* 103, 207-227.

Dearden, K. A., et al. 2002. What Influences Health Behavior? Learning from Caregivers of Young Children in Viet Nam. *Food & Nutrition Bulletin,* 23, 117-127.

Department of Health 2009. Report on Health and Plans I & Ii for 2009. Can Tho City: Department of Health.

Department of Labour Invalids and Social Affairs 2010. Poverty Alleviation Handbook Can Tho City: People's Committee of Can Tho.

DiGiacomo, S. M. 1999. Can There Be a "Cultural Epidemiology"? *Medical Anthropology Quarterly,* 13, 436-457

Dittmann, S. 2001. Vaccine Safety: Risk Communication - a Global Perspective. *Vaccine,* 19, 2446-2456.

Djilas, M. 1957. *The New Class: An Analysis of the Communist System*, Praeger New York.

DONRE 2009. Factual Report on Environmental Quality from the Years 1999-2008 , City of Can Tho (1999-2008). Can Tho.

Douglas, M. 2002. *Purity and Danger: An Analysis of the Concepts of Pollution and Taboo*, Routledge.

DSO of Cai Rang 2010. Niên Giám Thống Kê 2009 (Statistical Yearbook 2009). Can Tho: Cai Rang District Statistics Office (DSO).

DSO Phong Dien 2010. Niên Giám Thống Kê 2009 (Statistical Yearbook 2009). Can Tho: Phong Dien District Statistics Office (DSO).

DSW (German Foundation for World Population) 2011. Health Spending in Vietnam: The Impact of Current Aid Structures and Aid Effectiveness. *In:* Koenig, S. H., Mareike (ed.). Action for Global Health.

Duong, T., et al. 2009. Bottled Drinking Water Microbial Infection: Upsetting Testing Results (Nước Uống □ óng Chai Nhiễm Vi Sinh: Kiểm □ ến □ âu, Rầu □ ến □ ấy). *Tuoitre Online*, 02/04/2009.

Dutton, P., et al. 2011a. Handwashing with Soap - Two Paths to National-Scale Programs. Lessons from the Field: Vietnam and Indonesia. *Global Scaling Up Handwashing Project.* The World Bank.

Dutton, P., et al. 2011b. The Power of Primary Schools to Change and Sustain Handwashing with Soap among Children: The Cases of Vietnam and Peru. *WSP: Technical Paper.* The World Bank.

Ehlert, J. 2011. *Living with Flood. Local Knowledge in the Mekong Delta, Vietnam,* Berlin, LIT Verlag.

Elahi, K. Q. & Danopoulos, C. P. 2004. Microcredit and the Third World: Perspectives from Moral and Political Philosophy. *International Journal of Social Economics,* 31, 643-654.

Elmendorf, M. L. & Isely, R. B. 1983. Public and Private Roles of Women in Water Supply and Sanitation Programs. *Human Organization,* 42, 195-204.

Erik Swyngedouw 2009. The Political Economy and Political Ecology of the Hydro-Social Cycle. *Journal of Contemporary Water Research & Education*, 56-60.

Falola, T. & Heaton, M. M. 2006. *Endangered Bodies: Women, Children, and Health in Africa*, Africa World Press.

Farmer, P. 2005. *Pathologies of Power: Health, Human Rights, and the New War on the Poor*, Univ of California Press.

Farthing, M. 2000. Diarrhoea: A Significant Worldwide Problem. *International Journal of Antimicrobial Agents,* 14, 65-69.

Feachem, R. G., et al. 1983. Diarrhoeal Disease Control: Reviews of Potential Interventions. *Bulletin of the World Health Organization,* 61, 637.

Few, R. & Tran, P. G. 2010. Climatic Hazards, Health Risk and Response in Vietnam: Case Studies on Social Dimensions of Vulnerability. *Governance, Complexity and Resilience,* 20, 529-538.

Fewtrell, L., et al. 2005. Water, Sanitation, and Hygiene Interventions to Reduce Diarrhoea in Less Developed Countries: A Cystematic Review and Meta-Analysis. *The Lancet Infectious Diseases,* 5, 42-52.

Fforde, A. 2013. Vietnam in 2012: The End of the Party. *Asian Survey,* 53, 101-108.

Fischer, T. K., et al. 2005. Health Care Costs of Diarrheal Disease and Estimates of the Cost-Effectiveness of Rotavirus Vaccination in Vietnam. *Journal of Infectious Diseases,* 192, 1720-1726.

Fisher, E. B., et al. 2011. Behavior Matters. *American Journal of Preventive Medicine,* 40, e15-e30.

Fitzwater, S., et al. 2011. Infectious Diarrhea. *In:* Selendy, J. M. H. (ed.) *Water and Sanitation-Related Diseases and the Enviornment: Challenges, Interventions and Preventive Measures.* first ed. New Jersey: John Wiley & Sons, Inc.

Fleßa, S. 2003. Gesundheit Und Gesundheitswesen in Vietnam Health and Health Care in Vietnam. *Gesundheitswesen,* 65, 336-342.

Foley, E. 2009. *Your Pocket Is What Cures You: The Politics of Health in Senegal,* Rutgers University Press.

Food Safety and Hygiene Unit 2011. Communication Plan: Month of Aaction for Food Quality, Safety and Hygiene. *In:* Health, D. o. (ed.). Can Tho.

Forsberg, L. T. 2011. The Political Economy of Health Reform in Vietnam. *Working paper 2011 for the Oxford Princeton Global Leaders Program.* Oxford University.

Fortier, F. 2012. Viet Nam's Food Security: A Castle of Cards in the Winds of Climate Change. *Kasarinlan: Philippine Journal of Third World Studies,* 26, 89-120.

Foucault, M. 2003. *The Birth of the Clinic: An Archaeology of Medical Perception,* Routledge.

Frewer, L. J., et al. 1994. The Interrelationship between Perceived Knowledge, Control and Risk Associated with a Range of Food-Related Hazards Targeted at the Individual, Other People and Society. *Journal of Food Safety,* 14, 19-40.

Fritzen, S. A. 2007. Legacies of Primary Health Care in an Age of Health Sector Reform: Vietnam's Commune Clinics in Transition. *Social Science & Medicine,* 64, 1611-1623.

Gainsborough, M. 2001. Political Change in Vietnam: In Search of the Middle Class Challenge to the State.

Gainsborough, M. 2010a. Vietnam. *In:* Dizard, J., et al. (eds.) *Countries at the Crossroads: An Analysis of Democratic Governance.* Rowman & Littlefield.

Gainsborough, M. 2010b. *Vietnam. Rethinking the State,* New York, Chiang Mai, Zed Books Ltd, Silkworm Books.

Gammeltoft, T. 1999. Body and Health. *Women's Bodies Women's Worries: Health and Family Planning in a Vietnamese Rural Community.* Curzon Press.

Gatrell, A. C. 2005. Complexity Theory and Geographies of Health: A Critical Assessment. *Social Science & Medicine,* 60, 2661-2671.

Gaudine, A., et al. 2009. Developing Culturally Sensitive Interventions for Vietnamese Health Issues: An Action Research Approach. *Nursing & Health Sciences,* 11, 150-153.

Geist, P. & Gates, L. 1996. The Poetics and Politics of Re-Covering Identities in Health Communication. *Communication Studies,* 47, 218-228.

General Statistics Office 2009. General Poverty Rates by Residence and Region. General Statistics Office of Vietnam.

Gerring, J. 2004. What Is a Case Study and What Is It Good For? *American Political Science Review,* 98, 341-354.

Gillespie, J. 2001. Self-Interest and Ideology: Bureaucratic Corruption in Vietnam. *The Australian Journal of Asian Law,* 3, 1-36.

Glass, R. I., et al. 2006. Rotavirus Vaccines: Current Prospects and Future Challenges. *Lancet,* 368, 323-332.

GoV 2001. On the Classification of Urban Centers and Urban Management Levels *In:* Government of Vietnam (GoV) (ed.) *72/2001/ND-CP.* Hanoi.

GoV 2002. On the Financial Regime of Income Units *In:* Government of Vietnam (ed.) *10/2002/N□ -CP.*

GoV 2004. On the Transformation of State Companies into Joint-Stock Companies. *In:* Government of Vietnam (ed.) *187/2004/ND-CP.* Hanoi.

GoV 2005. On the Classification of Hospitals *In:* Government of Vietnam (ed.) *23/2005/TT-BYT.* Hanoi.

GoV 2006a. National Target Program for Rural Water Supply and Sanitation (2006 2010). Final Draft. Hanoi.

GoV 2006b. On the Defined Autonomy, Self-Responsibility for Performing Tasks, Organizating Structure, Staffing and Financing of Public Service Units *In:* Government of Vietnam (ed.) *43/2006/N□-CP.*

GoV 2007. On the Prevention and Control of Infectious Diseases *In:* Government of Vietnam (ed.) *03/2007/QH12.* Hanoi.

GoV 2008. On Health Insurance. *In:* Government of Vietnam (ed.) *25/2008/QH12.* Hanoi.

GoV 2009a. On Medical Examination and Treatment *In:* Government of Vietnam (ed.) *No 40/2009/QH12.*

GoV 2009b. On the Grading of Urban Centers. *In:* Vietnam, G. o. (ed.) *42/2009/ND-CP.* Hanoi.

GoV 2010a. On the Declaration, Information and Reporting of Infective Diseases. *In:* Vietnam, G. o. (ed.) *48/2010/TT-BYT.* Hanoi.

GoV 2010b. On the Standards, Functions and Duties of the Village Health Workers. *In:* Vietnam, G. o. (ed.) *39/2010/TT-BYT* Hanoi.

GoV 2011. On National Criteria for Commune Clinics for the Period 2011-2020. *In:* Vietnam, G. o. (ed.) *3447 / QD-BYT.* Hanoi.

GoV, et al. 2006. National Target Programme for Rural Water Supply and Sanitation - Phase Ii (2006-2010).

Graham, J. & Selendy, J. 2011a. Sanitation and Hygiene: Taking Stock after Three Decades. *In:* Selendy, J. (ed.) *Water and Sanitation Related Diseases and the Environment: Challenges, Interventions and Preventive Measures.* Jonh Wiley & Sons, Inc.

Graham, J. & Selendy, J. 2011b. Tackling the Water Crisis: A Continuing Need to Address Spatial and Social Equity. *In:* Selendy, J. (ed.) *Water and Sanitation Related Diseases and the Environment: Challenges, Interventions and Preventive Measures.* Jonh Wiley & Sons, Inc.

Grimwood, K. & Lambert, S. B. 2009. Rotavirus Vaccines. *Human Vaccines,* 5, 57-69.

GSO 2008. *Result of the Survey on Household Living Standards 2008,* Hanoi, General Statistics Office of Vietnam.

GSO 2010a. *The 2009 Vietnam Population and Housing Census - Annex,* Hanoi, General Statistics Office of Vietnam.

GSO 2010b. *Result of the Survey on Household Living Standards 2010,* Hanoi, General Statistics Office of Vietnam.

GSO 2011a. Multiple Indicator Cluster Survey 2011, Final Report. Hanoi: General Statistics Office of Vietnam.

GSO 2011b. Statistical Yearbook of Vietnam 2010. Hanoi: General Statistics Office of Vietnam.

GSO 2012a. General Poverty Rate by Residence and by Region. *In:* Integrated Statistics Department (ed.) 30.08.12 ed. Hanoi: General Statistics Office of Vietnam.

GSO 2012b. Statistical Yearbook of Vietnam 2011. Hanoi: General Statistics Office of Vietnam.

GSO 2013. *Statistical Handbook 2012,* Hanoi, General Statistics Office of Vietnam.

GTZ & Zimbabwe National Family Planning Council 1994. Information Education and Communication (Iec): Reference Manual for Health Programme Managers. 2 ed. Harare, Zimbabwe: Ministry of Health and Child Welfare.

Guénel, A. 2004. Malaria, Colonial Economics and Migrations in Vietnam.

Guerrant, R. L., et al. 2002. Magnitude and Impact of Diarrheal Diseases. *Archives of Medical Research,* 33, 351-355.

Ha Mi. 2013. Why Do Vietnam's Patients Bribe Their Doctors? *BBC Vietnamese,* 10.07.13.

Ha Nguyen Thi Hong, et al. 2002. Household Utilization and Expenditure on Private and Public Health Services in Vietnam. *Health Policy and Planning,* 17, 61-70.

Ha Van. 2010a. Pollution - Tragedy from Waste and Wastewater. *Can Tho online,* 24.08.2010.

Ha Van. 2010b. Residential Security Solutions for People Living Along the Rivers. *Can Tho online,* 24.09.2010.

Hall, P. A. & Taylor, R. C. R. 1996. Political Science and the Three New Institutionalisms. *Political Studies,* XLIV, 936 - 957.

Hampel, J. 2006. Different Concepts of Risk - a Challenge for Risk Communication. *International Journal of Medical Microbiology,* 296, 5-10.

Han Sun Sheng & Vu Kim Trang 2008. Land Acquisition in Transitional Hanoi, Vietnam. *Urban Studies,* 45, 1097-1117.

Hanh Nguyen 2007. Fly: A Factor That Transmits Diarrhea. *Health for a Cultural Village.* Hanoi: MoH.

Harms, E. 2011. *Saigon's Edge: On the Margins of Ho Chi Minh City,* University of Minnesota Press.

Harriss, K. & Salway, S. 2009. Long-Term Ill-Health, Poverty and Ethnicity. *Ethnicity and Inequalities in Health and Social Care,* 2, 39-48.

Harrits, G. S. 2011. More Than Method?: A Discussion of Paradigm Differences within Mixed Methods Research. *Journal of Mixed Methods Research,* 5, 150 166.

Heller, L., et al. 2003. Environmental Sanitation Conditions and Health Impact: A Case-Control Study. *Revista da Sociedade Brasileira de Medicina Tropical,* 36, 41-50.

HELVETAS & NCERWASS 2010. The Sodis Story in Vietnam: Safe, Easy, Clean Drinking Water. Hanoi: HELVETAS, NCERWASS.

HEMA & UNICEF 2011. Study on the Correlation between Sanitation, Household Water Supply, Mother's Hygiene Behaviors for Children under 5 and the Status of Child Nutrition in Vietnam. Hanoi.

Hénock Blaise, N. Y. & Dovie, D. B. K. 2007. Diarrheal Diseases in the History of Public Health. *Archives of Medical Research,* 38, 159-163.

Herbst, S., et al. 2009. Perceptions of Water, Sanitation and Health: A Case Study from the Mekong Delta, Vietnam. *Water Science & Technology,* 60, 699-707.

Hien, N. T., et al. 1995. The Pursuit of Equity: A Health Sector Case Study from Vietnam. *Health Policy,* 33, 191-204.

Hoang Xuan Thanh, et al. 2008. *Urbanization and Rural Development in Vietnam's Mekong Delta: Livelihood Transformations in Three Fruit-Growing Settlements,* Earthprint.

Hofmann, B. 2011. On the Concepts Disease, Illness and Sickness. *In:* Halvor Nordby, et al. (eds.) *Social Aspects of Illness, Disease and Sickness Absence.* Oslo: Oslo Academic Press, Unipub Norway.

Hoque, B. A., et al. 2006. Rural Drinking Water at Supply and Household Levels: Quality and Management. *International Journal of Hygiene and Environmental Health,* 209, 451-460.

Howie, C. 2002. Doing Research in the Mekong Delta, Vietnam, and Doing a Phd in the England Are Not the Same Things: Some Reflections on the Tensions of Serving Two Masters. *RGS/IBG Annual Conference.* Belfast.

HSPI 2012a. Analysis of Current Situation and Reccomended Revisions to Some Allowance Schemes for Government Permanent Staff and Employees in the Health Sector. Hanoi: HSPI (Health Strategy and Policy Institute).

HSPI 2012b. Develop Rural Health Insurance Towards Equity and Sustainability to Ensure Health Care for Rural Population: End-Term Result Evaluation (2010). Hanoi: HSPI (Health Strategy and Policy Institute).

HSPI 2012c. Evaluating Private Health Sector Participation in Health Insured Examination and Treatment in Hanoi, Da Nang and Ho Chi Minh City. Hanoi: HSPI (Health Strategy and Policy Institute).

Hue Hoa. 2011. There Are Many Concerns. *Can Tho online*, 18.07.2011.

Hunar□, M. á., et al. 1999. *Health Ecology: Health, Culture and Human-Environment Interaction*, Psychology Press.

IHPH 2011a. Results of Testing the Sanitation of Clean Water, Eating and Drinking Water and Household Latrines, in 2010. Ho Chi Minh City: Ministry of Health (MoH).

IHPH 2011b. Results of Testing the Sanitation of Clean Water, Eating and Drinking Water and Household Latrines, in 2011. Ho Chi Minh City: Ministry of Health (MoH).

IHPH 2012. Health Statistics on the Incidence of Infectious Diseases (2005-2011) for the Southern Provinces of Vietnam. Ho Chi Minh City: MoH.

Inocencio, A. B., et al. 1999. Determination of Basic Household Water Requirements. *Discussion Paper Series.* Philippine Institute for Development Studies.

International Center for Environmental Management (ICEM) 2007. Analysis of Pollution from Manufacturing Sectors in Vietnam. Indooroopilly, Queensland, Australia.

International Labour Organization. 2012. Vietnam Overview of Schemes: Health Certificates for the Poor and Ethnic Minorities. Available: http://www.ilo.org/dyn/ilossi/ssimain.viewScheme?p_lang=en&p_scheme_id=1082&p_geoaid=704 [Accessed 06.03.2013].

Irwin, A. & Wynne, B. 1996. *Misunderstanding Science?: The Public Reconstruction of Science and Technology*, Cambridge University Press.

Jenkins, C. N. H., et al. 1996. Health Care Access and Preventive Care among Vietnamese Immigrants: Do Traditional Beliefs and Practices Pose Barriers? *Social Science & Medicine,* 43, 1049-1056.

Jensen, P. K., et al. 2002. Domestic Transmission Routes of Pathogens: The Problem of in-House Contamination of Drinking Water During Storage in Developing Countries. *Tropical Medicine & International Health,* 7, 604-609.

Jensen, P. K., et al. 2004. Is There an Association between Bacteriological Drinking Water Quality and Childhood Diarrhoea in Developing Countries? *Tropical Medicine & International Health,* 9, 1210 - 1215.

Jewitt, S. 2011. Geographies of Shit: Spatial and Temporal Variations in Attitudes Towards Human Waste. *Progress in Human Geography,* 35, 608-626.

JMP. 2012a. Annexes of the Working Groups' Proposals in Water, Sanitation, Hygiene and Equity. Available: www.wssinfo.org/fileadmin/user_upload/resources/ANNEXES_WG_reports.pdf.

JMP. Jmp Process on Global Post-2015 Monitoring. Stocholm World Water Week - 2012, 2012b Stocholm. Joint Monitoring Program (JMP) of the WHO and UNICEF.

JMP Vietnam 2012a. Estimates for the Use of Improved Drinking-Water Sources. Joint Monitoring Program (JMP) of the WHO and UNICEF.

JMP Vietnam 2012b. Estimates for the Use of Improved Sanitation Facilities. Joint Monitoring Program (JMP) of the WHO and UNICEF.

Jones, K. & Moon, G. 1987. *Health, Disease, and Society: A Critical Medical Geography*, Routledge/Thoemms Press.

Jones, K. & Moon, G. 1991. Medical Geography. *Progress in Human Geography,* 15, 437.

Joralemon, D. 2010. *Exploring Medical Anthropology*, Pearson Education, Inc., .

Joshi, D., et al. 2011. Health, Hygiene and Appropriate Sanitation: Experiences and Perceptions of the Urban Poor. *Environment and Urbanization,* 23, 91-111.

Kaika, M. 2003. Constructing Scarcity and Sensationalising Water Politics: 170 Days That Shook Athens. *Antipode,* 35, 919-954.

Kallis, G. & Coccossis, H. 2003. Managing Water for Athens: From the Hydraulic to the Rational Growth Paradigm. *European Planning Studies,* 11, 245-261.

Karanis, P. 2006. A Review of an Emerging Waterborne Medical Important Parasitic Protozoan. *Jpn. J. Protozool. Vol,* 39.

Karim, L. 2008. Demystifying Micro-Credit the Grameen Bank, Ngos, and Neoliberalism in Bangladesh. *Cultural Dynamics,* 20, 5-29.

Kasperson, R. E. & Kasperson, J. X. 2005. *The Social Contours of Risk: Publics, Risk Communication and the Social Amplification of Risk*, Earthscan.

KBR (Kellogg Brown & Root Pty Ltd.) 2009. Socialist Republic of Viet Nam: Water Sector Review Asian Development Bank (ADB).

Kearns, R. & Moon, G. 2002. From Medical to Health Geography: Novelty, Place and Theory after a Decade of Change. *Progress in Human Geography,* 26, 605.

Kearns, R. A. 1993. Place and Health: Towards a Reformed Medical Geography. *The Professional Geographer,* 45, 139-147.

Kelly-Hope, L. A., et al. 2008. Temporal Trends and Climatic Factors Associated with Bacterial Enteric Diseases in Vietnam, 1991–2001. *Environmental Health Perspectives,* 116, 7.

Kerkvliet, B. J. T. 2001. An Approach for Analysing State-Society Relations in Vietnam. *Journal of Social Issues in Southeast Asia (SOJOURN),* 16.

Kerkvliet, B. J. T. 2003. Authorities and the People: An Analysis of State-Society Relations in Vietnam. *In:* Luong, H. V. (ed.) *Postwar Vietnam: Dynamics of a Transforming Society.* Oxford: Rowman & Littlefield.

Kerkvliet, B. J. T. 2005. *The Power of Everyday Politics. How Vietnamese Peasants Transformed National Policy,* Ithaca, Cornell University Press.

Keusch, G. T., et al. 2006. Diarrheal Diseases. *In:* Jamison, D. T., et al. (eds.) *Disease Control Priorities in Developing Countries.* 2nd ed. Washington (DC): World Bank.

Khe, N. D., et al. 2002. Primary Health Concept Revisited: Where Do People Seek Health Care in a Rural Area of Vietnam? *Health Policy,* 61, 95-109.

Kieu Linh. 2012. Poor Foreign Investment Health. *Vietnam Investment Review.*

Kieu Minh. 2009. Why Not Criminal Violation of Food Safety and Hygiene? *VietBao (Vietnam News),* 20.04.2009.

Kim, S. Y., et al. 2009. Cost-Effectiveness of Rotavirus Vaccination in Vietnam. *BMC Public Health,* 9, 29.

King, B. 2010. Political Ecologies of Health. *Progress in Human Geography,* 34, 38–55.

King, V. T. 2008. The Middle Class in Southeast Asia: Diversities, Identities, Comparisons and the Vietnamese Case. *International Journal of Asia Pacific Studies (IJAPS),* 4, 75-122.

Knudsen, L. G., et al. 2008. The Fear of Awful Smell: Risk Perceptions among Farmers in Vietnam Using Wastewater and Human Excreta in Agriculture. *The Southeast Asian Journal of Tropical Medicine and Public Health,* 39, 341-52.

Köster, U. 2008. *Gesundheit, Wasser Und Hygiene. Eine Fallstudie Aus Dem Mekong Delta, Vietnam (Health, Water and Hygene. A Case Study from the Mekong Delta, Vietnam).* Diploma Thesis, Rheinische Friedrich-Wilhelms-Universität Bonn.

Krause, M. 2008. The Political Economy of Water and Sanitation Services in Colombia. *Water Politics and Development Cooperation.* Springer.

Ladinsky, J. L., et al. 1987. The Influence of Traditional Medicine in Shaping Medical Care Practices in Vietnam Today. *Social Science & Medicine,* 25, 1105-1110.

Laverack, G. & Dap, D. H. 2003. Transforming Information, Education and Communication in Vietnam. *Health Education,* 103, 363-369.

Le Kien. 2011. Trade Villages Get Polluted: Life Expectancy Reduce 10 Years. *Tuoi Tre online*, 08.11.2011.

Le Thanh Ha. 2010. Management of Drug Prices: The State Must Have Hands! *Tuoi Tre Online*, 21.04.10.

Leatherman, T. 2005. A Space of Vulnerability in Poverty and Health: Political-Ecology and Biocultural Analysis. *ETHOS* [Online], 33.

Levine, M., et al. 1981. Duration of Infection-Derived Immunity to Cholera. *Journal of Infectious Diseases,* 143, 818-820.

Lieberman, S. S. & Wagstaff, A. 2009. *Health Financing and Delivery in Vietnam: Looking Forward,* Washington, DC, The World Bank.

Lim, M. L. & Wallace, M. R. 2004. Infectious Diarrhea in History. *Infectious disease clinics of North America,* 18, 261-274.

Lock, M. 1993. Cultivating the Body: Anthropology and Epistemologies of Bodily Practice and Knowledge. *Annual Review of Anthropology,* 22, 133-155.

Lock, M. 2001. The Tempering of Medical Anthropology: Troubling Natural Categories. *Medical Anthropology Quarterly,* 15, 478-492.

Loftus, A. J. 2005. *A Political Ecology of Water Struggles in Durban, South Africa.* PhD thesis, University of Oxford.

London, J. 2008a. Reasserting the State in Viet Nam: Health Care and the Logics of Market-Leninism. *Policy and Society,* 27, 115-128.

London, J. D. 2008b. Reasserting the State in Viet Nam Health Care and the Logics of Market-Leninism. *Policy and Society,* 27, 115-128.

Lupton, D. 2012a. *Medicine as Culture: Illness, Disease and the Body*, SAGE Publications Limited.

Lupton, D. 2012b. Theoretical Perspectives on Medicine and Society *Medicine as Culture: Illness, Disease and the Body.* 3rd ed.: SAGE Publications Limited.

Luxemburger, C., et al. 2001. Risk Factors for Typhoid Fever in the Mekong Delta, Southern Viet Nam: A Case-Control Study. *Transactions of the Royal Society of Tropical Medicine and Hygiene,* 95, 19-23.

Manderson, L. 1987. Blame, Responsibility and Remedial Action:Death , Disease and the Infant in Early Twentieth Century Malaya. *In:* Owen, N. G. (ed.) *Death and Disease in Southeast Asia.* Asian Studies Association of Australia, Oxford University Press.

Mann, G. 2009. Should Political Ecology Be Marxist? A Case for Gramsci's Historical Materialism. *Geoforum,* 40, 335-344.

MARD 2003. Guidelines on Information, Education and Communication for Rural Water Supply and Environmental Sanitation. *In:* CERWASS (ed.). Hanoi.

MARD 2008a. The Monitoring and Evaluation Indicator Set for Clean Rural Water Supply and Environmnetal Sanitation. *In:* (MARD), M. f. A. a. R. D. (ed.).

MARD 2008b. The Monitoring and Evaluation Indicator Set for Clean Rural Water Supply and Environmnetal Sanitation. Hanoi.

MARD 2010. National Rural Clean Water Supply and Sanitation Strategy up to Year 2020

MARD & MoC 2000. National Rural Clean Water Supply and Sanitation Strategy up to the Year 2020. Hanoi.

Marr, D. G. 1992. Vietnam (World Bibliographical Series, Vol. 147). Oxford.

Mayer, J. D. 1996a. The Political Ecology of Disease as One New Focus for Medical Geography. *Month*, 441-456.

Mayer, J. D. 1996b. The Political Ecology of Disease as One New Focus for Medical Geography. *Progress in Human Geography,* 20, 441-456.

McIntosh, W. A. 1996. Food and Nutrition as Social Problems. *Sociologies of Food and Nutrition.* New York: Springer.

Medical Centre of Co Do 2011. Water Supply, Sanitation and Hygiene Statistics. *In:* Department of Health (ed.). Can Tho.

Minh Nguyen Thang & Popkin, B. M. 2003. Income and Health Dynamics in Vietnam: Poverty Reduction, Increased Health Inequality. *Population (english edition),* 58, 253-264.

Mintz, E., et al. 2001. Not Just a Drop in the Bucket: Expanding Access to Point-of-Use Water Treatment Systems. *Journal Information,* 91.

MoH 2004. On Promulgating the Regulation on the Title of Healthy Family, Healthy Neighborhood and Healthy Village or Area Certificate. *1635/2004/QD-BYT.*

MoH 2005. On the Hygiene Standards for Various Types of Latrines. *08/2005/QD-BYT* Hanoi.

MoH 2006. Health Metrics Network: Vietnam Health Information System Review and Assesment. *In:* Duong, H. L. (ed.).

MoH 2007a. Instruction for Diagnosis and Treatment of Cholera and Dengue Fever for Hospitals - According to Decision No 4178/Qd-Byt/2007. Hanoi: Government of Vietnam.

MoH 2007b. Vietnam National Strategy on Preventive Medicine to 2010 and Orientations Towards 2020 & Master Plan on Development of Vietnam's Health Care System up to 2010 with a Vision to 2020 Hanoi: Government of Vietnam.

MoH 2008. On Guiding the Functions, Tasks, Powers and Organizational Structure and Staffing of Food Hygiene and Safety Department under the Department of Health of the Provinces and Cities Directly under the Central Government. *12 /2008/TTLT-BYT-BNV*. Hanoi.

MoH 2009a. Instuctions of Treating Water and Sanitation During the Flooding Season. Hanoi: Ministry of Health (MoH).

MoH 2009b. National Technical Regulations on Drinking and Domestic Water Quality. *In:* General Department of Preventive Medicine and the Environment (ed.). Hanoi: Ministry of Health (MoH).

MoH 2009c. On Guiding the Management of Diarrhea in Children. *4121/Q□-BYT*.

MoH 2010a. Five-Year Health Sector Development Plan: 2011 - 2015. Hanoi: Government of Vietnam.

MoH 2010b. On Prescribed Standards, Functions and Duties of Village Workers. *39/2010/TT-BYT*

MoH 2011. National Data on Infectious Disease Prevalence (2002-2011). Hanoi.

MoH 2012a. National Data on Infectious Disease Prevalence (2001-2010). Hanoi.

MoH 2012b. National Health Statistics on Infectious Diseases (2001-2010). Hanoi.

MOH, et al. 2007. On the Implementaton of State Management of Drug Prices. *11/2007/TTLT-BYT-BTC-BCT*. Hanoi.

Molle, F. & Hoanh, C. T. 2008. Implementing Integrated River Basin Management: Lessons from the Red River Basin, Vietnam. Institut de Recherche pour le Developpement, Mekong Program on Water Environment and Resilience, International Water Management Institute.

Mollinga, P. P. 2008. Water, Politics and Development: Framing a Political Sociology of Water Resources Management. *Water Alternatives,* 1, 7-23.

MONRE & UNDP 2008. Health, Water Supply, Sanitation and the Poor. *In:* Nguyen Trung Thang, et al. (eds.). Hanoi: United Nations Development Program (UNDP) and Ministry of Natural Resources and the Environment (MONRE).

Morris, G. 2010. New Approaches to Problem Framing in Environmental Health: Application to Water. *Public health,* 124, 607-612.

Morris, G. P., et al. 2006. Getting Strategic About the Environment and Health. *Public health,* 120, 889-903

Morsy, S. 1979. The Missing Link in Medical Anthropology: The Political Economy of Health. *Reviews in Anthropology,* 6, 349-363.

Movik, S. & Mehta, L. 2010. Liquid Dynamics: Accessing Water and Sanitation in an Uncertain Age. Symposium Report *Working Paper* Brighton: STEPS Centre.

Mylott, E. 2009. Urban-Rural Connections: A Review of the Literature. *Collections* [Online]. Available: http://ir.library.oregonstate.edu/xmlui/bitstream/handle/1957/10574/Urban-RuralConnectionsLitReview.pdf?sequence=1 [Accessed 15.09.2013].

Myrick, R. 1996. *Aids, Communication, and Empowerment: Gay Male Identity and the Politics of Public Health Messages,* Harrington Park Press New York/London.

National Assembly of the Socialist Republic of Vietnam 2010. On Food Safety. *55/2010/QH12.* Hanoi.

National Center of Preventive Health 2007. Process for the Treatment of Dangerous Acute Diarrhea. *Health for a cultural village.* Hanoi: MoH.

National Institute of Nutrition & UNICEF 2011. Summary Report: General Nutrition Survey 2009 - 2010. Hanoi: MoH.

Nations, M. K. & Monte, C. M. 1996. "I'm Not Dog, No!": Cries of Resistance against Cholera Control Campaigns. *Social science & medicine,* 43, 1007-1024.

Nga Nguyen, et al. 2011. Vietnam: A Handwashing Behavior Change Journey for the Caretakers' Program. *WSP (Water and Sanitation Program): Global Scaling Up Handwashing Project.*

Nghiem Tran Dung 2010. Presentation Titled: Social Health Insurance in Viet Nam. *In:* Health Insurance Department (ed.). Hanoi: Ministry of Health of Vietnam.

Nguyen Ha 2011. The Principal-Agent Problems in Health Care: Evidence from Prescribing Patterns of Private Providers in Vietnam. *Health Policy and Planning,* 26, i53-i62.

Nguyen Khanh Phuong, et al. 2009. An Evaluation of Initial Impacts of Hospital Financing Autonomy Policy on Provision of and Payment for Healthcare Services. Available: http://en.hspi.org.vn/vclen/trang-chu [Accessed 13.09.12].

Nguyen, T. A., et al. 2007. Diversity of Viruses Associated with Acute Gastroenteritis in Children Hospitalized with Diarrhea in Ho Chi Minh City, Vietnam. *Journal of Medical Virology,* 79, 582-590.

Nguyen Thang, et al. 2006. Poverty, Poverty Reduction and Poverty Dynamics in Vietnam. *Chronic Poverty Report 2008-09 - Background Paper*. Chronic Poverty Research Center.

Nguyen Thi Kim Tien, et al. 1997. Preliminary Results of Epidemiological Study on Risk Factors Associated to the Prolongation of Diarrheal Duration in Children under 5 Years of Age in the Community (Cai Be - Tien Giang). Ho Chi Minh City: Pasteur Institute, Center of Preventive Medicine.

Nguyen Thi Phuong Loan 2010a. Legal Framework of the Water Sector in Vietnam. *In:* Center for Development Research (ed.) *ZEF Working Paper No. 52*. Bonn: University of Bonn.

Nguyen Thi Phuong Loan 2010b. Problems of Law Enforcement in Vietnam: The Case of Wastewater Management in Can Tho City. *In:* Center for Development Research (ed.) *ZEF Working Paper No. 53*. Bonn: University of Bonn.

Nichter, M. 1996a. Drink Boiled Cooled Water: A Cultural Analysis of a Health Education Message. *In:* Nichter, M. & Nichter, M. (eds.) *Anthropology & International Health: South Asian Case Studies*. Routledge.

Nichter, M. 1996b. Health Social Science Research on the Study of Diarrheal Disease: A Focus on Dysentery *In:* Nichter, M. & Nichter, M. (eds.) *Anthropology & International Health: South Asian Case Studies*. Routledge.

Nichter, M. 1996c. Vaccinations in the Third World. A Consideration of Community Demand. *In:* Nichter, M. & Nichter, M. (eds.) *Anthropology & International Health: South Asian Case Studies*. Routledge.

Nichter, M. & Nichter, M. 1996a. *Anthropology & International Health: South Asian Case Studies*, Routledge.

Nichter, M. & Nichter, M. 1996b. Education by Appropriate Analogy. *In:* Nichter, M. & Nichter, M. (eds.) *Anthropology & International Health: South Asian Case Studies*. Routledge.

Nutbeam, D. 2000. Health Literacy as a Public Health Goal: A Challenge for Contemporary Health Education and Communication Strategies into the 21st Century. *Health Promotion International,* 15, 259-267.

O'Rourke, D. 2004. *Community-Driven Regulation: Balancing Development and the Environment in Vietnam*, The MIT Press.

Office of Health of Phong Dien 2011. Poverty Statistics for 2011, by Commune. Can Tho.

Ohtsuka, R. & Ulijaszek, S. J. 2007. *Health Change in the Asia-Pacific Region*, Cambridge University Press

Okumura, J., et al. 2002. Drug Utilisation and Self-Medication in Rural Communities in Vietnam. *Social Science & Medicine,* 54, 1875-1886.

OLISA Cai Rang 2011. Poverty Statistics for 2011, by Ward. Can Tho: Office of Labour, war Invalids and Social Affairs (OLISA).

Otero, I., et al. 2010. Water Scarcity, Social Power and the Production of an Elite Suburb: The Political Ecology of Water in Matadepera, Catalonia. *Ecological Economics,* In Press, Corrected Proof.

Özdemir, S., et al. 2011. Rainwater Harvesting Practices and Attitudes in the Mekong Delta of Vietnam. *Journal of Water, Sanitation and Hygiene for Development,* 01, 171 - 177.

Panter-Brick, C., et al. 2006. Culturally Compelling Strategies for Behaviour Change: A Social Ecology Model and Case Study in Malaria Prevention. *Social Science & Medicine,* 62, 2810-2825.

Parfitt, T. W. 2002. *The End of Development?: Modernity, Post-Modernity and Development*, Pluto press London.

PATH 2012. Controlling Diarrheal Disease in Vietnam. Hanoi: PATH.

Pattanayak, S., et al. 2006. The Use of Willingness to Pay Experiments: Estimating Demand for Piped Water Connections in Sri Lanka. *World Bank Policy Research Working Paper.*

Paulson, S., et al. 2003. Locating the Political in Political Ecology: An Introduction. *Human Organization,* 62, 205-217.

Peet, R. & Hartwick, E. 1999. *Theories of Development,* New York, The Guilford Press.

Peet, R. & Watts, M. 2002. *Liberation Ecologies: Environment, Development and Social Movements*, Routledge.

Pham Kim 2007. Acute Diarrhea Caused by Food Poisoning. *Health for a cultural village.* Hanoi: MoH.

PHC Binh Thuy 2011. 'Sanitation and Clean Water': Information for the Local Staff in Organizations and Unions. Can Tho.

PHC Cai Rang 2011a. Annual General Reports of Preventive Health Programs for 2008 - 2011. *In:* Department of Health (ed.). Can Tho

PHC Cai Rang 2011b. Collection of Cdd Program Reports, by Ward.

PHC Cai Rang 2011c. Water Supply and Sanitation Reporting for 2011. Can Tho.

PHC Can Tho City 2011a. Children's Malnutrition Rates for Can Tho (2000 - 2010).

PHC Can Tho City 2011b. Monthly Statistical Data on the Number of Diarrhoea Cases in Can Tho City (2008 - 2011). Can Tho.

PHC Can Tho City 2011c. Results of Water Quality from Mini-Supply Stations from Rural Communes in Phong Dien and Cai Rang Districts. CERWASS.

PHC Can Tho City 2011d. Water Quality Results from the Water Provided by the Ctwc. Can Tho: Can Tho Water Company (CTWC).

PHC Can Tho City 2011e. Water Quality Results from the Water Provided by the Water Company in Cai Rang Can Tho: Water Company - Cai Rang banch.

PHC Ninh Kieu 2011. Water, Sanitation and Hygiene Statistics, by Ward. Can Tho: Department of Health.

PHC O Mon 2011a. Preventive Medicine Activity in the First Semester and Plan for the End of the Year. *Summary report.* Can Tho.

PHC O Mon 2011b. Report of Preventive Health Activities for 2011 and Future Plans *In:* Department of Health (ed.). Can Tho.

PHC O Mon 2011c. Water Supply and Sanitation Reporting for 2011. Can Tho.

PHC Phong Dien 2011. Summary of the Preventive Health Activities for 2009 and 2010. Can Tho.

Potter, R., et al. 2012. *Key Concepts in Development Geography*, SAGE Publications Limited.

Prime Minister of Vietnam 2004. On the Credit for the National Strategy of Rural Clean Water Supply and Sanitation. *62/2004/QD-TTg.* Hanoi.

Priwitzer, K. 2012. *The Vietnamese Health Care System in Change: A Policy Network Analysis of a Southeast Asian Welfare Regime*, Institute of Southeast Asian Studies.

Reis, N. 2012. *Tracing and Making the State: Policy Practices and Domestic Water Supply in the Mekong Delta,* Berlin, Münster, Wien, Zürich, London, Lit Verlag.

Reis, N. & Mollinga, P. P. 2009. Microcredit for Rural Water Supply and Sanitation in the Mekong Delta - Policy Implementation between the Needs for Clean Water and 'Beautiful Latrines'. *In:* Center for Development Research, U. o. B. (ed.) *ZEF Working Paper Series.* Bonn: University of Bonn.

Reis, N. & Mollinga, P. P. 2012. Water Supply or 'Beautiful Latrines'? Microcredit for Rural Water Supply and Sanitation in the Mekong Delta, Vietnam. *ASEAS - Austrian Journal of South-East Asian Studies,* 5, 10 - 29.

Renaud, F. G. & Kuenzer, C. 2012. *The Mekong Delta System*, Springer Netherlands.

Rheinländer, T., et al. 2010. Hygiene and Sanitation among Ethnic Minorities in Northern Vietnam: Does Government Promotion Match Community Priorities? *Social Science & Medicine,* 71, 994-1001.

Richmond, C., et al. 2005. The Political Ecology of Health: Perceptions of Environment, Economy, Health and Well Being among Namgis First Nation. *Health & place,* 11, 349-365.

Roberts, M., et al. 2003. *Getting Health Reform Right: A Guide to Improving Performance and Equity*, Oxford University Press.

Rogaly, B. 1996. Micro-Finance Evangelism,'Destitute Women', and the Hard Selling of a New Anti-Poverty Formula. *Development in Practice,* 6, 100-112.

Rosenstock, I. M., et al. 1988. Social Learning Theory and the Health Belief Model. *Health Education & Behavior,* 15, 175-183.

Ryan, E. T. 2011. The Cholera Pandemic, Still with Us after Half a Century: Time to Rethink. *PLoS Negl Trop Dis,* 5, e1003.

Sakata, S. 2006. Mass-Organizations as Active Participants in Poverty Reduction in Vietnam. *IDE ASDEP Series*, 46-63.

Santosham, M., et al. 2010. Progress and Barriers for the Control of Diarrhoeal Disease. *The Lancet,* 376, 63-67.

Saravanan, V. & Gondhalekar, D. 2013. Water Supply and Sanitation as a 'Preventive Medicine': Challenges in Rapidly Growing Economies. *Water International,* 38, 867-874.

Saravanan, V., et al. 2011. Global Change, Wastewater and Health in Fast Growing Economies. *Current Opinion in Environmental Sustainability.*

Scheper-Hughes, N. & Lock, M. M. 1987. The Mindful Body: A Prolegomenon to Future Work in Medical Anthropology. *Medical anthropology quarterly,* 1, 6-41.

Schlipköter, U. & Flahault, A. 2010. Communicable Diseases: Achievements and Challenges for Public Health. *Public Health Reviews,* 32, 90-119.

Schuler, S. R., et al. 2006. Constructions of Gender in Vietnam: In Pursuit of the 'Three Criteria'. *Culture, Health & Sexuality,* 8, 383-394.

Schuurman, F. J. 2000. Paradigms Lost, Paradigms Regained? Development Studies in the Twenty-First Century. *Third World Quarterly,* 21, 7-20.

Scott, S., et al. 2006. Doing Fieldwork in Development Geography: Research Culture and Research Spaces in Vietnam. *Geographical Research,* 44, 28–40.

Sijbesma, C., et al. 2010. Case Study on Sustainability of Rural Sanitation Marketing in Vietnam. *wsp (water and sanitation program): Technical Paper (Global Scaling Up Sanitation Project).*

Simon, D. 2008. Urban Environments: Issues on the Peri-Urban Fringe. *Annual Review of Environment and Resources,* 33, 167-185.

Singer, M. 1990. Reinventing Medical Anthropology: Toward a Critical Realignment. *Social science & medicine,* 30, 179-187.

Singer, M., et al. 1992. Why Does Juan Garcia Have a Drinking Problem? The Perspective of Critical Medical Anthropology. *Medical Anthropology,* 14, 77-108.

Smith, S. A. E. 2002. *Water First: A Political History of Hydraulics in Vietnam's Red River Delta.* PhD, Australian National University.

SNV 2010. Study of Rural Water Supply Service Delivery Models in Vietnam. Netherlands Development Organization (SNV).

Sobsey, M. D. 2002. Managing Water in the Home: Accelerated Health Gains from Improved Water Supply. Available: http://www.who.int/water_sanitation_health/dwq/WSH02.07.pdf [Accessed 08.09.2013].

Soussan, J., et al. 2005. Joint Gov - Donor Sector Review on Rural Water Supply, Sanitation and Health in Viet Nam. Sector Status Report. Hanoi.

Statistical Division of Cai Rang district 2010. Statistical Yearbook: 2009. *In:* Department of Statistics (ed.). Can Tho City.

Statistical Division of Phong Dien district 2010. Statistical Yearbook: 2009. *In:* Department of Statistics (ed.). Can Tho City.

Statistical Office of Can Tho City 2009. *Statistical Yearbook Can Tho City 2009,* Can Tho City, Socialist Office of Can Tho City.

Statistical Office of Can Tho City 2011. *Statistical Yearbook Can Tho City 2010,* Can Tho City, Socialist Office of Can Tho City.

Stephenson, L. S., et al. 2000. Malnutrition and Parasitic Helminth Infections. *Parasitology,* 121, 23-38.

Strecher, V. J., et al. 1986. The Role of Self-Efficacy in Achieving Health Behavior Change. *Health Education & Behavior,* 13, 73-92.

Stumpf, M. J. 2012. Housing and Urbanization: A Socio-Spatial Analysis of Resettlement Projects in Hồ Chí Minh City. *Independent Study Project (ISP) Collection* [Online]. Available: http://digitalcollections.sit.edu/isp_collection/1284.

Sugita, E. W. 2004. *Domestic Water Use, Hygiene Behavior, and Children's Diarrhea in Rural Uganda.* PhD thesis, University of Florida.

Susanne, K. 2006. "Poor Whiteism", White Maternal Mortality, and the Promotion of Public Health in South Africa: The Department of Public Health's Endorsement of Contraceptive Services, 1930 - 1938. *In:* Falola, T. & Heaton, M. M. (eds.) *Endangered Bodies: Women, Children, and Health in Africa.* Africa World Press.

Swyngedouw, E. 1997. Power, Nature, and the City. The Conquest of Water and the Political Ecology of Urbanization in Guayaquil, Ecuador: 1880 - 1990. *Environment and Planning A,* 29, 311-332.

Swyngedouw, E. 2008. Where Is the Political? . Available: http://www.socialsciences.manchester.ac.uk/disciplines/politics/research/hmrg/activities/documents/Swyngedouw.pdf [Accessed 07.11.2012].

Taylor, P. 2004. Redressing Disadvantage or Re-Arranging Inequality? Development Interventions and Local Responses in the Mekong Delta. *In:* Taylor, P. (ed.) *Social Inequality in Vietnam and the Challenges to Reform.* Singapore: Institute of Southeast Asian Studies.

Taylor, R. & Rieger, A. 1984. Rudolf Virchow on the Typhus Epidemic in Upper Silesia: An Introduction and Translation. *Sociology of Health & Illness,* 6, 201-217.

Than Tung, K. A. 2012. Risky Treatment. *Thanh Nien News online*, 13.07.2012.

Thang, T. D. 2002. *Field Survey and Laboratory Studies on Salt Water Contamination Issues in the Mekong Delta.* Asian Institute of Technology.

Thanh Nien news. 2012. Medical Bribery Commonplace in Vietnam: A Survey *Thanh Nien news*, 14.09.2012.

Thanh Nien online. 2010. "Hot" Hot Season Diseases. *Thanh Nien online*, 29.03.2010.

Thanh, V. V. 2009. Hygiene and Food Safety Management: A "Squad" Type ... Three "Divisions". *Tuoi Tre online*, 21/04/2009.

Thapar, N. & Sanderson, I. R. 2004. Diarrhoea in Children: An Interface between Developing and Developed Countries. *The Lancet,* 363, 641-653.

The Prime Minister of Vietnam 1994. On Clean Water and Rural Sanitation Assurance. *200-TTg.*

The World Bank (WB) & International Development Association (IDA) 2006. Ida at Work: Sanitation and Water Supply. Improving Services for the Poor.

Thompson, C. M. 2003. Medicine, Nationalism, and Revolution in Vietnam: The Roots of Medical Collaboration to 1945. *East Asian Science, Technology, and Medicine*, 114-148.

Thompson, T., et al. 2003. Providing Clean Water, Keeping Water Clean: An Integrated Approach. *International Journal of Environmental Health Research,* 13, 89-94.

Trach, D., et al. 1997. Field Trial of a Locally Produced, Killed, Oral Cholera Vaccine in Vietnam. *Lancet,* 349, 231-235.

Trading Economics. 2012. *Vietnam Gdp Annual Growth Rate* [Online]. Available: http://www.tradingeconomics.com/vietnam/gdp-growth-annual.

Tran Giuu DS 2007. Using Chloramine B to Disinfect Water for Daily Activities. *Health for a cultural village.* Can Tho: MoH.

Tran Hong Phuoc Tai. 2009. *Assessment of Domestic Water Quality in Hung Phu Ward, Cai Rang District, Can Tho City.* Master's degree, Can Tho University.

Tran Van Tien, et al. 2011. A Health Financing Review of Viietnam with a Focus on Social Health Insurance: Bottlenecks in Institutional Design and Organizational Practice of Health Financing and Options to Accelerate Progress Towards Universal Coverage. The World Health Organization (WHO).

Tran Vu 2007. Six Steps for Hand Washing - to Save Lives. *Health for a cultural village.* Hanoi: MoH.

Trostle, J. A. 2005. *Epidemiology and Culture*, Cambridge University Press.

Trumper, R. & Phillips, L. 1995. Cholera in the Time of Neoliberalism: The Cases of Chile and Ecuador. *Alternatives: Global, Local, Political,* 20, 165-193.

Tuan Tran Van; Thi Mai Dung; Neu, I. D., M.J. 2005. Comparative Quality of Private and Public Health Services in Rural Vietnam. *Health Policy and Planning,* 20, 319-327.

Tung, T. & Chau, L. 2013. Vietnam Street Food Still Unsafe: Studies *Thanh Nien News*, 01.08.13.

Turshen, M. 1977. The Political Ecology of Disease. *Review of Radical Political Economics,* 9, 45-60.

UNDP 2011. Social Services for Human Development: Viet Nam Human Development Report 2011. Hanoi, Viet Nam: United Nations Development Programme (UNDP).

UNICEF 2008a. Knowledges Attitudes and Practices of Child and Woman Health Care, Water Sanitation and Hygiene, Results from Survey in 4 Project Communes *An Giang Provincial Child Friendly Project.*

UNICEF 2008b. Results of Survey on Knowledge, Attitudes and Practices of Child and Woman Health Care, Water Sanitation and Hygiene, Results from Survey in Four Project Communes. *Provincial Child Friendly Project (PCFP) An Giang* Ho Chi MInh City: UNICEF.

UNICEF. 2011. An Analysis of the Situation of Children and Wash Sector in Vietnam. Available: http://www.unicef.org/sitan/files/SitAn-Viet_Nam_2010_Eng.pdf [Accessed 13.09.2012].

UNICEF 2012a. An Analysis of the Situation of Children in an Giang Province. *Provincial Child Friendly Programme (PCFP),*

Unite for Children. Hanoi: UNICEF Vietnam Country Office.

UNICEF 2012b. Pneumonia and Diarrhoea: Tackling the Deadliest Diseases for the World's Poorest Children. New York: United Nations Children's Fund (UNICEF).

UNICEF & WHO 2009. Diarrhoea: Why Children Are Still Dying and What Can Be Done.

United Nations 2007. Universal Declaration of Human Rights. *Dignity and Justice for All of Us.* 60th Anniversary Special Edition ed.: United Nations.

United Nations. 2010. Press Release of High-Level Plenary Meeting of the General Assembly : Un Summit Concludes with Adoption of Global Action Plan to Achieve Development Gols by 2015. Available: http://www.who.int/pmnch/media/membernews/2010/20100922_un_closingpr.pdf [Accessed 12.09.2012].

Urry, J. 2003. *Global Complexity*, Wiley.

Van Man, N., et al. 2005. Epidemiological Profile and Burden of Rotavirus Diarrhea in Vietnam: 5 Years of Sentinel Hospital Surveillance, 1998–2003. *Journal of Infectious Diseases,* 192, S127 - S132.

Van Nguyen, K., et al. 2013. Antibiotic Use and Resistance in Emerging Economies: A Situation Analysis for Viet Nam. *BMC Public Health,* 13, 1158.

Varis, O. 2008. Poverty, Economic Growth, Deprivation, and Water: The Cases of Cambodia and Vietnam. *AMBIO: A Journal of the Human Environment,* 37, 225-231.

VBSP 2011. Statistical Information on Micro-Credit Loans Provided for Water Supply and Sanitation in the Period 2005 - 2010 in Can Tho. Can Tho: Vietnam Social Policy Bank (VSPB).

Vian, T., et al. 2012. Confronting Corruption in the Health Sector in Vietnam: Patterns and Prospects. *Public Administration and Development,* 32, 49-63.

Vietnam Environment Protection Agency 2004. Country Report: On Land-Based Pollution in Vietnam. Hanoi: Center for Marine Environmental Survey Research & Consultation.

Vietnam News. 2007. Licencing of Food Found to Be Too "Open". *Vietnam News*, 16.08.2007.

Vietnews. 2012. Prime Minister Dung Urges the Country for a Route to Health Insurance for Everyone. *Vietnews*, 13.09.2012.

Vo Thanh Danh 2008. Household Switching Behavior in the Use of Groundwater in the Mekong Delta, Vietnam. Singapore: Economy and Environment Program for Southeast Asia (EEPSEA) and the International Development Research Centre.

Vo Thi Yen Phi. 2010. *Quantitative Microbial Risk Assessment for Faecal Management – Health Consequences in the Mekong Delta, Vietnam.* Erlangung des Doktorgrades (Dr. rer.nat.) PhD thesis, Rheinischen Friedrich-Wilhelms-Universität Bonn.

Wagner, E. G., et al. 1959. Water Supply for Rural Areas and Small Communities/Edmund G. Wagner, Jn Lanoix.

Wahlberg, A. 2006. Bio-Politics and the Promotion of Traditional Herbal Medicine in Vietnam. *Health:,* 10, 123-147.

Waibel, G. 2010. State Management in Transition: Understanding Water Resources Management in Vietnam. *In:* Center for Development Research (ed.) *ZEF Working Paper Series.* Bonn: University of Bonn.

Waibel, G., et al. 2012. Water Governance under Renovation? Concepts and Practices of Iwrm in the Mekong Delta, Vietnam. *In:* Renaud, F. G. & Kuenzer, C. (eds.) *The Mekong Delta System. Interdisciplinary Analyses of a River Delta.* Dordrecht: Springer.

Waibel, G. & Glück, S. 2013. More Than 13 Million: Mass Mobilisation and Gender Politics in the Vietnam Women's Union. *Gender & Development,* 21, 343-361.

Wallerstein, N. & Bernstein, E. 1988. Empowerment Education: Freire's Ideas Adapted to Health Education. *Health Education & Behavior,* 15, 379-394.

WaterAid Australia & International Water Centre 2008. Sharing Experiences: Sustainable Sanitation in South East Asia and the Pacific. Brisbane, Australia.

Weiss, G. L. & Lonnquist, L. E. 2003. *The Sociology of Health, Healing, and Illness*, Prentice Hall.

WHO 1987. Communication: A Guide for Managers of National Diarrhoeal Disease Control Programmes. Planning, Management and Appraisal of Communication Activities. *In:* WHO (ed.).

WHO (ed.) 1997. *Guidelines for Drinking-Water Quality: Surveillance and Control of Community Supplies, 2nd Edition*, Geneva.

WHO 2000. World Health Report 2000: Health Systems : Improving Performance. Geneva: World Health Organization.

WHO 2001a. The Role of Ministries of Health in Reducing Disease Burden Due to Water, Sanitation and Hygiene Related Illnesses. WHO Regional Office for South East Asia.

WHO. 2001b. Water-Related Diseases: Malnutrition. Available: http://www.who.int/water_sanitation_health/diseases/malnutrition/en/ [Accessed 06.05.2011].

WHO 2005. Core Indicators 2005: Health Situation in the South-East Asia and Western Pacific Regions. WHO.

WHO 2008. Country Health Information Profile. Available Online at Http://Www2.Wpro.Who.Int/Nr/Rdonlyres/7903fa6f-96c5-4778-Bfe9-D981b82c7715/0/Vtn_Data_Bank.Pdf.

WHO. 2009. Diarrhoeal Disease Available: http://www.who.int/mediacentre/factsheets/fs330/en/index.html [Accessed 27.07.2012].

WHO. 2011. Enterohaemorrhagic Escherichia Coli (Ehec). Available: http://www.who.int/mediacentre/factsheets/fs125/en/index.html [Accessed 27.07.2012].

WHO. 2012a. Country Health Information Profiles: Viet Nam. Available: http://www.wpro.who.int/countries/vnm/36VTNpro2011_finaldraft.pdf [Accessed 06.07.2012].

WHO 2012b. Un-Water Global Analysis and Assessment of Sanitation and Drinking-Water (Glaas) 2012 Report: The Challenge of Extending and Sustaining Services. Geneva, Switzerland: WHO.

WHO. 2012c. Viet Nam: Health Profile. Available: http://www.who.int/gho/countries/vnm.pdf [Accessed 03.07.2012].

WHO. 2012d. Water, Sanitation and Hygiene Links to Health. Available: http://www.who.int/water_sanitation_health/publications/facts2004/en/ [Accessed 05.07.2012].

WHO 2012e. World Health Statistics 2012. Geneva: World Health Organization.

WHO. 2012f. World Malaria Report: Vietnam Available: http://www.who.int/malaria/publications/country-profiles/profile_vnm_en.pdf [Accessed 07.01.13].

Wilbers, G. 2012. Personal Communication. Bonn, Germany: United Nations University.

Witter, S. 1996. 'Doi Moi'and Health: The Effect of Economic Reforms on the Health System in Vietnam. *The International journal of health planning and management,* 11, 159-172.

Wolpe, P. R. 1985. The Maintenance of Professional Authority: Acupuncture and the American Physician. *Social Problems,* 32, 409-424.

World Bank (WB) 2006. Vietnam Environment Monitor 2006. Water Quality in Vietnam with a Focus on the Cau, Nhue-Day and Dong-Nai River Basins. Manila: World Bank (WB),.

World Bank (WB) 2008. Review and Analysis of the Pollution Impacts from Vietnamese Manufacturing Sectors. The World Bank (WB).

World Bank (WB) 2010. An Evaluation of World Bank Support, 1997 - 2007: Water and Development *IEG Study Series.* Washington D.C.

World Bank (WB). 2011. Mortality Rate (Per 1000 Live Births) of under 5 Year-Olds in Vietnam. *Country Indicators* [Online]. Available: http://data.worldbank.org/indicator/SH.DYN.MORT/countries/1W-VN?display=graph [Accessed 13.04.2012].

World Bank (WB) 2013. Vietnam Poverty Assessment 2012 : Well Begun, Not yet Done: Remarkable Progress on Poverty Reduction and the Emerging Challenges. World Bank (WB).

Wright, J., et al. 2004. Household Drinking Water in Developing Countries: A Systematic Review of Microbiological Contamination between Source and Point-of-Use. *Tropical Medicine & International Health,* 9, 106-117.

Wrigley, T. 2007. Microbial Counts and Pesticide Concentrations in Drinking Water after Alum Flocculation of Channel Feed Water at the Household Level, in Vinh Long Province, Vietnam. *Journal of Water and Health,* 5, 171-178.

Yin, R. K. 2003. *Case Study Research: Design and Methods, Third Edition. Applied Social Research Methods Series, Vol.5,* London, Sage.

Young, B. & Briscoe, J. 1988. A Case-Control Study of the Effect of Environmental Sanitation on Diarrhoea Morbidity in Malawi. *Journal of epidemiology and community health,* 42, 83-88.

Socio-political and Cultural Determinants of Diarrheal Disease in the Mekong Delta. From Discourse to Incidence

ANNEX

I. Trajectory of fieldwork methodology

Contextualisation

Within the first two months of research, interviews were held with district-level organisations in six of the nine districts of Can Tho City[175] (hospitals, Preventive Health Centres, district offices of health under the People's Committee, etc). In addition, representatives of provincial and higher-level authorities that were responsible for water supply and sanitation, environmental protection and health were also interviewed (including DONRE, CERWASS, Institute of Public Health and Hygiene, medical universities, CIDS, WHO, UNICEF). At this stage, interviewees were not personally selected and their names were not made known to the researcher before the actual interview took place. As will be described below, a representative would be assigned by the organisation to participate in the interview based on the topics of discussion, which had to be predesigned and presented beforehand for review by state authorities.

The typical duration of each interview was between 45 min and 1.5 hours, as most interviewees would claim to be too busy or too tired to stay longer. A list of questions/prompts was always used as a guide for the issues to be raised. During this first stage of research, the interview topics were generic and similar for all the informants. In practice, the depth of the discussion would much depend on the respondent's interest and expertise. By the end of the fieldwork period, it increasingly the case information was triangulated through newly identified sources as well as follow-up interviews.

Language barriers that the researcher could not overcome herself called for the hiring of a research assistant. All the interviewing and the communication with local authorities were made possible through the work of the research assistant, who also translated Vietnamese documents. This constituted both an indispensable help and a research constraint, as will be explained below. The use of a voice-recorder that would allow accurate transcription and easily reviewable original statements was faced with discomfort from interviewees. Even in the few cases where respondents did not explicitly disapprove of its use, they would keep a rather "stiff upper lip" during the discussions. Therefore, its use was abandoned after the first few interviews, as it was proving more of a research

175 Those were the districts of: Cai Rang, Ninh Kieu, Phong Dien, O Mon, Binh Thuy and Co Do.

obstacle than a facilitator. The difficulties in acquiring detailed and accurately documented oral information were only surpassed to a substantial degree through the extensive training of the assistant and her gradual familiarisation with the research topic and the demands of the researcher herself.

After 27 semi-structured interviews, a first overview of the institutional structure and its functions around health care, prevention of disease, water provision and sanitation in the region was assembled. Interviewees and secondary data verified the relevance and importance of the research problem, namely diarrheal disease. During this phase, the contrast between areas that were developing an urban character and those remaining essentially rural became increasingly evident and developed as an issue worth examining. Through an initial analysis of the results, a selection was made of the two districts where research would go further in-depth.

Selected districts

Within the selected districts of Cai Rang and Phong Dien, 21 more semi-structured interviews took place. Interviewees mostly consisted of civil society representatives (Women's Union, Farmer's Union, Youth Union, Red Cross offices, etc) but also cadres of health-related offices, departments of education, economic and social policy[176]. Finally, some interviews took place with workers in the healthcare sector at commune and ward clinics as well as with teachers and caretakers in elementary schools and kindergartens.

In this round of interviews, the questions were more tailored to the different interviewees, more focused and less explorative. Triangulation of previously gathered information was possible and some patterns in the discourse patterns were already becoming evident. From a practical standpoint, research became easier because it focused on a smaller area, where relations with locals could be built. Some offices were visited for the second time and familiarity between the researcher and the informants gradually increased. Moreover, some explorative "drive-around" the communes and hamlets was allowed by the authorities. This offered useful observations about the livelihoods and the particular characteristics of rural and urban spaces, while at the same time enriching the photographic material. More importantly, the researcher could obtain a better idea of the different areas within each district for the future selection of study-sites for the household survey.

---

176 Namely, these were the district-level offices of education, offices of health, preventive health centres, offices of labour and social affairs, office of agriculture and rural development (Phong Dien) and offices of industry and economy (Cai Rang).

Household Survey

The choice to conduct a household survey with a standardised questionnaire was a research decision shaped by the characteristics of the field. While the preferred approach would be an equally high number of in-depth interviews with targeted residents of these two selected localities, this method had to be re-considered. In depth interviewing was thought of as a way to explore people's perceptions, voice their concerns and document their realities in relation to topics of health, disease, water and sanitation. It would also provide the opportunity to closely observe their household practices, habits and current situation with regard to these issues. Despite the adequacy of the method, access to households was not possible without a research permit. In order to obtain such a permit, a pre-set list with the addresses of individual interviewees and a predefined set of questions was required. Interaction between a foreign researcher and local cadres or citizens was confined and restricted by this "official research permit" regulation and thus the researcher often lacked trustworthy key informants who would be willing and able to guide the selection of those households (according to certain criteria such as poverty, profession, location). Under these conditions, the only way to obtain permission for interviewing citizens would be a random selection of households and a pre-decided questionnaire, something that is not very different from a household survey.

Household surveys, fortunately, were a research process very familiar to the Vietnamese authorities, which makes it is easier to pass bureaucratic and procedural obstacles. Therefore, although it was initially viewed as a complementary method, the household survey proved to be the perfect "Trojan horse" for observations and conversations with people in the research study-sites. The process was well-known to local officials and administering the survey with their facilitation proved simple once central approval was obtained. A large number of households were visited and, apart from the collection of quantitative information, "off-research" time was spent with local cadres and people from the localities, which basically ensured unlimited and daily access to the selected hamlets and communes.

Sample selection and characteristics

Whereas the selection of districts and communes was based on an extensive round of observations, local literature study and interviews with district-level authorities, the selection of the hamlets and areas for the household survey was mostly based on the advice and help of local cadres who were very knowledgeable of the area's specificities, such as the extent of the available water supply and sanitation infrastructure; often, they could even could provide information for each household in their jurisdiction. Generally, the involvement of local cadres in the organisation and supervision of the survey was an official requirement (see also section 3.3), which introduced a bias but also facilitated the research process. It was often the case, for example, that the consulting cadre would lead the survey to households whose members would have a public office position, with the claim that people working for the state are more likely to tolerate the survey procedure. Even if the above was true, the selection of such households is also believed to have presented a bias in the direction of receiving "correct" answers, or those in line with regulations and social imperatives; this was especially the case if a household is connected directly to the party-state apparatus. As a result, some answers might have been biased towards the recommended or legal way of doing things and not the practices or ideas that people actually adopt.

The final decision about which households to visit was left to the researcher and was mostly based on a desired representation of the distinction between purely rural and distinctively urban locations. The second requirement set by the researcher was sampling a mix of poor, middle-class and better-off households. In total, 25 households from the sample were officially classified as poor or nearly-poor and the remaining 106 were not. Within this set, and by judging from each household's belongings, infrastructure and livelihood sources, a representation of the "average household" was attempted; in particular, the goal was to avoid interviewing households that seemed overly wealthy. The percentage of those in an extremely poor situation did not exceed ¼ of the sample. The third requirement was to examine both households that had direct access to river water and those which did not. In the rural case, the sample included mostly households that are located near a surface water source (47) while for the remainder this was either not true or no related information was gathered (22). In the urban case there was a "natural" division between the two selected areas. The visited households located in the central Yen Hoa area did not have access to surface water (29), while those located in Yen Binh area (33) were located near the river where the floating market activities take place (26). About half of these houses were actually "floating", as is described in detail in section 4.3.

The gender and the age of the respondents were left to chance because the researcher could not control which member of the family would be available at the time of the interview. In total, more women (83) than men (48) were interviewed. Concerning the age of the sampling, most were fairly equally distributed among the age group 36 -55 years (45%) and over-56 years old (43%), with only 11.5% of the respondents being younger than 35 years old. Finally, the education level varied significantly, with 17 respondents being illiterate, 47 having attended elementary school, 27 being junior high-school graduates, 38 having finished secondary high-school and only one interviewee having gone through higher education.

Questionnaire

The questionnaire used for the household survey was a shortened and slightly modified version of a questionnaire designed by researchers Simon Benedikter, Ute Köster and Phạm Thị Trung Ngọc[177] for previously conducted research in Can Tho. The questionnaire is published and available in the Master thesis of Ute Köster (2008). Making use of this pre-designed and pre-tested research tool with formulated categories (i.e. water storage types, water supply sources, wastewater disposal options, diarrhoea symptoms etc) allowed for time economy by avoiding repetition in piloting. The questions were translated into Vietnamese and re-tested during the training of the local enumerators in order to ensure its clarity and contextual fit. The selection and adjustment of some questions was necessary in order to suit the particular objectives of this research. In detail, 24 of the 43 questions were carried over exactly from the original questionnaire (Köster, 2008), nine were slightly changed and ten questions were newly introduced.

In the selection and formulation of questions, attention was paid to keep the questionnaire short and manageable enough to finish within 45 minutes. Maintaining already existing and creating more open-ended questions allowed the opportunity to prompt discussion with the interviewees. Descriptive information from these open-ended questions was used to form new categories which were included later in the survey analysis (see Codebook in Annex). Other type of information obtained through the household-survey discussions was used as complementary qualitative data, to be combined with field notes, observations and photographic material.

Training survey assistants

Apart from the full-time research assistant/translator that worked full time with the researcher, two additional enumerators were recruited especially for the administering of the household survey (female university students). In order to train the enumerators, we held two training sessions of four hours each, during which survey questions were discussed and the desired approach was explained,

---

[177] A resulting journal publication of 2009: Herbst, S., et al. 2009. Perceptions of Water, Sanitation and Health: A Case Study from the Mekong Delta, Vietnam. *Water Science & Technology*, 60, 699-707.

stressing the need for subtlety, respect and patience. Before the enumerators began their work independently, each was required to participate in about ten survey interviews acting as the researcher's translator in order to clearly exemplify the desirable manner of going about with the survey questions. Overall, the training drew attention to the following issues:

- Providing an introductory overall presentation of the research project to the participants, shortly explaining the survey's purpose, and getting their consent.

- Not giving the questionnaire to the respondents to fill in but asking questions openly, in order to avoid any predisposition created by the wording or the pre-defined categories. This also covered the skill of fitting answers into the multiple-choice options or keeping notes and creating new categories.

- Allowing dialogue and expression of personal opinion by the respondents, even beyond the strict boundaries of the survey questions. Constantly keeping notes on additional information provided from the respondents

- Oral and written reporting at the end of each day, including a description of the visited households and respondents, a run-through of the questionnaires filled in and discussion of any uncertainties (blanks, open-ended answers) or difficulties faced.

In total, the number of survey interviews led by the researcher herself was 61 (of the 131), with the remaining 70 conducted by the trained enumerators. At the end of each interview, a small gift was offered to each household as an appreciation of their time and willingness to be part of this research project. The gift constituted of a bag with some basic essentials for a household (a pack of sugar, coffee or tea and some bars of hand-washing soap) which constitute a basic symbolic and functional gesture of gratitude, as recommended by the local authorities.

Overall, the survey allowed the research to deal with local realities and strengthen the findings on issues that were beforehand only discussed in terms of existing policy by official representatives of the state. Previous observations and their implications were crystallising through the accumulated interview time and the research gained momentum. However, it must be stressed that many of the respondents seemed confused about whether they should talk, what they should say, and were generally hesitant to open up in conversation, especially in the presence of local cadres (see also section 3.3)

In-depth household interviews

The presence of the researcher in the same hamlets and areas for more than a month as part of undertaking the household survey resulted in the building of trust between her and the local authorities. This consequently allowed for a number of in-depth household interviews to be organised. Nevertheless, the involvement of the local cadres in selecting the households and their attendance at interviews was outside of the researcher's control. That being said, all nine in-depth interviews lasted from one to two hours, during which the presence of the local cadre was less intrusive than in the household survey. In fact, the researcher was often left alone with the interviewees after the first 20 minutes, allowing for discussions to expand and for more "difficult" questions to be asked.

The examined issues were mostly focusing on the preventive communication approach and the influence it has on the perceptions of people. One of the sample selection criteria was for interviewees to be mothers of young children. The secondary criterion was for respondents to have (also) undertaken micro-credit loans or subsidies for the improvement of their sanitation situation. As a result, four young mothers were interviewed in the rural hamlets of Phong Dien district, one of which had also taken up a loan for sanitation. In the urban Le Binh ward of Cai Rang district, there is no loan policy being implemented but, as local informants claimed, there are households that face sanitation problems:

> "In Cai Rang, there is no policy that gives loans; people build their toilets on their own and by now 99% have toilets. But there are people who need to repair their toilets but have no money to do so. Those who are classified as poor are more taken care of than those who might be a bit better-off. This is because only the poor get state support to build and repair the toilets in their house; the rest have to manage on their own" (Local informant from Cai Rang, 20.12.11, personal communication).

This was seen as an interesting case of non-access to social policy and thus, apart from the four households with young mothers in Phong Dien district, one of the selected households in Le Binh also had a sanitation facility that needed repair.

Interviews in targeted offices

After the rounds of interviews described above and an exercise comparing official statements with people's opinions and with issued policies, the data presented certain gaps and mismatches. Moreover, various unanswered questions emerged from divergences discovered between collected answers and the study's refined objectives. This indicated the need for more research in order to clarify and triangulate information. Specifically, this led to interviewing in a selection of 19 state offices and organisations in the wider case study area of Can Tho[178]. Additionally, interviews with representatives from six high-level departments and research institutes in Ho Chi Minh City and Hanoi were conducted[179]. The method used in this stage was also semi-structured interviews facilitated by an interview guide. In parallel to these scheduled visits, some additional informal meetings were held with fellow researchers, NGO representatives and local experts, whose knowledge and experiences brought about rich discussions and cross-referenced the findings.

II. Figures

Figure 1: The MEME (Multiple Exposures Multiple Effects) model

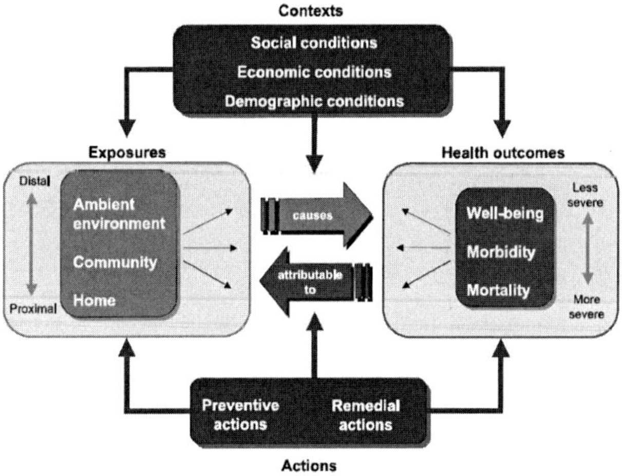

Adopted by Briggs (2003)

[178] These were: CERWASS, CIDS, the Food Safety Unit, PHC of Can Tho, the DoPI and the CHECC of Can Tho, as well as the district hospitals in Cai Rang and Phong Dien, the public pharmacies within these hospitals, local clinics and health stations within the above districts, water supply companies of Can Tho City and the Cai Rang branch, rural water stations in the communes of Phong Dien, and finally the district level Women's Union offices.

[179] These were: the IHPH, the WHO and the Pasteur Institute in Ho Chi Minh City, as well as the Institute of Hygiene and Epidemiology, the Department of Preventive Medicine, the VIHEMA and the HSPI of the MoH which are located in Hanoi.

Figure 2: The treatment process that water companies follow

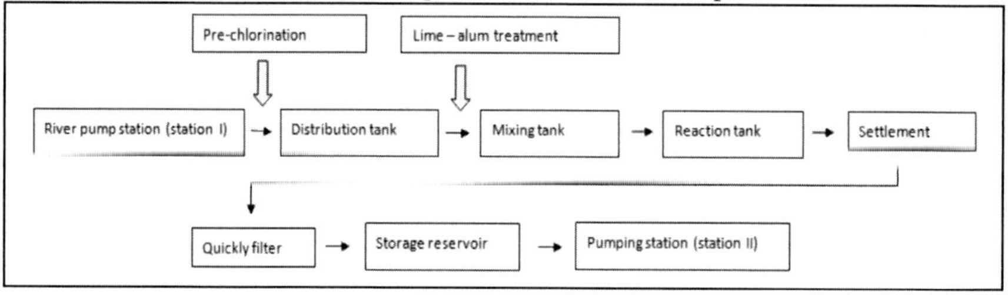

Source: Head of water factory in Cai Rang district, personal communication

IV. Boxes

Box 1: New indicators and targets for re-defining "improved" water and sanitation proposed by the Joint Monitoring Program of UNICEF and the WHO

For water supply: For a basic water service in the household, drinking water should be simply collected from an "improved" source (proxy for both availability and quality), within 30 minutes per trip (accessibility). For an intermediate/higher water service, the criteria to be fulfilled are:

(i) Drinking water collected from a source that supplies 50 litres per capita per day year-round (with daily or weekly interruptions in supply); (ii) requiring no more than 10 minutes to collect; (iii) with no detectable E. coli in a 100 ml sample; (iv) the combined expenditures on water, sanitation and hygiene will cost no more than 5% of the disposable household income.

For sanitation: A proper sanitation:

(i) Separates excreta from human contact and ensures that excreta does not re-enter the immediate household environment; (ii) is safe (protects the user from risks such as vermin, falling into the pit); (iii) is durable; (iv) belongs to one household or is a shared toilet within or nearby the plot shared by no more than 5 families or 30 people, whichever is fewer, and used by people who know each other; (v) is accessible at all times (seven days a week, 24 hours a day), (vi) is accessible to all members of household, including those with disabilities, (vii) protects users from culturally-inappropriate exposure or invasion of privacy.

Additional parameters include aspects of affordability and community-wide sanitation by the abolishment of open defecation and adequate treatment of excreta before they are disposed.

(JMP, 2012b)

Box 2: Official instructions for collecting data on clean water supply of households in Can Tho (MARD, 2008a, CERWASS, 2011b, CERWASS, 2011e)

Hygienic water (NƯỚC SẠCH) definition: Hygienic is the water used directly or after filtration satisfying the quality requirements: colourless, odourless, with no strange taste, can be used for drinking after boiling. This definition is also quantitative, and should be combined with the observations that follow the instructions below:

Tap water: water that is collected from a faucet (in the house or public tap water) supplied from a water supply centre station. The water resource must be not polluted, treated hygienically for the supply of people via a pipe system.

Rain water: collected in tanks or jugs (clay). Rain water is collected from a tile roof (red one), steel roof, and concrete ceiling (after the discharge of dirt before collection) and leaded into the pottery jugs which are also washed before water collection. Tanks and clay jugs must have covering and an installed tap or the use of mugs to get the water is required.

Mineral water or surface water: water that is being collected from the stream or a spring and is lead to the household by conduit; surface water that is not polluted by human or animal waste, chemicals, pesticides, industrial waste material, or handicraft village waste.

Dug wells (water from shallow layer) with a covering, floor, water extraction tool and filtering material: dug-wells must be located at least 10m far from a barn or any other source of pollution. The well has to be made out of bricks or rocks and the drop pipe has to be at least 3 meters deep. The floor around the well has to be covered with concrete or bricks without cracks.

Deep drilled wells (using drilling machine): The well should be located far from latrines, cattle barns, or other sources of pollution at least 10m. The floor of and around the well has to be built with concrete or bricks without cracks.

Considering data collection on hygienic water:

Data is collected at the hamlet level by observing the type of water supply (based on the criteria such as colour, odour, and strange traces), checking the quality of the construction and the current operational status of it (the way people use it):

If a household uses two or more of waterworks (infrastructure) at the same time, only the source mostly used will be recorded into the statistic records to assess whether households use clean water. If households have to buy clean water regularly from a boat or a mobile water truck, the source of this water (drilling well or tap water) is determined and recorded accordingly.

For the hamlet level: reporting is done by observing methods and by interviewing and collecting statistical data from each household. For the commune/district/Province level: representative data sources can be selected (normally selecting from 20% to 30% of the population in the commune or surveying the total population)

Box 3: Sanitation regulations and definitions in Vietnam

Houses' sanitation should technically ensure the following requirements: Isolating the faeces, preventing their spread and strictly preventing their contact with humans, animals and insects, being able to kill pathogens in the faeces (viral, bacterial, protozoan eggs, worms) and not polluting the surrounding environment. Specific regulations exist for the construction of each type of latrine to qualify as hygienic. For the two prominent types (septic tank latrine and pour-flush latrine) it is suggested accordingly:

Septic tank latrines: should be constructed to process waste in a 3-compartment tank, with the sub-tank not sinking or falling, its lid being sealed and not have any cracks, with no odour or water leaks. There should be a flush and a ventilation pipe. Regarding its maintenance, the flush should have intense flow and enough water. There should be no mosquito larvae in the flush water tank. The toilet should be odourless; the room should be clean, without slippery moss and without paper trash around. The toilet paper should be placed through a hole (if it is for consumption) or placed in trash cans (if it has been used already). There should be no flies or insects in the toilet room; it should be clean and tidy. Latrines must be housed and protected from rain. Sewage must enter drains or sewage pits and not flow freely around.

Pour-flush latrines: should not be built in flooded areas and should be at least 10 meters away from drinking water sources. The sub-tank should not be sinking (above the ground at least 20cm) and its lid should have no cracks. The floor should be flat and not cause stagnation of water. There should be a flush. [...] Regarding its use and preservation, there should be enough and intense water flowing from the flush container and it should be free of mosquito larvae. There should be no bad odours; the room should be clean, without any slippery moss or paper trash. The toilet-paper should be flushed down (if the paper is bio-degradable) or placed in trash bins. There should be no flies or insects in the room; it should be clean and tidy, with a roof and protected from rainwater.

(CERWASS, 2011b, MoH, 2005, CERWASS, 2011a, CERWASS, 2011d)

Box 4: The way out of sanctioning: the case of bottled water and ice

In order for a water-bottling company to get officially registered and be allowed to begin operation, a two-step process of sampling and testing has to take place[180]:

---

[180] Officer in the checking department of the Food Safety Unit in Can Tho 16.12.11, personal interview

- The company sends a sample of the produced water to the Food Safety Unit, together with a description of the purifying technology that the company is using.

- If the analysis of this sample assures it is adequate for human consumption (according to national water quality standards)[181], staff from the Unit will re-sample and analyze the water produced by the company, making sure that the results from the two samples coincide. However, this visit does not happen unannounced as the company is notified of it beforehand.

- After the successful crosschecking of the samples, the company is free to operate without any further requirements.

- Snap-checks might take place abruptly, but this is not necessary happening to all companies.

- Even when standards are found not to be met, the Food Safety Unit has no sanctioning power and can only give advice for better compliance.

- The only authority able to actually impose fines is the Department of Health, representatives of which would have to visit again the company and confirm the violation of food safety standards taking place.

Box 5: Selection of legal excerpts on preventive health education

Connecting communication and education with awareness-raising:

"[...] to accelerate communication and education work so as to raise public awareness about the importance and benefits of preventive medicine; to foster knowledge and skills in the people, families and community so that they can proactively prevent and combat diseases and improve their health, prevent and combat lifestyle-related diseases and change their behaviours in order to build a healthy lifestyle in their community; to encourage people not to smoke, reduce the number of smokers, especially among adolescents and children" (MoH, 2007b: 84)

"Food hygiene and safety has gained concern from authorities at different levels and the public response. Propaganda, education activities as well as surveillance, monitoring, inspection on food hygiene and safety have been conducted effectively with intersectoral collaboration. These activities have contributed to raise the public awareness and reduce the number of poisoning cases" (MoH, 2007b: 102).

Connecting communication and education to the control of infectious disease:

"Article 10: Everyone is entitled to access to information, education and communication on prevention and control of infectious diseases" (GoV, 2007: 58) ... "Requirements on information, education and communication on prevention and control of

[181] Water quality parameters checked include concentrations of total coliform, Clostridium, Streptococcus, and total bacteria, as well as Pd, Mg, Fe, and Ca, to name a few.

infectious disease: (1) to be accurate, clear, easily understandable, practical and timely. (2) To be suitable to target groups, cultural and national traditions, social morality, religions and beliefs and traditional practices and customs" (GoV, 2007: 59).

Using communication and education to promote water and sanitation for disease prevention:

"Article 13: Education establishments are responsible for providing learners with education about sanitation for prevention and control of infectious diseases, including personal hygiene, sanitation in daily life and working activities and environmental sanitation. Health care units of education establishments are responsible for providing public information on sanitation for disease prevention, examining and supervising environmental sanitation and food safety and hygiene and applying measures for preventing and controlling infectious diseases" (GoV, 2007).

"The quality of drinking water has been ensured. The proportion of households using clean water and hygienic latrines is increasing. This is the result of the 'Cultural and Healthy Village' movement which is being scaled up and developed, the inter-sectoral collaboration and the community response in the movement of 'The entire population unites and builds a cultural life' " (MoH 2007: 103).

V. Pictures

Picture 1: Basic types of designs for case-studies

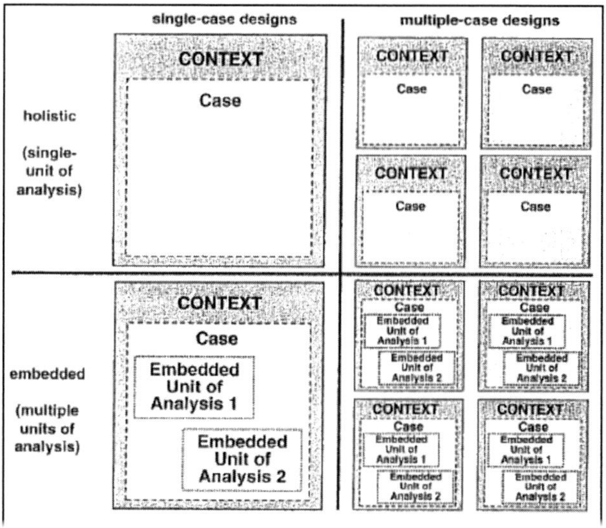

Adopted by Yin (2003).Cited source: COSMOS corporation

Picture 2: Map of Phong Dien from the district's statistical yearbook (2010).

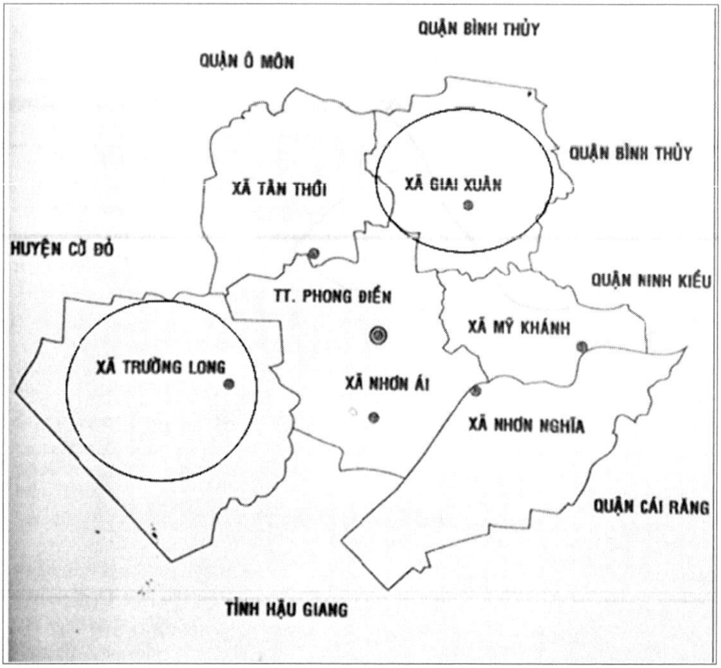

The map is showing the commune boarders and their centres, with the central town as a separate entity (TT Phong Dien). The circle indicates the case-study communes (Xa Giai Xuan and Xa Truong Long

III. Tables

Table 1: Example of the questionnaire used for the survey on poverty status

Revenue	Total income	Total expenditures
1. Crop Production (including product sales and consumer products for household)		
• food crops		
• Industrial plants		
• Fruit trees		
• Crop by-products (coal, leaves, tree tops, straw, wood ....)		

- Other planting products (seedlings, ornamental plants ....)

2. Livestock (including product sales and consumer products for household)

- Cattle
- Poultry
- Other products (eggs, milk, cocoons, honey farming, seed)
- Animal by-products (faeces, feathers, leather...)

3. Agricultural service activities
4. Forestry (including product sales and consumer products for the household) and forestry services
5. Fisheries ((including product sales and consumer products for the household) and Fishery Service
6. The business activities of non-agricultural services (including product sales and consumer products for household)
7. Salaries and wages
8. Other amounts (including items on revenue gathering, gifts, remittances from outside, interest savings, home rentals, pensions, grants preferential treatment of persons)

TOTAL

Total household income (= total income of question 4 – total expenditures of question 4)

Average income / person / month (= total income in question 5.1 / demography of households / 12 months)

CONCLUSION (Mark x in appropriate boxes)

POOR HOUSEH0LD

Rural : < = 400,000 / person / month

Urban: < = 500,000 / person / month

NEAR POOR HOUSEHOLD

Rural: > 400,000/person / month and < = 520,000 / person / month Urban:> 500,000 VND / person / month and < = 650,000 / person / month

Source: (OLISA Cai Rang, 2011), translated.

Table 2: Reported cases of diarrhoea from various agencies, accumulating statistics to the indicated administrative levels

Source	Years	Accumulated per administrative level	Average annual cases	Reference documents
MoH	2001-2011	National	**925893**	(MoH, 2012a)
IHPH	2005 – 2011	Regional (20 Southern provinces)	**220476**	(IHPH, 2012)
Children's Hospital	2009 - 2010	Regional (various provinces of the South) – children diagnosed	**12670**	(Can Tho Regional Paediatrics Hospital, 2011a)
Children's Hospital	2009 - 2010	Regional (various provinces of the South) – children inpatients	**2562**	(Can Tho Regional Paediatrics Hospital, 2011b)
Reported for the Province				
MoH	2007 - 2010	Province (Can Tho City)	**17990**	(MoH, 2012a)
PHC of CTC	2008 - 2011	Province (Can Tho City)	**2090**	(PHC Can Tho City, 2011b)
PHC of CTC	2011	Province (Can Tho City) - children	**10**	(PHC Can Tho City, 2011f)
General Hospital of CTC	2006 - 2011	Province (Can Tho City)	**1528**	(General Hospital of Can Tho City, 2011)
Reported for the district of O Mon				
O Mon hospital	2010 - 2011	District of O Mon	**931**	(General Hospital of O Mon, 2011)
O Mon PHC	2010 - 2011	District of O Mon	**868**	(PHC O Mon, 2011a)
PHC of CTC	2010 - 2011	District of O Mon	**1350**	(PHC Can Tho City, 2011b)
Reported for the district of Phong Dien				

Phong Dien hospital	2010 - 2011	District of Phong Dien	**346**	(General hospital of Phong Dien, 2011)
Phong Dien PHC	2010	District of Phong Dien	**76**	(PHC Phong Dien, 2011)
PHC of CTC	2010 - 2011	District of Phong Dien	**1270**	(PHC Can Tho City, 2011b)
Reported for the district of Binh Thuy				
Bihn Thuy PHC	2009 - 2011	District of Binh Thuy - children	**562**	(PHC Binh Thuy, 2011)
PHC of CTC	2009 - 2011	District of Binh Thuy	**1558**	(PHC Can Tho City, 2011b)
Reported for the district of Cai Rang				
Cai Rang PHC	2007 – 2011	District of Cai Rang	**377**	(PHC Cai Rang, 2011a)
PHC of CTC	2008 - 2011	District of Cai Rang	**1839**	(PHC Can Tho City, 2011b)
Reported for the district of Co Do				
Co Do PHC	2010 – 2011	District of Co Do	**976**	(Medical Centre of Co Do, 2011a)
PHC of CTC	2010 - 2011	District of Co Do	**997**	(PHC Can Tho City, 2011b)

Based on collected reports and statistics from health institutions, 2011

Table 3: Household survey results from the PATH project, on water treatment methods in Co Do and Vinh Thanh districts

Methods	Ever heard of	Ever used*	Used yesterday**	Used (almost) every day the past month**
Boiling the water	100.0	99.8	69.7	65.2
Alum	97.8	69.1	7.9	6.7
Filter water using cloth, or net filter	91.2	50.7	5.8	7.2
Allow water to settle and decant	83.9	69.1	10.7	11.2

Chlorine/bleach tablet or liquid	19.5	34.3	4.4	4.4
Mineral pot (purifying device)	9.2	30.1	78.6	78.6

Note: * Among household who ever used this method, ** Among households who ever used the method . Data by (Abt Associates Inc., 2011) for PATH project. Design by author.

Table 4: Water supply sources for the districts of Can Tho (excluding Ninh Kieu) according to CERWASS-provided information for 2011

		% of people using hygienic water (%)		Deep drilled (dd) well			Clay jugs with stored rainwater			River/lake water		Piped-supply water	
Distr	Pop.	Pop. using hygienic water	%	# dd wells	# dd wells hyg. water	Pop. using hyg. water from dd wells	# clay jugs	# clay jugs with hyg. rain-water	Pop. using hygienic rain-water from clay jugs	# surface water sources treated hygienically	# people using surface water	# private taps	# People w. taps
Vinh Thanh	104.867	62.028	59,15	6.479	4.458	23.380	1.947	1.812	7.367	5	26	6.953	31.255
Thot Not	126.828	86.657	68,33	2.590	2.502	11.852	123	114	466	2.403	5.613	15.603	68.726
Co Do	114.138	93.856	82,23	8.824	8.647	42.614	900	776	3.045	108	452	10.612	47.745
Thoi Lai	116.909	84.953	72,67	11.764	10.238	49.894	476	362	1.442	288	868	7.234	32.749
O Mon	100.269	74.038	73,84	7.292	6.992	34.524	284	263	960	2.190	5.213	7.216	33.341
Binh Thuy	40.380	27.467	68,02	1.802	1.802	9.059	243	243	640	0	0	4.202	17.768

Phong Dien *	98.450	67.683	68,75	6.410	6.168	29.552	1.014	988	3.766	2.596	9.694	7.866	34.365
Cai Rang *	76.711	59.649	77,76	2.791	2.583	13.019	295	276	1.245	1.721	6.861	8.914	38.524
total	778.552	556.331	71,46	47.95 2	43.39 0	213.894	5.282	4.834	18.93 1	9.311	28.72 7	68.60 0	304.473
total (2010)	778.552	538.824	69,21	47.95 2,0	43.39 0	213.894	5.276	4.834	18.93 1	9.303	28.72 7	64.58 5	286.966

* Case-study districts. Source: (CERWASS, 2011a, CERWASS, 2010)

Table 5: Reported rural and urban population in Can Tho City from the Statistical Yearbook and by CERWASS

Yearbook of Can Tho:	Urban 2006	Rural 2006	Total 2006	Urban 2009	Rural 2009	Urban 2011	Rural 2011	Total 2011	CERWASS 2010[182]:
Ninh Kieu	212.095	-	212.095	244.065	-	249.451	-	249.451	-
O Mon	130.537	-	130.537	130.274	-	131.972	-	131.972	100.269
Binh Thuy	93.839	-	93.839	111.306	-	116.349	-	116.349	40.380
Cai Rang	78.708	-	78.708	86.328	-	88.432	-	88.432	76.711

182 Reporting on rural and parts of urban districts

Thot Not	23.528	172.413	195.941	159.461	-	161.563	-	1[illegible]1 563	126.828
Vinh Thanh	13.374	139.363	152.737	17.302	95.586	17.458	96.900	1[illegible]4 358	104.867
Co Do	26.047	153.091	179.138	12.979	111.266	13.071	111.718	1[illegible]4 789	114.138
Thoi Lai	- - -	- - -	- - -	10.643	110.678	10.735	111.517	1[illegible]2 252	116.909
Phong Dien	-	104.072	104.072	10.746	88.921	10.828	89.198	1[illegible]0 026	98.450
Total	578.128	568.939	1.147.067	783.104	406.451	799.859	409.333	1.2[illegible]9.192	556.331

Based on data by Can Tho Statistica Office (2007, 2011, 2009) and CERWASS (2011[illegible])

Table 6: Results from hygiene and water quality checks in water factories (serving>500hh) in 10 provinces of the Delta

Testing the general hygiene in water factories	2010	2011
Total water factories in the area	1610	6515
Total water factories were checked	1171	3525
Total testing checks in a water factory	2954	3003
Total testing checks that showed non compliance with general hygiene	748	522
Percentage of non-compliance in the total of factories	63, 87%	[illegible]4,81%

checked		
Total facilities that were tested for a second time and were still found to not comply	2	0
2. Results from water samples	2010	2011
Total water samples are tested	3077	4645
Total water samples that complied with hygienic standards	2251	3868
Percentage of water samples that reached hygienic standards	73,16%	83,27%
Total water samples that did not reach hygienic standards	826	777
- of which, how many did not reach physical and chemical indicators	619	614
- of which how many were due to microbiological indicators	300	163

Source: (IHPH, 2011a, IHPH, 2011b)

Table 7: Sanitation information for the districts of Can Tho, provided by CERWASS Can Tho

		% of hh using hygienic toilet:		% hh having hygienic toilet		1. septic tank latrine		2. pour-flush latrines		3. two-vault composting		4. pit latrine with aeration		5. other
	# hh	hh using hyg. toilet	% of total	hh hygienic toilet	% of total	# latrines	# hyg. latrines	# latrines	# hyg. latrines	# latrines	# hyg. latrines	# latrines	# hyg. latrines	# latrines
Vinh Thanh Thot	23.080	11.852	51,4	11.385	49,33	9.463	9.463	1.827	1.826	30	27	69	69	11.228
Not	28.534	15.510	54,3	14.211	49,8	12.414	12.333	1.878	1.878	0	0	0	0	13.024
Co Do Thoi	25.806	10.524	40,8	10.144	39,31	4.188	4.188	5.804	5.676	0	0	297	280	15.282
Lai	27.221	7.787	28,6	7.364	27,05	5.347	5.204	2.073	2.057	0	0	103	103	19.434
O Mon Binh	23.327	8.025	35,9	7.845	35,14	5.177	5.159	2.607	2.573	23	23	90	90	14.297
Thuy	9.878	4.386	44,4	4.240	42,92	3.974	3.974	266	266	0	0	0	0	5.492

Phong Dien *	22.998	8.102	35,2	7.834	34,06	6.019	6.017	1.603	1.603	58	58	156	156	14.563
Cai Rang *	18.479	12.975	70,2	12.064	65,28	9.363	9.248	2.831	2.816	0	0	0	0	5.504
Total of 2011	178.323	80.461	45,1	75.087	42,11	55.946	55.586	18.889	18.695	111	108	715	698	98.824
total of 2010	178.323	77.716	43,6	73.807	41,39	55.946	55.586	17.609	17.415	111	108	715	698	100.169

* study districts

1. septic tank latrine
2. pit pour-flush latrine (THẤM DỘI NƯỚC)
3. two-departments composting latrine (HAI NG□N)
4. sink with aeration latrine (CHÌM CÓ ỐNG THỐNG HƠI)

Source: (CERWASS, 2011a, CERWASS, 2010)

Table 8: Sanitation information from 10 Provinces of the Mekong Delta

Data provided by IHPH Ho Chi Minh City		2010	2011	Average
General information	Total households (in the study area)	5.904.427	4.042.074	
	Total latrines	5.534.034	2.929.496	
	Total hygienic latrines	3.738.730	2.156.207	
	Percentage of hygiene	67,56%	73,6	
	Number of hygienic latrines that newly built in the report duration	65.619	52.307	
	Number of latrines becoming unhygienic latrines in the report duration	108.927	98.125	
Details of the specific type of latrines				
Septic latrines	Total latrines	3.641.083	1.651.401	
	Number of hygienic latrines	2.707.845	1.452.951	
	Percentage of hygienic latrines (compared to total septic latrines)	74,37%	87,98%	81,17%
	Number of newly built hygienic latrines in the report duration	46.935	38.676	
	Number of latrines becoming unhygienic latrines in the report duration	20.254	13.156	

	Percentage of septic latrines % (compared to total households)	61,67%	40,86%	51.26%
Pour-flush latrines= NHÀ TIÊU THẤM DỘI NƯỚC	Total latrines	1.083.602	909.408	
	Number of hygienic latrines	882.754	743.490	
	Percentage of hygienic latrines (compared to total pit pour water latrines)	81,46%	81,76	
	Number of newly built hygienic latrines in the report duration	18.336	14.257	
	Number of latrines becoming unhygienic latrines in the report duration	8.604	8.366	
	Percentage of pit latrines % (compared to total households)	18,35%	22,50%	20.43%
Two vault compost latrines= NHÀ TIÊU HAI NG□N	Total latrines	64.698	50.155	
	Number of hygienic latrines	51.591	37.493	
	Percentage of hygienic latrines (compared to total two compartments latrines)	79,74%	74,75	
	Number of newly built hygienic latrines in the report duration	215	212	
	Number of latrines becoming unhygienic latrines in the report duration	1.743	745	
	Percentage of two-vault compost latrines % (compared to total households)	1,10%	3,04%	2.07%
Pit latrines with	Total latrines	118.467	63.051	

aeration = NHÀ TIÊU CHÌM CÓ ỐNG THÔNG HƠI	Number of hygienic latrines	96.540	45.159	
	Percentage of hygienic latrines (compared to total pit latrines with aeration)	81,49%	71,62	
	Number of newly built hygienic latrines in the report duration	959	266	
	Number of latrines becoming unhygienic latrines in the report duration	695	3155	
	Percentage % of pit latrines with aeration (compared to total households)	3,25%	3,82%	3.54%
Other kinds	Number of latrines	626.184	503.564	
	Percentage % (compared to total number of households)	31,10%	12,46%	21.78%

(IHPH, 2011a, IHPH, 2011b)

Table 9: Microbial water quality standards for drinking and daily use water in Vietnam

	Parameter	Unit	Maximum limit	Testing method
Drinking water	Total Coliform	Bacterial/100ml	0	TCVN 6187 – 1, 2: 1996 (ISO 9308 – 1,2 – 1990) or SMEWW 9922

	E.coli or thermo-tolerant coli-form	Bacterial/ 100ml	0		TCVN 6187 – 1, 2: 1996 (ISO 9308 – 1,2 – 1990) or SMEWW 9922
Domestic water	Total Coli-form	Bacterial/ 100ml	50*	150**	TCVN 6187 – 1, 2: 1996 (ISO 9308 – 1,2 – 1990) or SMEWW 9922
	E.coli or thermo-tolerant coli-form	Bacterial/ 100ml	0*	20**	TCVN 6187 – 1, 2: 1996 (ISO 9308 – 1,2 – 1990) or SMEWW 9922

* Applies for water provision units. ** Applies for water exploitation of individual, household (piped water supply through simple treatment e.g. drilled wells, dug wells, rain-tank, gravity pipeline). According to the National Technical Regulations (MoH, 2009b)

Table 10: Number of loans for WSS from the VSPB for the years 2005 – 2010

	Total (2005-2010)		2005		2006		2007		2008		2009		2010	
	hh	#	hh	#	hh	#	hh	#	hh	#	hh	#	hh	#
Thốt Nốt	4.629	25.338	0	0	906	4.260	1.452	7.662	2.271	13.416	0	0	0	0
Thới Lai	2.372	9.492	0	0	0	0	0	0	0	0	672	2.688	1.700	6.804
Cờ □ỏ	7.218	32.482	0	0	302	1.000	1.174	4.688	2.254	9.015	2.307	10.708	1.181	7.071
V□nh Thạnh	4.732	32.031	0	0	222	994	1.052	5.822	1.067	7.239	1.358	10.284	1.033	7.692
Phong □iền	6.229	34.593	0	0	435	1.710	842	3.323	2.144	10.500	2.003	13.600	805	5.460
Total	**25.180**	**133.936**	**0**	**0**	**1.865**	**7.964**	**4.520**	**21.495**	**7.736**	**40.170**	**6.340**	**37.280**	**4.719**	**27.027**

Notes (by the issuing authority): These numbers include loans for water supply network connection and for building toilets / Only give loans to hh in rural areas (communes) / In 2009 Thot not changed from rural to urban district and Co Do split to create Thoi Lai and Co Do in 2009

(Unit: households / million)

Data source: (VBSP, 2011)

Annex

Table 1: Analysis of the IEC material acquired by three types of organizations, according to the number of times selected recommendations were mentioned

Selected recommendations	CHECC	pPHC	dPHC	Overall	Average CHECC	Average pPHC	Average dPHC	Average overall
1. Cook food well and boil water	8	2	3	13	1	0,67	0,6	0,81
2. Wash hands clean before having meals, when preparing food	6	2	3	11	0,75	0,67	0,6	0,69
3. Wash hands after using the toilet	6	1	3	10	0,75	0,33	0,6	0,62
4. Do not eat fish and seafood, especially not raw	5	0	2	7	0,62	0	0,4	0,44
5. Use a hygienic toilet	2	2	3	7	0,25	0,67	0,6	0,44
6. Do not exercise open defecation	5	2	2	9	0,62	0,67	0,4	0,56
7. Use clean water for cooking	4	2	1	7	0,67	0,67	0,2	0,44
8. Use chloramine B or alum to disinfect water	5	2	2	9	0,62	0,67	0,4	0,56
9. When someone in the family gets acute diarrhoea, inform the nearest health care centre	6	1	2	9	0,75	0,33	0,4	0,56
10. Do not eat raw vegetable	4	1	0	5	0,5	0,33	0	0,31

11. Avoid eating out in mass servings like in weddings etc.	2	0	1	3	0,25	0	0,2	0,19
12. Keep your latrines clean, have enough water and soap	3	1	0	4	0,37	0,33	0	0,25
13. When having diarrhoea, one must throw powdered lime or Chloramine B with water to flush the toilet (magazine on food poisoning)	3	0	1	4	0,37	0	0,2	0,25
14. Don't throw garbage or dead animals into the rivers, lakes and ponds	3	2	1	6	0,37	0,67	0,2	0,37
15. Control the spread of flies (magazine – on flies)	1	1	0	2	0,12	0,33	0	0,12

Table 12: Analysis of semi-structured interviews with preventive health offices in Can Tho, based on the mention of selected issues around diarrheal disease understandings

Issues that were discussed /brought up after or without prompt by the interviewer	ministry	provincial	district	commune /ward	hamlet/area
1. the high prevalence of diarrhoea in the region	75%	20%	25%	25%	0
2. the distinction between different epidemiological causes and knowledge on the symptoms	44%	0	30%	0	0
3. the general connections between water, sanitation and diarrhoea	69%	80%	65%	75%	50%
4. the importance of in-the-house behaviours for the prevention of diarrhoea	56%	40%	70%	50%	50%
5. the importance of hand-washing to be promoted as a prevention measure	31%	40%	25%	25%	0%
6. the connection between diarrhoea and malnutrition, exhaustion and other health impeding conditions	31%	20%	20%	0	0
7. the different stages of diarrhoea and the recommended treatments	37%	60%	50%	100%	100%

8. The role of IEC in enhancing understandings around disease and changing behaviours other than WSS improvements	56%	40%	60%	50%	0
9. Knowledge of diarrheal disease pathways (faeces, fingers, water, food, people, digestive system)	50%	60%	30%	25%	0
Total score	50%	40%	42%	39%	22%

ZEF Development Studies

edited by Solvay Gerke and Hans-Dieter Evers (Center for Development Research (ZEF), University of Bonn)

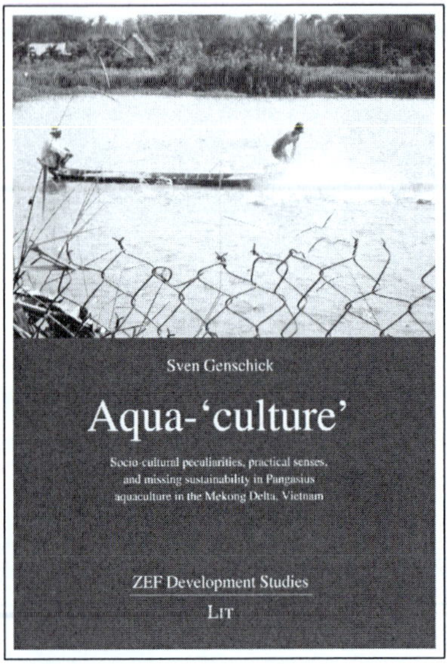

Sven Genschick

Aqua-'culture'

Socio-cultural peculiarities, practical senses, and missing sustainability in Pangasius aquaculture in the Mekong Delta, Vietnam

Water pollution in Pangasius aquaculture endangers its economic success and meaning for rural development in the Mekong Delta. With the help of Bourdieu´s theory of practice, the author considers the interplay of subjective and objective structures to conclude on the conduct of practices in Pangasius cultivation. The study shows that economic dependencies in a global commodity production system have led to a transformation process that most aquaculturists cannot cope with. The discrepancy between the ideal and real situation can no longer be ignored otherwise the downward trend continues.

Bd. 26, 2014, 280 S., 29,90 €, br.,
ISBN 978-3-643-90485-0

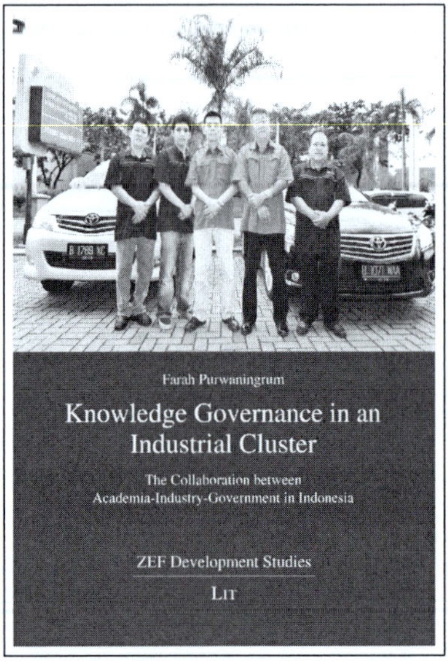

Farah Purwaningrum

Knowledge Governance in an Industrial Cluster

The Collaboration between Academia-Industry-Government in Indonesia

This book explains why there persists a divergence of academia-industry- government inter-linkage in the Indonesian science system. This divergence constrains the capacity of the science system in localising knowledge from the supply chain linkage. The study shows the centralised character of the Indonesian science system. The Jababeka Industrial Cluster is shaped by the supply chain linkage and, thus, lacks the capacity of a knowledge cluster. The horizontal collaboration between academia-industry is restricted and limited.

Bd. 27, 2014, 296 S., 39,90 €, br.,
ISBN 978-3-643-90508-6

LIT Verlag Berlin – Münster – Wien – Zürich – London

Auslieferung Deutschland / Österreich / Schweiz: siehe Impressumsseite